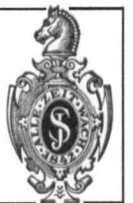

Klaus J. Zülch

Atlas of Gross Neurosurgical Pathology

With 379 Figures

Springer-Verlag Berlin
Heidelberg GmbH 1975

KLAUS JOACHIM ZÜLCH, Professor Dr., Max-Planck-Institut für Hirnfor-
schung, Abteilung für Allgemeine Neurologie, D-5000 Köln 91, Ostmer-
heimer Straße 200

ISBN 978-3-642-65730-6   978-3-642-65728-3 (eBook)

DOI 10.1007/978-3-642-65728-3

ISBN 978-3-540-06480-0 Springer-Verlag Berlin · Heidelberg · New York

ISBN 978-0-387-06480-2 Springer-Verlag New York · Heidelberg · Berlin

Typsetting, printing, and bookbinding by Universitätsdruckerei H. Stürtz AG, Würzburg

Preface

This Atlas is one of a series devoted to neurosurgical and neurological conditions and is complementary to *Atlas of the Histology of Brain Tumors* (Springer-Verlag, Berlin-Heidelberg-New York 1971), which was the first in the atlas series. The Atlas is based on the *Handbuch der Neurochirurgie*, Vols. I and III (Springer 1956, 1959) but, whereas this is a comprehensive reference work, the present book is intended to give the practicing neurosurgeon, neuroradiologist, neuropathologist and neurologist the concise information they need for diagnostic purposes concerning the aspect, site, and malignancy of tumors and other space-occupying lesions in the brain. The schematic diagrams showing the sites of predilection of these tumors, as well as a prognosis based on the degree of malignancy, will be most useful here.

The early chapters discuss the general rules governing displacements due to space-occupying lesions and the manifestations of brain herniations. Other neurosurgical conditions, such as localized inflammatory processes, edema and obstructive hydrocephalus, are dealt with in brief chapters; in this case I have chosen to show some of the rarer conditions rather than all the common lesions. In spite of probable future changes in terminology and classification, we have retained the classification used in the *Atlas of Histology of Brain Tumors*.

The intention was to present as many gross morphological conditions as possible and to keep the accompanying text short and precise. However, in describing the anatomical details I have tried to consider the problems facing the neurosurgeon, with which I am familiar through daily contact and close cooperation over many years. I have tried to reinforce these impressions by considering the books and chapters by H. OLIVECRONA (*Handbuch der Neurochirurgie*, Vol. IV, Springer 1967), L. G. KEMPE (Springer 1968/70), G. GURDJIAN (Williams and Wilkins 1952; 3rd edit. 1970), G. MERREM (*Lehrbuch der Neurochirurgie*, VEB, 3rd edit. 1969). As additional and more detailed sources of information, I recommend the German, English and Italian version of my short book on *Brain Tumors* (Springer Publishers, New York) and the relevant chapters in the *Handbuch der Neurochirurgie*, Vols. I and III.

This atlas does not cover the pathology of trauma except for certain kinds of hemorrhage. Trauma *per se* will be subject of a subsequent atlas. Vertebral pathology seemed to be too remote from the contents of this atlas and has therefore not been considered.

V

I am most grateful to Dr. J. MILHORAT of Philadelphia, and Dr. W. BOEHM of Atlanta for undertaking the translation, and also to Drs. M. FUKUI (Fukuoka), H. D. MENNEL (Köln), T. SATO (Sapporo), E. SCHARRER (Köln), and E. SIMON (Poznan), for their help in the reclassification of our tumor collection. Finally, I thank Herr und Frau GÖLDNER for their technical assistance in my scientific work over the past twenty years.

Prof. em. JOSEPH EVANS has been kind enough to give me his advice and help during the editorial work. I should also like to thank Springer-Verlag for the excellent layout and quality of this book.

Köln, November 1974   K. J. ZÜLCH

Contents

Contents

Increased Intracranial Pressure, Generalized or Focal, and its Consequence—Mass-Movements and Herniations

General Rules for Displacement due to Space-Occupying Lesions

Consideration must first be given to rules of displacement within the intracranial space since they differ from those of the primarily elastic body cavities, such as the thorax and the abdomen. This is due to the rigid wall of the intracranial space, the skull, aptly described as a "closed box" in the English literature. The addition of volume—i.e., a space-occupying lesion—results in a displacement of other substances within this space. When a tumor develops, the volume of cerebrospinal fluid or blood must be reduced, or the brain itself must either undergo atrophy or (because it is essentially non-compressible) be forced out of the skull through the foramen magnum (Fig. 1). As the space-occupying lesion evolves, the adjacent ventricles are first distorted and compressed and then the reserve spaces of the arachnoidal sulci and cisterns (Fig. 2) are filled with brain tissue. In this manner, local "herniations" into the cisterns (Figs. 3–12) occur.

Although the external skull is rigid in adults, it is elastic in children. Because of this, hydrocephalus occurring in the first years of life is followed by a secondary enlargement of the head.

In older individuals there is less brain to compete with as a result of atrophy (Fig. 7) —which commences in the 25th year of life— so that the volume of the "reserve spaces" filled with cerebrospinal fluid (i.e., the arachnoidal sulci, the cisterns and the ventricles) is greater than in the 25-year-old. Thus, the tumor will have evolved to a greater size before general signs of increased intracranial pressure appear in the aged since greater volume can be assimilated by the enlarged CSF spaces after the cerebrospinal fluid has been forced out. This is true for the frontal areas and for the temporoparietal areas—not, however, for the frontobasal or temporobasal regions or for the occipital lobe since atrophy rarely occurs in these areas.

Certain anatomical features within the skull are of importance. For example, the falx which separates the two hemispheres and which is fixed posteriorly to the tentorium can be only moderately shifted at its "deeper" edge anteriorly (Figs. 3, 4), and is thus a fairly rigid structure. It should also be noted that the falx lies posteriorly directly on the splenium of the corpus callosum (Figs. 11, 16, 22) so that any mass displacement here is impossible unless the corpus callosum is first depressed downward (Fig. 9). In the frontal area, on the other hand, where the falx lies well above the rostrum of the corpus callosum considerable lateral displacement of the brain is possible (Fig. 11).

Furthermore, it should be noted that unobstructed axial displacements—i.e., from in front toward the posterior fossa (Fig. 1) and vice versa (Fig. 39)—are possible. In more laterally situated lesions (for example in the temporal lobe) such a shift of brain tissue towards the posterior fossa is more difficult because of the position of the tentorium and because a right angle must be negotiated in order to permit the displaced brain to proceed via the tentorial hiatus into the posterior fossa (Fig. 12, II).

If these fundamental rules of displacement are applied to specific space-occupying lesions, a tumor located in the *frontal* region (Fig. 12 I) may result in an unobstructed *lateral* displacement of brain tissue into the anterior midline in the region of the septum pellucidum. *Axial* displacements from in front towards the posterior fossa are also easily possible. This is the reason for the frequent appearance of a cerebellar pressure cone (Figs. 39, 42, 43) at the onset of a space-occupying lesion in the frontal lobe; in contrast, *lateral* displacements rarely (Fig. 12 I) occur more posteriorly in the region of the third ventricle or the posterior corpus callosum-quadrigeminal region in such lesions.

A *parietal* space-occupying lesion (Fig. 11) produces an initial displacement towards the base. At the base, the mass then encounters the large reserve spaces of the cisterns (Figs. 25, 26, 28) (cisterna basalis, ambiens) which can be filled. Displacements towards the frontal lobe and from there towards the *opposite side* are also possible. Towards the occipital region (Fig. 12 III), on the other hand, there is the cone-shaped tentorium and dura which provide an obstruction to tissue displacements because the occipital lobe is not affected by senile atrophy. As previously emphasized, in the case of a parietal space-occupying lesion a direct lateral shift is possible only if the corpus callosum has been depressed beforehand (Fig. 9). It was noted earlier that this cannot occur in the first stages of a parietal shift because the falx lies directly above the splenium of the corpus callosum (Fig. 11) and acts as a barrier. Thus, in the more posterior parts of the brain —i.e., in the area of the pars media and also around the third ventricle—displacements can occur (after depression of the corpus callosum); but parts of the brain around the anterior two-thirds of the cistern (Fig. 9) will also take part in these later shifts which will then also affect the septum.

The *temporal* space-occupying lesion acts (Figs. 12 II, 18–20) in a lateral direction primarily displacing the third ventricle so that it becomes rounded out due to its fixation at the infundibulum. The lateral shift of the lower basal ganglia is possible because its distance from the falx is greater, while a lateral displacement in the upper posterior parts of the cranial cavity is initially limited. The temporal tumor presses axially against the frontal lobe over the lesser sphenoid wing. However, at the same time it also exerts pressure against the posterior fossa by creating a hernia into the tentorial hiatus, first laterally, then with a change of direction of 90 degrees downwards towards the posterior fossa. All in all, this lateral shift produces its greatest effect more anteriorly (Fig. 25) or more posteriorly (usually more posteriorly) (Fig. 27), depending on the location of the tumor. In addition, it produces an *axial* effect primarily in a frontal direction (Figs. 19, 20). Axial effects in a posterior direction are less common (Fig. 12 II).

In the early phases an *occipital* space-occupying lesion can only displace brain tissue anteriorly against the temporal, parietal, and the frontal lobes. A lateral shift occurs only after a preceding displacement of brain tissue

anteriorly as far as the middle or anterior parts of the corpus callosum or at the level of the septum and to a lesser extent near the *more basally*-situated third ventricle (Fig. 12 III) (displacement against the temporal lobe has occurred). In this situation a *lateral* shift occasionally occurs quite far anteriorly because the space-occupying lesion in the occipital lobe lies mainly above the temporal lobe in the parieto-frontal axis.

Table 1; see also Figs. 8, 9, 13–17, 151, 199, 300, 323, 327, 328, 337, 341, 347, 351, 360, 368

Processes acting as space-occupying lesions are:	
Primary neoplasms	Hemorrhages
Metastases	Abscesses
Parasites	Circumscribed encephalitis
Arachnoidal cysts	Cerebral edema of any cause and similar conditions
	Hyperemia
	Hydrocephalus, obstructive

In essence, *all* space-occupying lesions fundamentally produce the *same* displacements. These depend, however, on the *volume* as much as on the *location* of the space-occupying lesion. The effective size of the displacing mass is ultimately determined by a combination of factors. These include not only the volume of the mass lesion itself (tumor, hemorrhage, etc.), but also secondary increases in adjacent *brain* volume due to infiltration of water. Tumor *type* may influence volume not only because tumors vary as to their speed of growth, but also because certain lesions tend to be associated with rather severe brain edema [e.g., glioblastomas and metastases (Figs. 10, 23), as well as abscesses (Fig. 338)].

A lesion of the frontal lobe which grows slowly is able to displace the falx gradually and can produce a more marked lateral shift than is possible if the lesion were of rapid development.

Thus, a small metastasis lying in the frontal area can lead to massive cerebral edema (Fig 10) of an entire hemisphere; in such situations, the point of maximum lateral displacement often does not correspond to the site of the primary tumor—a small parieto-occipital metastasis may cause extensive edema in the frontal lobe.

Cerebral edema is primarily a *time-dependent* reaction, requiring 24–36 hours to develop and the maximum cannot be expected until after the second and third day (see p. 202).

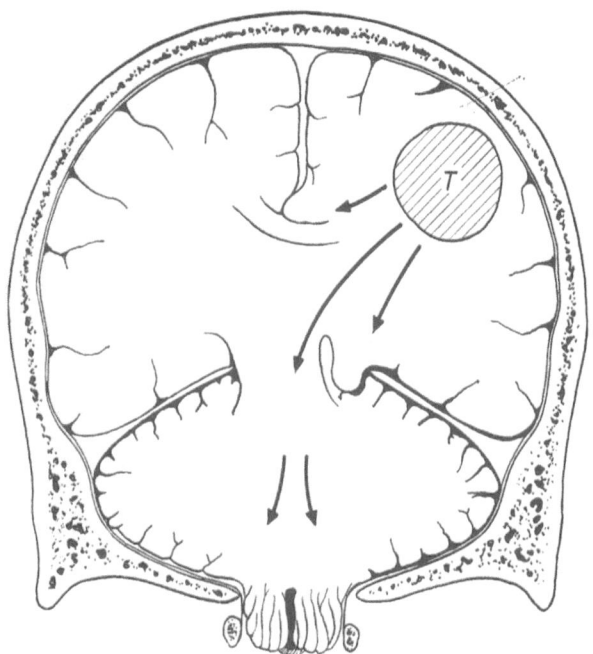

Fig. 1. Schematic drawing of the mass movements resulting from a parietal tumor. Superiorly the cingulate gyrus is being displaced to the opposite side. Near the midbrain a temporal pressure cone has been pushed into the posterior fossa. Inferiorly, the cerebellar tonsils and the medulla have been forced through the foramen magnum. Flattening of the convolutions overlying the tumor is also seen

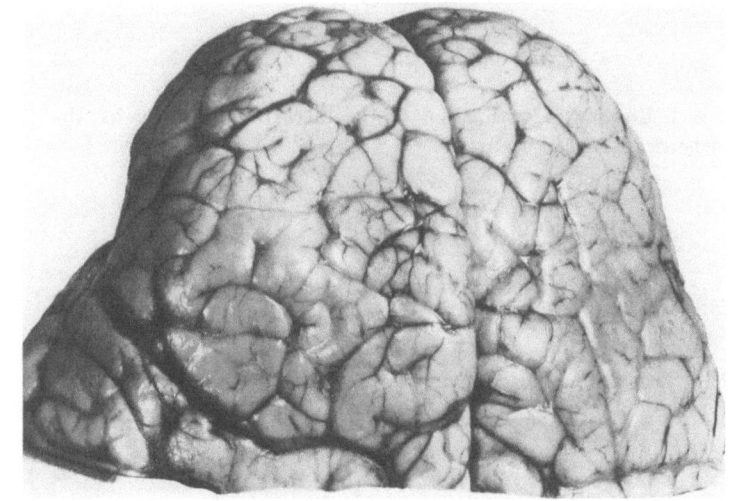

Fig. 2. Flattening of the convolutions and obliteration of the sulci in a case of obstructive hydrocephalus with a block in the posterior fossa. Such cortical changes with associated mass herniations are the characteristic pathological features of increased intracranial pressure

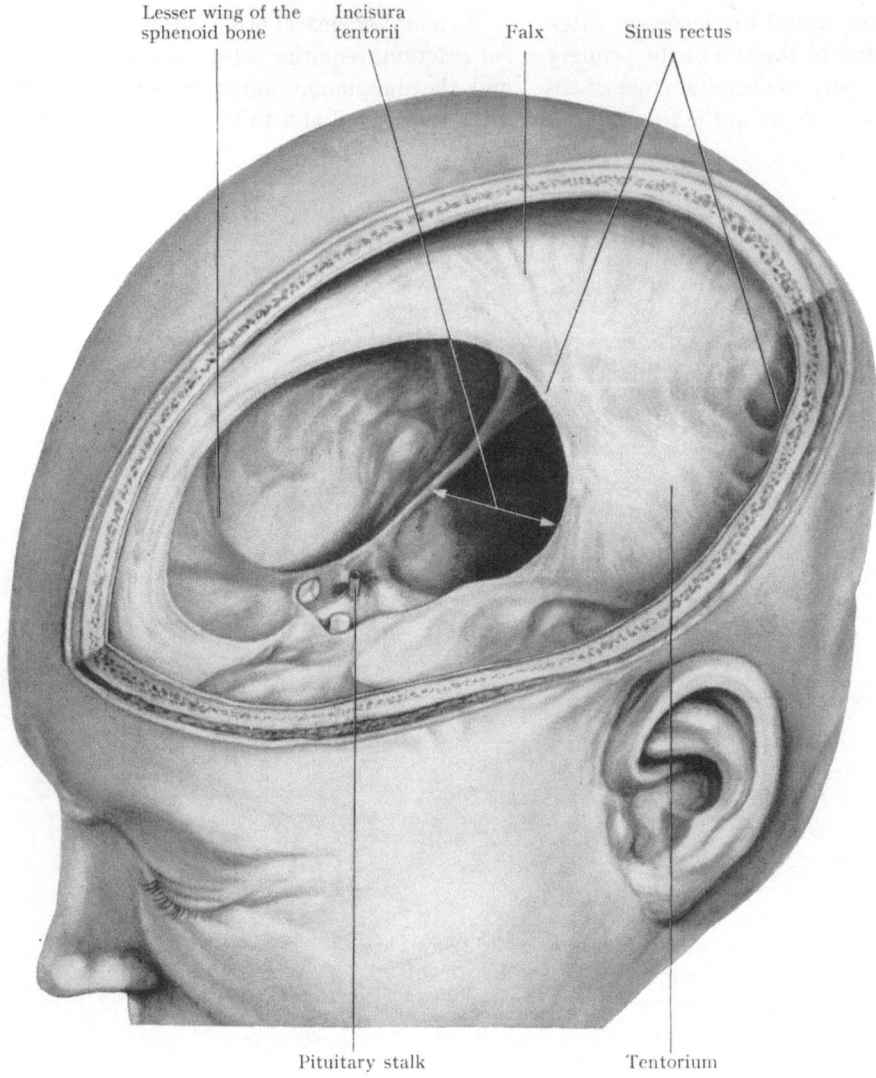

Fig. 3. Compartmentalization of the intracranial cavity by the falx and tentorium. The tentorial incisura is marked by arrows

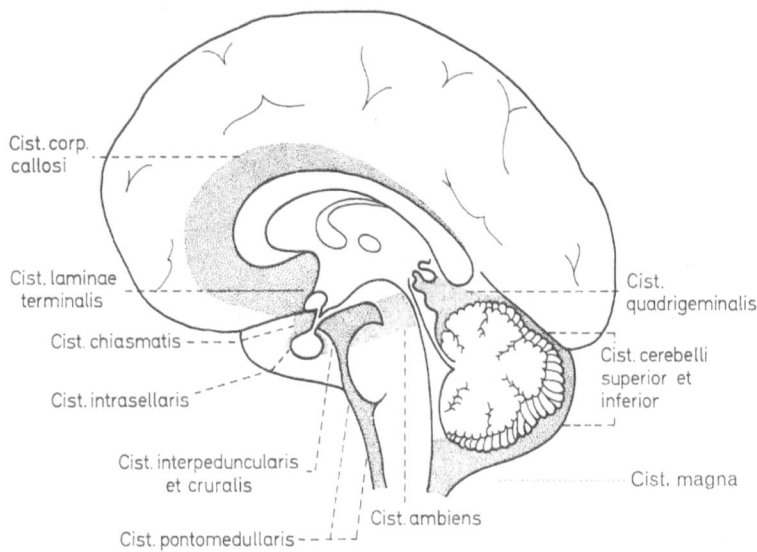

Fig. 4. The main cisterns of the brain in a sagittal section

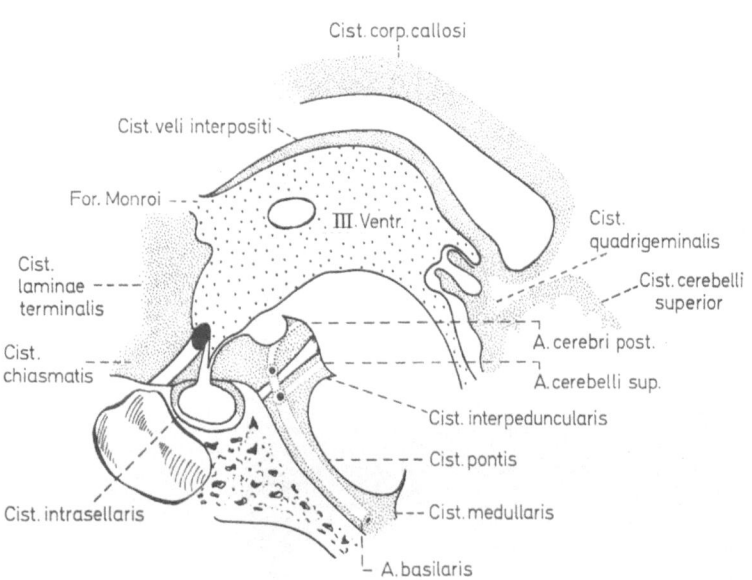

Fig. 5. Schema of the anatomical relationships of the third nerve to the posterior cerebral and the superior cerebellar arteries. Many cisterns are also well-illustrated (see labels above)

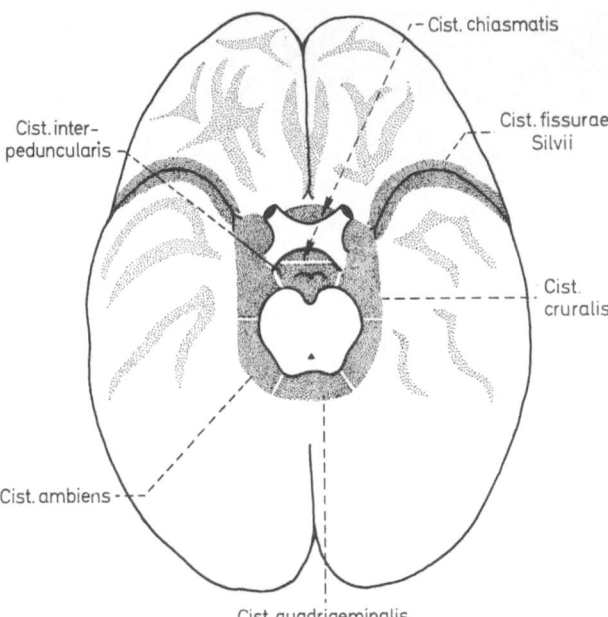

Cist. chiasmatis

Cist. inter-
peduncularis

Cist. fissurae
Silvii

Cist.
cruralis

Cist. ambiens

Cist. quadrigeminalis

Fig. 6. The main cisterns of the brain;
view from the base

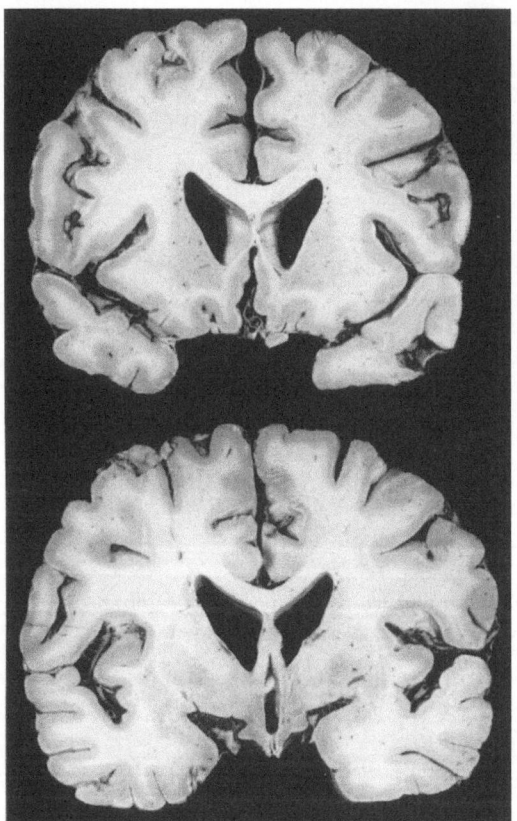

Fig. 7. Enlarged cisterns in a case of generalized
senile atrophy. The lateral cistern of the Sylvian
fissure, and the supracallosal and basal cisterns
are particularly prominent

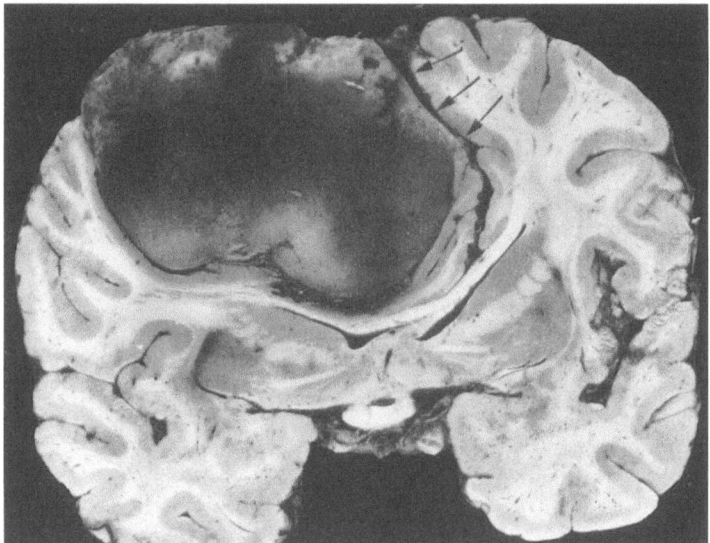

Fig. 8. Meningioma of the middle third of the sagittal sinus with marked displacement of the falx (arrows!) and shift to the opposite side. Note the distortion of the ventricular system. This huge tumor behaved as an exception from the rule, which is illustrated by Fig. 9

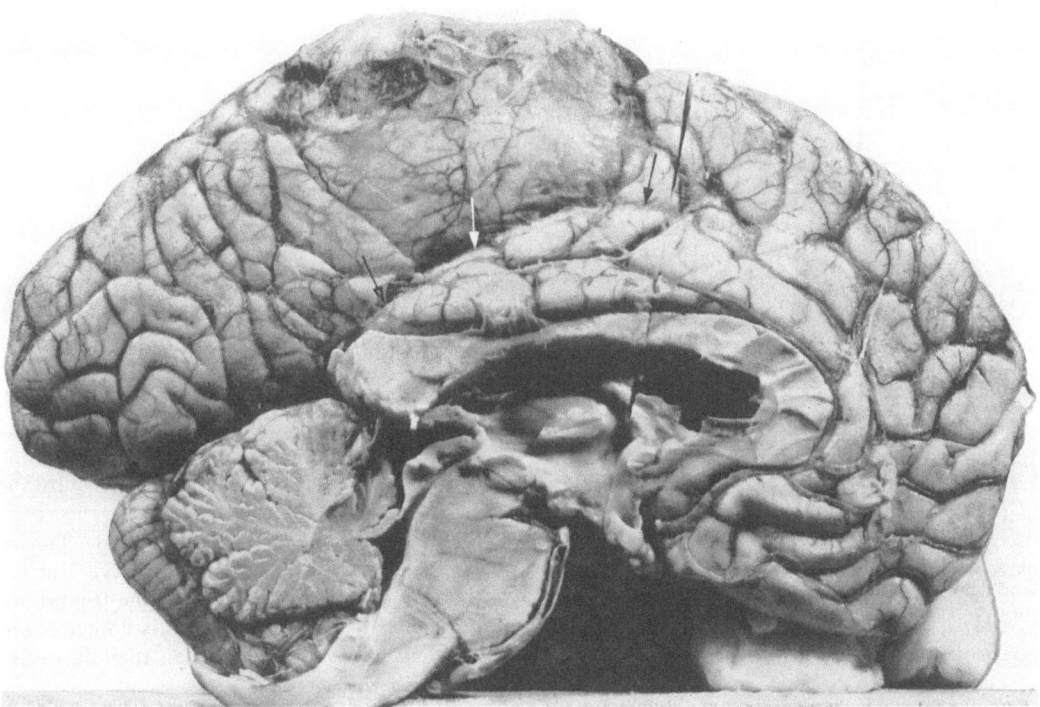

Fig. 9. Marked herniation of the cingulate gyrus (arrows!) under the falx in a meningioma of the middle third of the sagittal sinus. Note the difference from Fig. 22 where the posterior third of the gyrus is not herniated. Here, the extracerebral tumor has depressed the entire parietal lobe including the corpus callosum, thus permitting the observed herniation

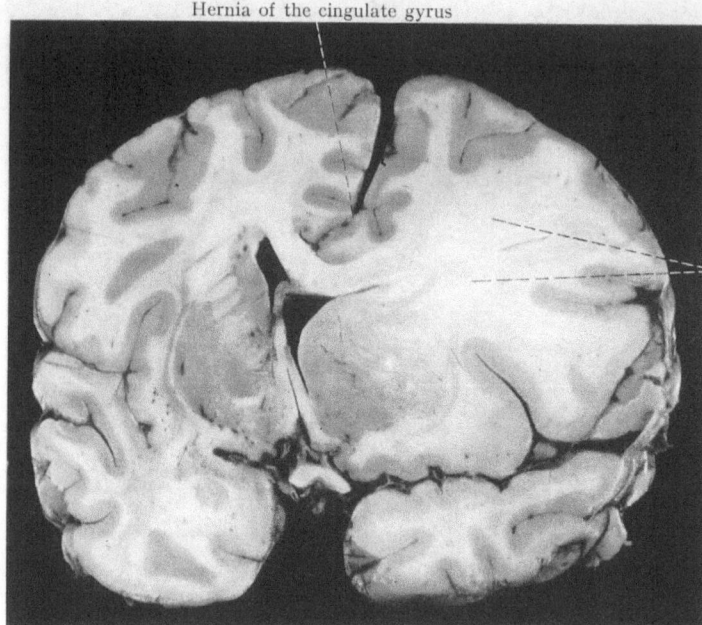

Fig. 10. Increase in volume of the left white matter by marked brain swelling adjacent to a frontobasal glioblastoma multiforme. Particularly marked cerebral displacement with herniation of the cingulate gyrus

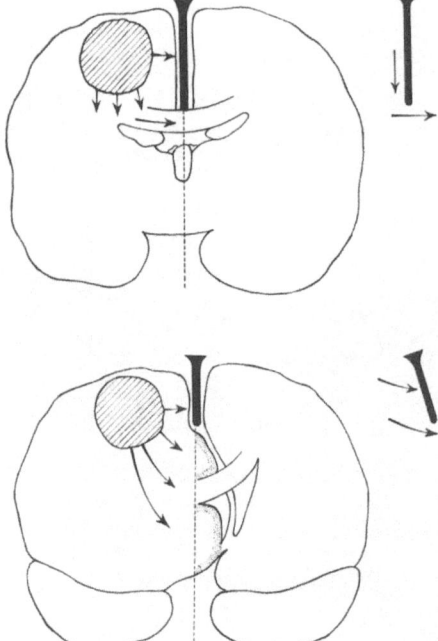

Fig. 11. Differences between mass shifts in the parietal area (top) and in the frontal area (bottom). Top: In the parietal area the falx lies adjacent to the corpus callosum and brain substance can be displaced laterally only after the corpus callosum has been depressed downwards. The falx can be moved only with difficulty. Bottom: Lateral displacement of brain in the frontal area is considerably easier, since the falx does not reach the corpus callosum. In addition the falx itself is more easily displaced

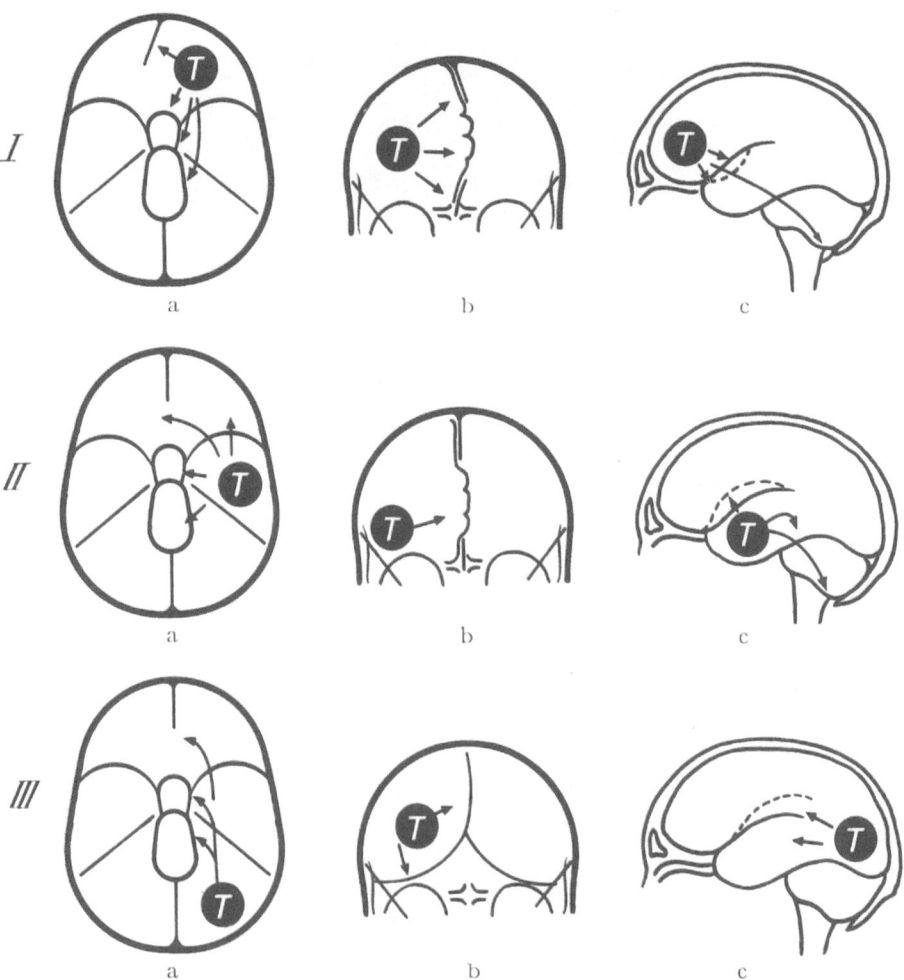

Fig. 12 I—III. Diagram of the most important mass shifts with frontal (I), temporal (II) and occipital (III) tumors. I. Here the frontal tumor presses on the falx so as to slant it, presses against the upper temporal lobe over the sphenoid wing and displaces the brain stem "axially" at an early stage. II. The temporal tumor presses against the frontal lobe and displaces the Sylvian fissure towards the front and upwards; the uncinate process, however, is pressed against the tentorial hiatus. Anteriorly this pressure is not sufficient to slant the falx. III. Since it lies in a cone-shaped space coated with dura, the occipital tumor must force the adjacent brain masses anteriorly where, however, the frontal parts of the brain may be readily displaced across the midline towards the opposite side. The Sylvian fissure is elevated. (From KAUTZKY and ZÜLCH, 1955)

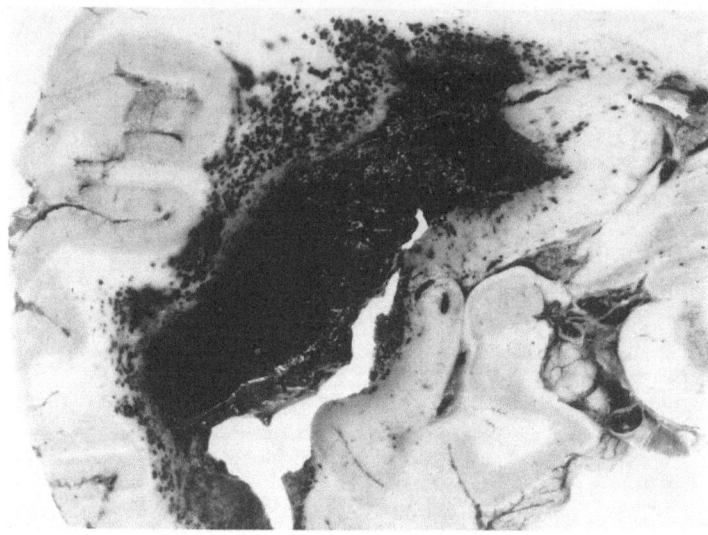

Fig. 13. Large hypertensive hemorrhagic mass in the basal ganglia displacing pulvinar, midbrain, and pineal gland

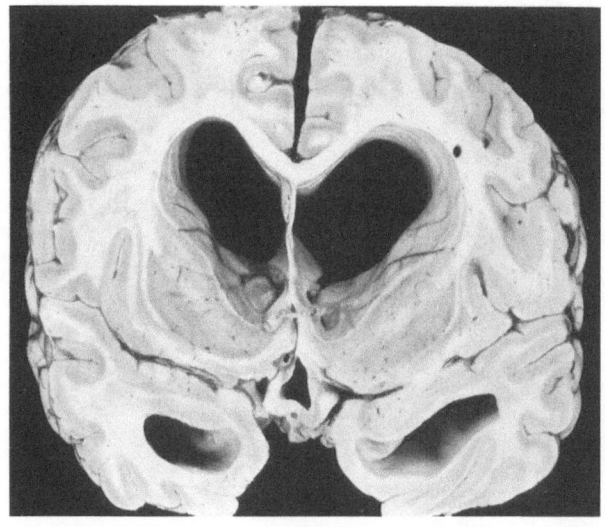

Fig. 14. Classical example of obstructive hydrocephalus secondary to a posterior fossa tumor. The septum pellucidum is not torn, yet the corpus callosum has been angulated on the lower edge of the falx

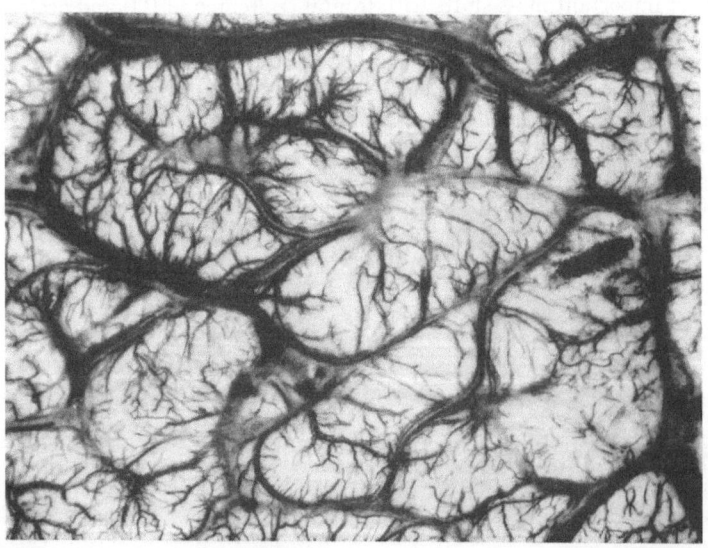

Fig. 15. Enormous degree of hyperemia in a case of fatal status epilepticus. Hyperemia contributed as an additional space-occupying factor

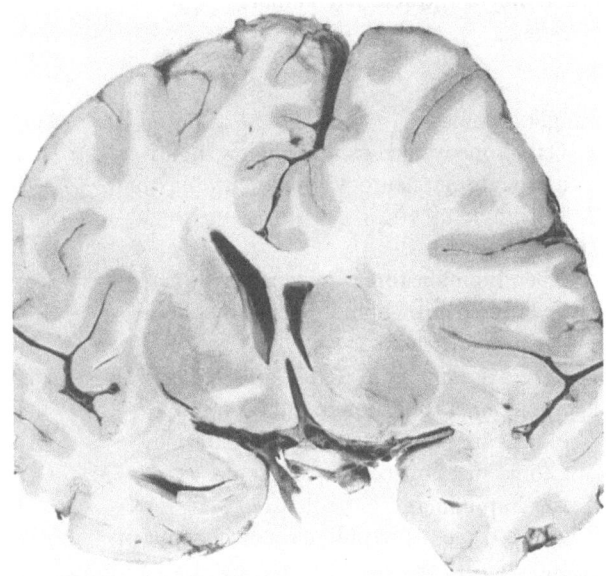

Fig. 16. Typical depression of one cerebral hemisphere by a subdural hematoma with corresponding shift of the midline structures including the ventricular system

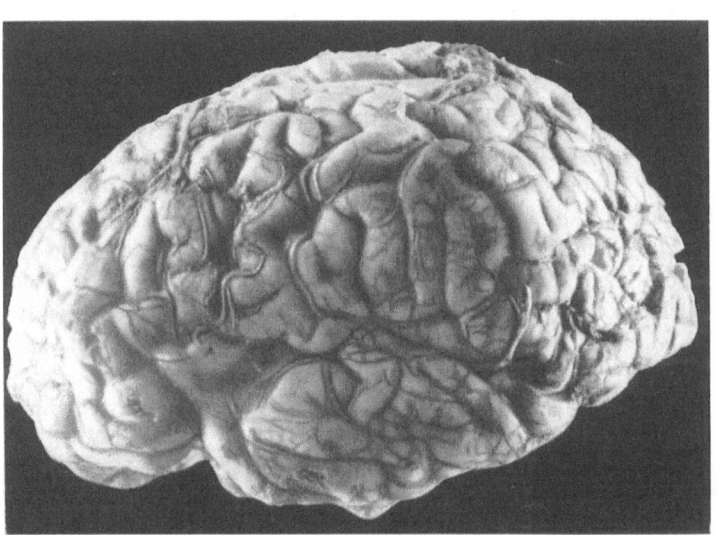

Fig. 17. Depression of the left hemisphere by a flat, frontal epidural hematoma

Synonyms of Intracranial Tumors

Gangliocytomas
Ganglioneuroma, ganglioglioma, neuro-astrocytoma, neurocytoma, neuroblastoma, Purkinjeoma etc.

Ependymomas
Ependymoblastoma, glioependymoma, ependymoepithelioma, ependymoglioma, "neuroepithelioma"

Ependymal Tumors in Tuberous Sclerosis
Spongioneuroblastoma, subependymal glomerate astrocytoma, subependymal glioma or giant-cell astrocytoma

Plexus Papillomas
Choroid plexus papilloma, epithelioma of the choroid plexus

Neuroepitheliomas

Retinoblastomas
Neuroepithelioma of the retina with or without rosettes

Astrocytomas
Fibrillary/protoplasmic/gemistocytic astro-cytoma, astrocytoma grade I—III, giant cell astrocytoma including astroblastoma

Oligodendrogliomas
Oligodendroblastoma and oligodendro-cytoma

Glioblastomas, malignant
Glioblastoma/spongioblastoma multiforme, giant-cell glioblastoma, astrocytoma grade IV, gliosarcoma

Spongioblastomas, polar
Pilocytic or piloid astrocytoma, astro-cytoma of juvenile type, optic nerve glioma, fusicellular oligodendrocytoma, "central neurinoma", polar glioma

Medulloblastomas
Neuroblastoma, isomorphic glioblastoma, neurogliocytoma (including medullo-myoblastoma)

Neurinomas
Schwannoma, neurilemoma, perineural fibroblastoma, neurofibroma

Meningiomas
Meningotheliomatous, fibrous (fibroblastic), transitional, psammomatous, angiomatous (angioblastic) meningiomas; endothelioma, exothelioma or mesothelioma of the dura mater; meningeal fibroblastoma, meningo-thelioma

Angioblastomas
Hemangioblastoma, capillary hemangio-blastoma, Lindau's cyst, disease or tumor, cerebellar angioma, angioreticuloma, cere-bellar hemangioendothelioma

Sturge-Weber's Disease
Capillary angiomatosis of the lepto-meninges

Sarcomas, various types
Reticulum cell sarcoma, reticulosarcoma, microglioma, microgliomatosis, retothelial sarcoma and other malignant lymphomas. Diffuse sarcomatosis of blood vessels, peri-adventitial diffuse sarcoma; sarcomatosis of the meninges, primary meningeal sarcoma-tosis; fibrosarcoma (circumscribed), spindle cell sarcoma.
Arachnoidal cerebellar sarcoma, circum-scribed arachnoidal cerebellar sarcoma

Sarcoma, monstrocellular
Circumscribed sarcoma of the blood vessels, gigantocellular or giant-cell glioblastoma

Pinealomas
Pineocytoma, pineoblastoma, germinoma of the pineal gland

Pituitary Adenomas
Acidophile (oxyphile), basophile, mixed, chromophobe adenoma

Craniopharyngiomas
Tumor or cyst of the hypophyseal duct or of Rathke's pouch, pituitary stalk tumor, Erdheim's tumor, adamantinoma or ameloblastoma of the pituitary region

Glomus Tumors
Carotid body tumor, glomus caroticum or jugulare tumor, paraganglioma, chemo-dectoma

Epidermoids — Dermoids — Teratomas
Epidermoid cyst, pearly tumor, cholesteatoma without hair. —
Dermoid cyst, cholesteatoma with hair

Cylindromatous Epitheliomas Cylindroma, adenoid cystic carcinoma

Cavernoma — Cavernous Angioma

Arteriovenous Angioma or Malformation (AVM)

1. The Space-Occupying Lesions

Displacement begins when the brain yields locally to the pressure of the growing tumor (Fig. 1). As this happens, the adjacent portions of the ventricles are deformed and the reserve space of the neighboring cisterns and overlying sulci is used up and filled with brain tissue (Fig. 2). The shift of the brain often exceeds the confines of the cisterns and indents the corresponding portion of the opposite hemisphere (Figs. 21, 22). The local increase in pressure does not confine itself to the homolateral hemisphere but may be transmitted to the opposite hemisphere where possible, as by displacement of tissue between the edge of the falx and the base (Figs. 16, 22). Finally, pressure is transferred from the structures above the tentorium to those beneath it (axial displacement; Fig. 1), leading to herniation of the cerebellar tonsils into the foramen magnum (Figs. 42, 43). 45). In tumors of the posterior fossa, upward displacement through the incisura tentorii is possible (Figs. 39, 40). Thus, well-recognized patterns of displacement exist due to space-occupying processes in various locations. These form the basis for localization by ventriculography or arteriography. An accurate analysis of a ventriculogram or arteriogram can only be carried out by someone who is thoroughly familiar with these rules of displacement. Herniations in those regions of brain adjacent to the cisterns —though small—may be visually very impressive and may show the *direction* of the displacement particularly well (Figs. 25–31).

The Forms of Internal Herniation. A thorough knowledge of the individual types of herniation into the cisterns is important for the anatomists. Displacements in the *cisterna supracallosa* mainly occur in the anterior portion (Figs. 16, 22); in the posterior portion they occur with any magnitude only following processes located dorsally which have first displaced the corpus callosum downward (Figs. 9, 184). The arteries of the median fissure (the peri-callosal and calloso-marginal arteries), which lie one over the other, will be displaced separately since the former lies in moveable tissue close to the corpus callosum, while the latter may be held in place by the falx. If the increase in volume of the two hemispheres is equal— hydrocephalus of the lateral ventricles—lateral displacement is absent. The corpus callosum will be pressed up from below (Fig. 14) against the falx, the lower edge of which causes a sharp pressure groove which can lead to virtual sagittal section of the corpus callosum (Figs. 49, 50, 362, 368, 370, 371).

In the *cisterna interpeduncularis and ambiens* portions of the adjacent temporal lobe gyri will be pressed downwards through the incisura tentorii (Fig. 25), displacing the midbrain to the opposite side (Figs. 32–35): "temporal" or "tentorial" pressure cone (Figs. 25–31). This can be demonstrated arteriographically by the downwards and medial displacement of the posterior cerebral artery, which can be stretched over the edge of the tentorium. Thus, flow can be reduced and hemorrhagic infarcts in the medial part of the occipital pole may develop as a result (Figs. 31, 33, 34).

Parts of the hippocampus and especially of the uncus are pressed into the basal cisterns (Figs. 25–27, 30, 31), forcing the peduncle towards the other side (Figs. 29, 32, 35) and compressing the third nerve (Figs. 46–48). In case of an extreme generalized increase in volume of one hemisphere, the brain can be pressed simultaneously into the cisterna supracallosa, interpeduncularis, cisterna cruralis and ambiens (Figs. 27–29); the different parts join one another in a ring-like form: the so-called "circular herniation" into the cisterns.

Conversely, the superior vermis can be pressed through the incisura into the supratentorial region (Figs. 39–41) from the posterior fossa (displacement from below upward; Fig. 39). This somewhat pyramidal-shaped part of the cerebellum can also squeeze the midbrain

(Figs. 36, 41) and the quadrigeminal region and bring about considerable morphological alterations. The posterior part of the third ventricle will be displaced upwards and anteriorly (kinking or "horse-tail" form of the aqueduct) in the pneumoencephalogram.

The best-known of all the changes occurring around the cisterns is the "cerebellar pressure cone", the herniation into the *cisterna magna*. The wedge-shaped invasion by the tonsils can reach grotesque proportions in young patients (most of the so-called Arnold-Chiari malformations?), because of the compliance of the bony canal.

We have subdivided the cerebellar pressure cone (Figs. 42, 43) into three stages according to severity:

1. Definite mark of a pressure groove on the tonsils.

2. Definite displacement of the tonsils.

3. Displacement of an elongated tonsillar cone (Fig. 43).

Since the three principal arteries of the brain lie in the three large cisterns (anterior c. art.—cisterna supracallosa; middle c. art.—cisterna fissurae Sylvii, posterior c. art.—cisterna interpeduncularis, cruralis and ambiens), a pronounced displacement of the brain into the cisterns (herniation) can cause infarct-like lesions at certain preferential sites (e.g., at the calcarine region from herniation into the cisterna ambiens; Figs. 31, 33, 34). In the case of chronic, generalized increased pressure tiny herniations of the brain force themselves into small dehiscences of the dura (mostly at the base) or into the burr holes (Fig. 44) used for ventricular puncture or ventriculography.

Manifestations of Brain Herniation. Herniation of important portions of the brain into the two most prominent physiological bottlenecks—incisura tentorii and foramen magnum (Fig. 1)—gives rise to certain clinical signs (temporal pressure cone; tonsillar pressure cone). Constriction of the midbrain tends to develop following space-occupying lesions of the temporoparietal lobes or the posterior fossa. In instances of compression from herniation into the cisterna interpeduncularis, cruralis and ambiens, the opposite border of the midbrain may be pressed against the tentorial edge and sustain an indentation (Fig. 32) with subsequent hemorrhagic softening (KERNOHAN's "tentorial

notch"; ipsilateral pyramidal syndrome). In addition to these compressions of the midbrain from without, due to herniation of portions of the brain into the incisura, compressions may also occur from within in tumors of the quadrigeminal plate; in this case the tumor pushes against the surrounding midbrain "like a cork in the neck of a bottle".

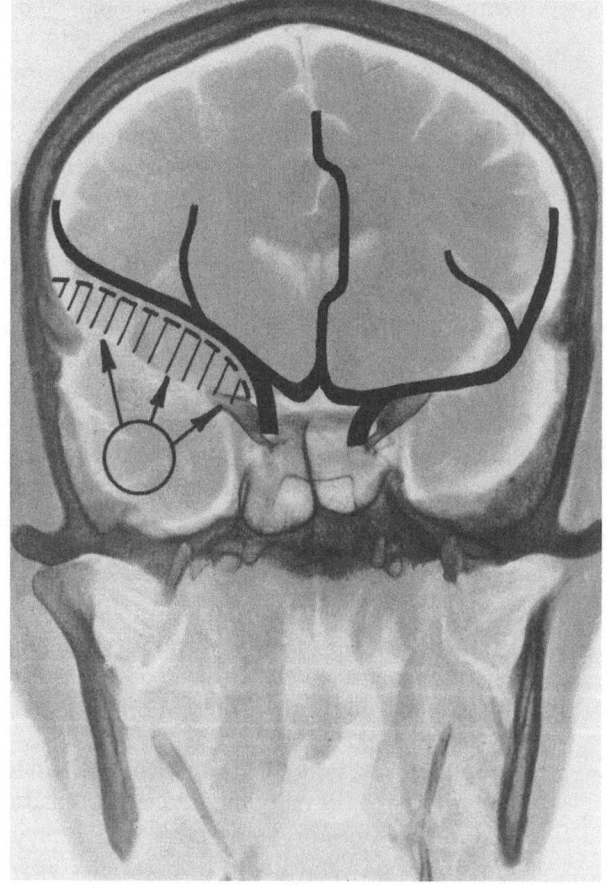

Fig. 18. Semi-schematic illustration of the action of a space-occupying lesion in the temporal fossa. The middle cerebral artery is stretched and elevated and the anterior cerebral arteries show a square-shaped ("parallel") shift (c.f. Fig. 20)

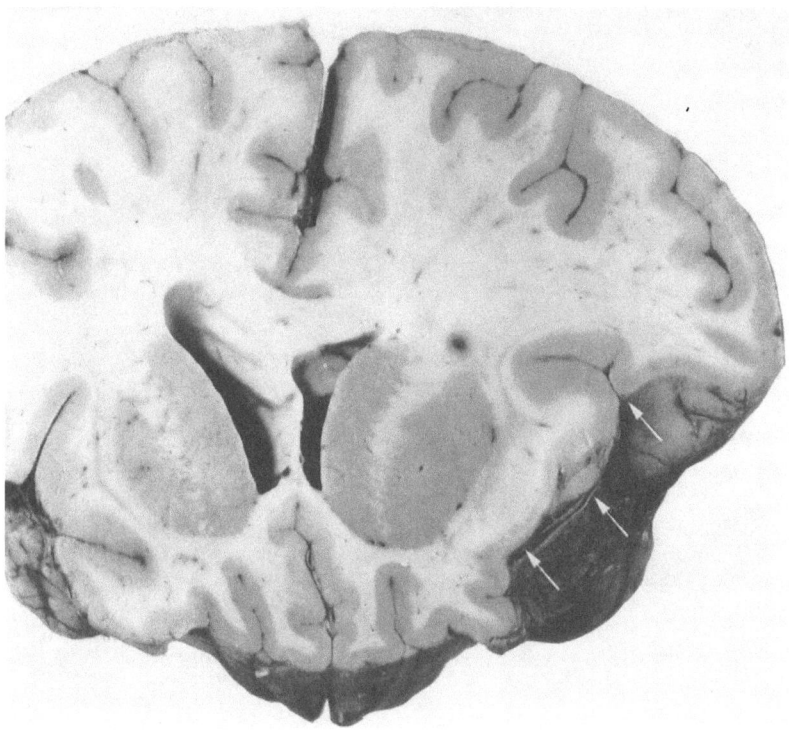

Fig. 19. A frontal section of the same case revealing the impressive excavation (see arrows) of the temporal lobe made by a space-occupying lesion in the middle cranial fossa

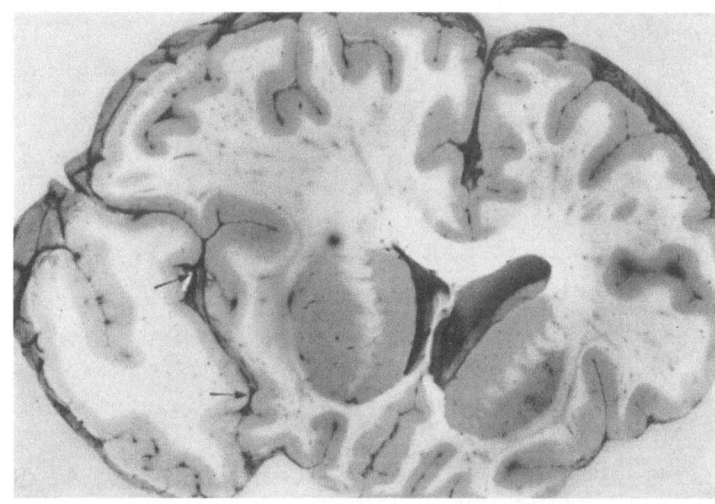

Fig. 20. Anatomical specimen demonstrating the principles outlined in Fig. 18 (arrows: Fissura Sylvii)

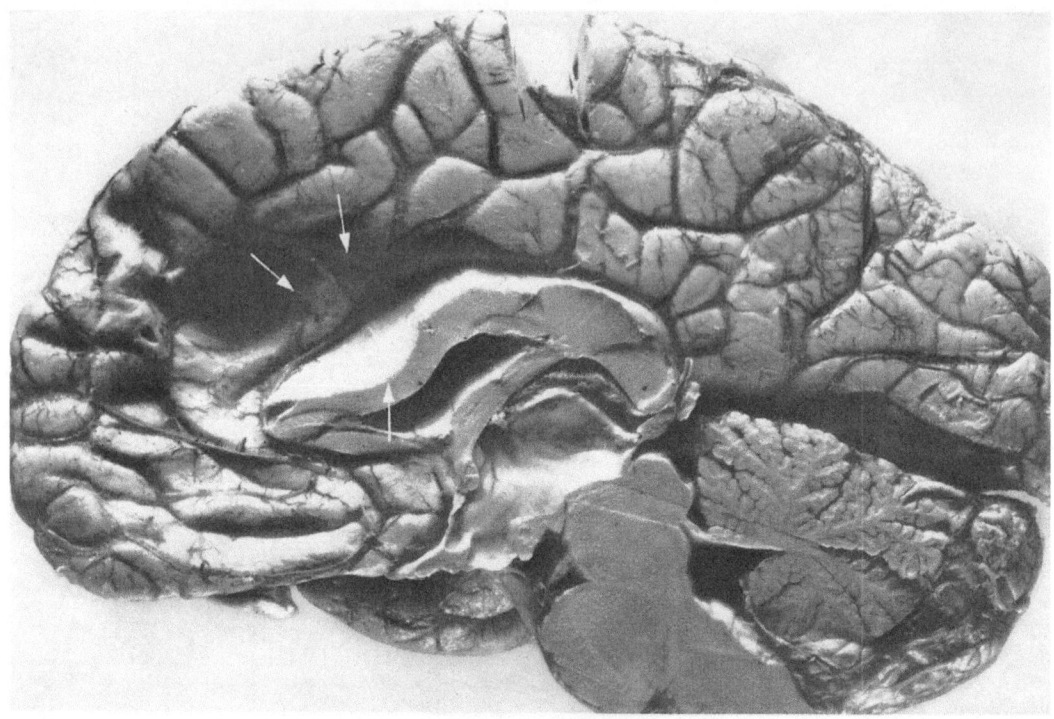

Fig. 21. Depression of corpus callosum and excavation of opposite cingulate gyrus in sub-falceal herniation (arrows!)

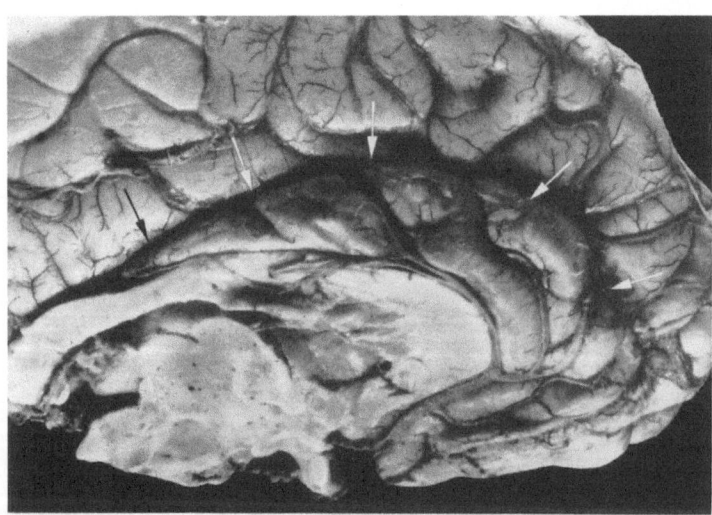

Fig. 22. Extensive mass-shifting and herniation beneath the falx to the opposite side. The arrows mark the lower border of the falx

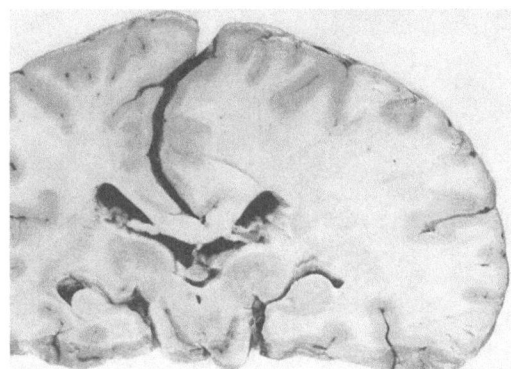

Fig. 23. In this case, note the marked displacement of an entire parietal lobe across the midline to the opposite side. This was explained by an abnormal, under-developed falx which offered no barrier to the observed displacement

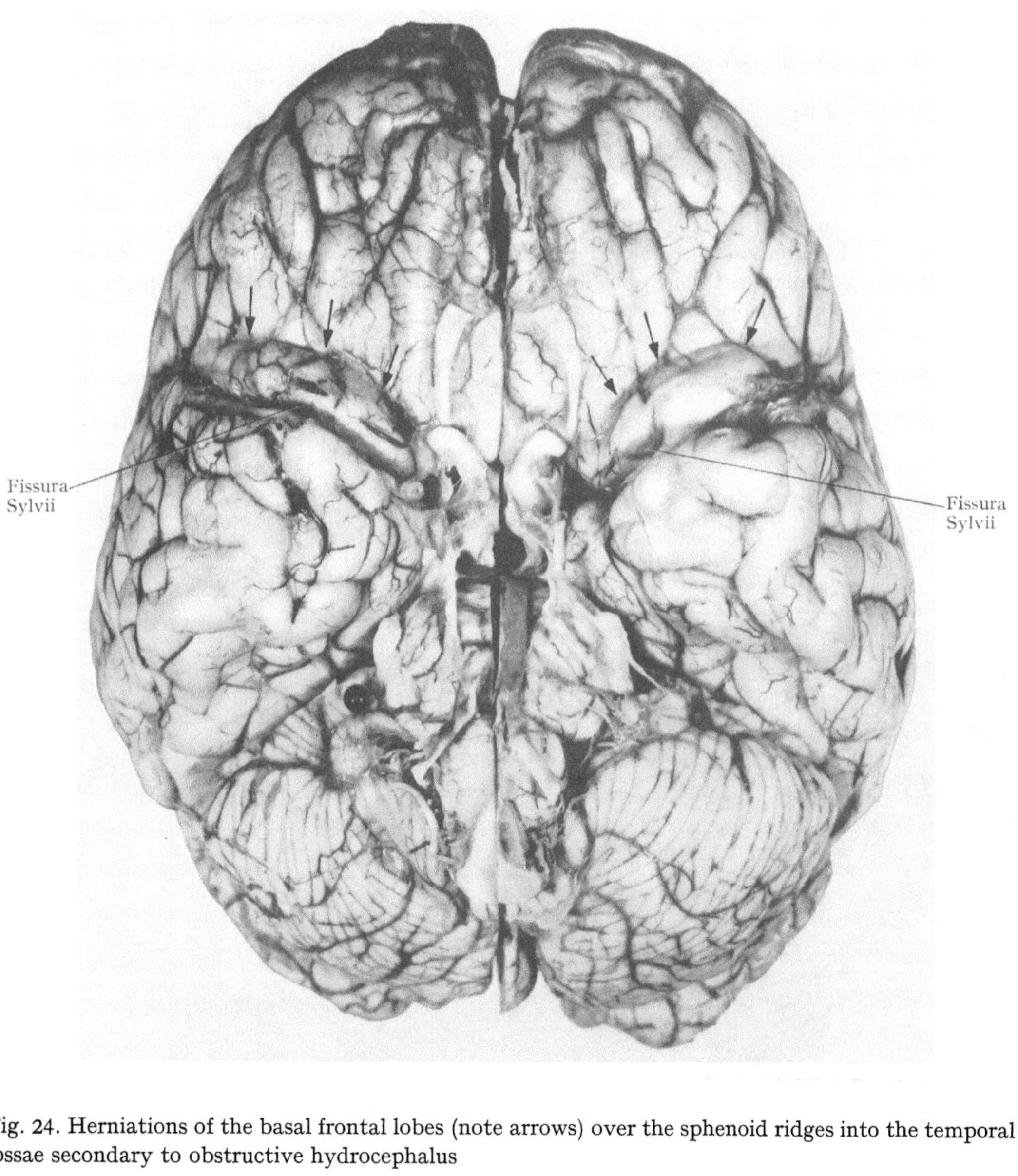

Fissura Sylvii

Fissura Sylvii

Fig. 24. Herniations of the basal frontal lobes (note arrows) over the sphenoid ridges into the temporal fossae secondary to obstructive hydrocephalus

17

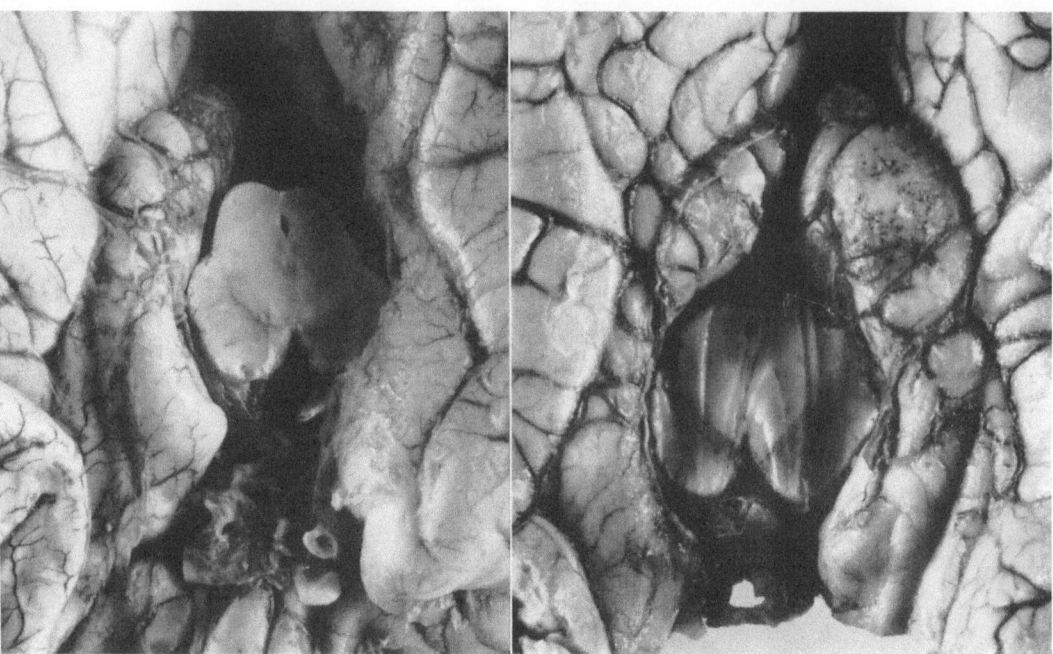

Fig. 25. Left: Transtentorial temporal herniation with displacement of the brain stem; there was also a sub-falceal herniation of the cingulate gyrus, thus forming a circular ring of herniated brain. Right: Bilateral herniation through the tentorial incisura with petechial hemorrhages. The brain stem shows only slight displacement

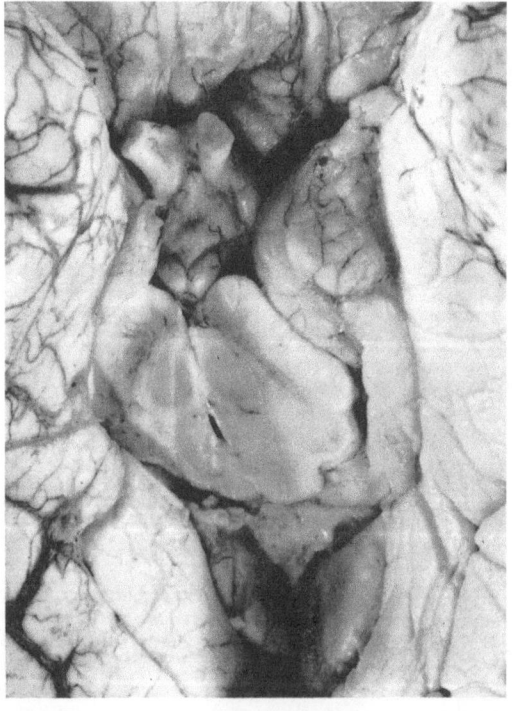

Fig. 26. Extensive herniation of tumor tissue into the tentorial hiatus in a temporomedial oligo-dendroglioma

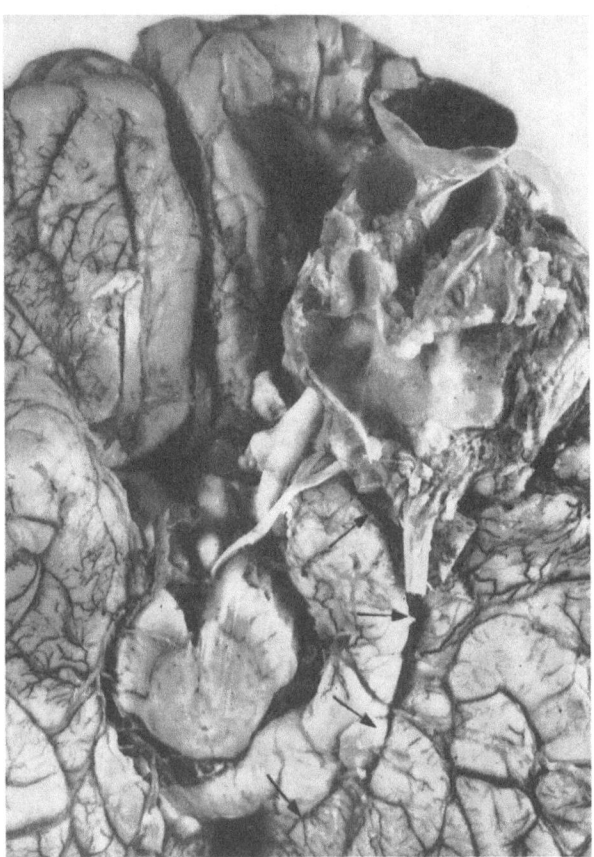

Fig. 27. Extensive tentorial pressure cone (arrows!) secondary to a large left sphenoid ridge meningioma. The lesion may be seen in the upper right corner

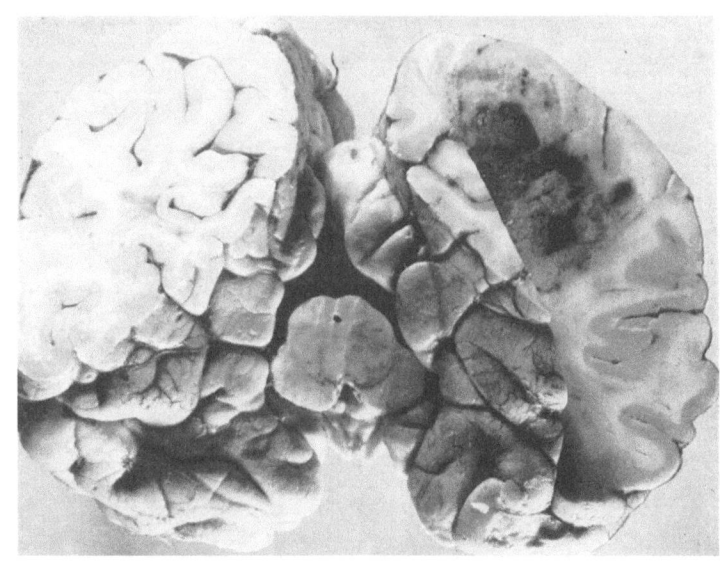

Fig. 28. Marked right-sided herniation through the tentorial incisura with only slight distortion of the midbrain. Only minor herniation has occurred on the left side. A right parietal glioblastoma can be seen in the cut-away section

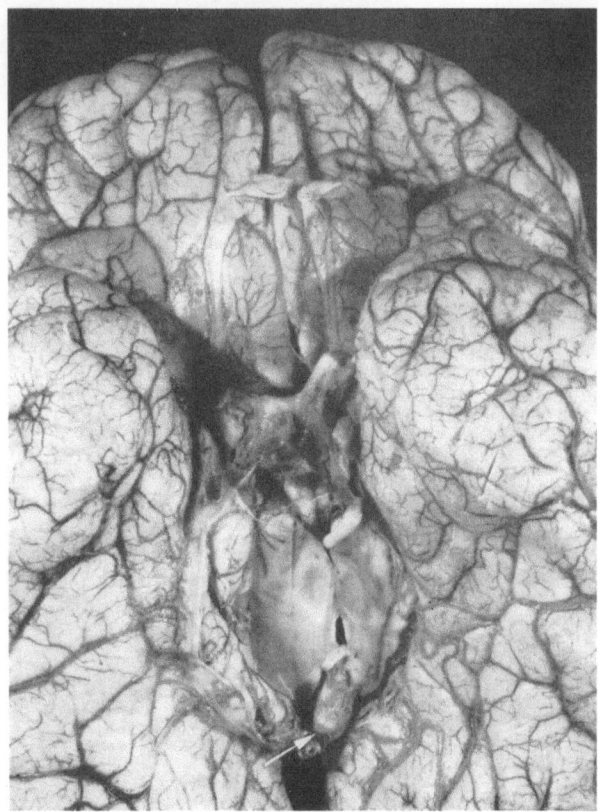

Fig. 29. Marked tentorial herniation displacing the midbrain and related structures. Note the "pineal shift" (**arrow**!)

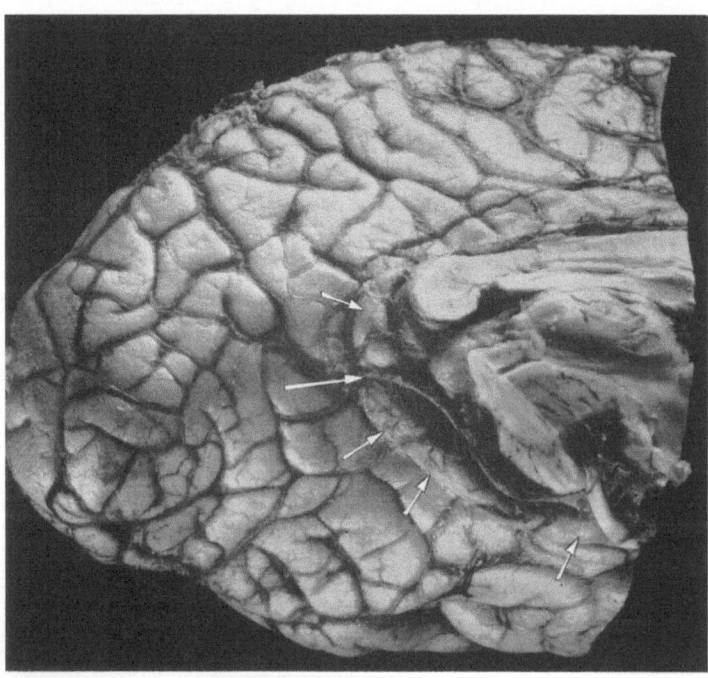

Fig. 30. An extensive temporal pressure cone (arrows!) which has compromised the posterior cerebral artery and has produced a small hemorrhagic infarct in the mediobasal occipital lobe

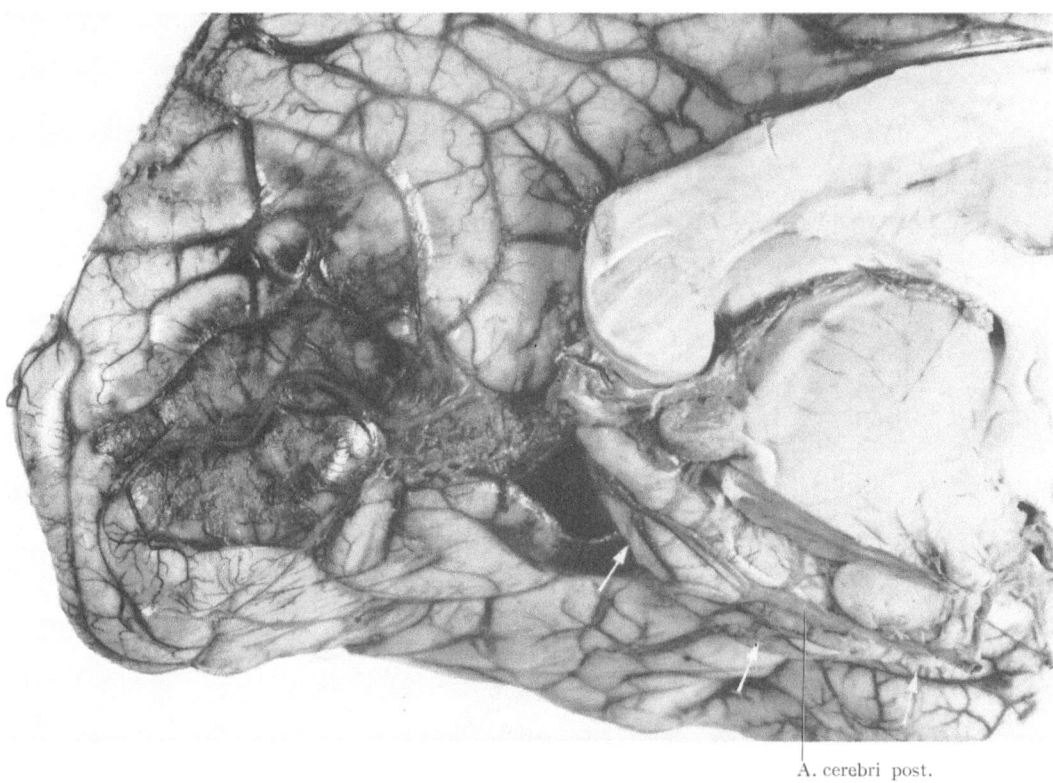

A. cerebri post.

Fig. 31. Marked temporal pressure cone which has displaced the posterior cerebral artery downwards and medially (seen also in the arteriograms!). The artery is stretched over the sharp tentorial edge which has resulted in a hemorrhagic infarction of the medial surface of the occipital lobe

Fig. 32. Deformation of mid-brain and adjacent cerebellum by a large temporal pressure cone. Note the notching and hemorrhage in the contralateral brain-stem. The arrow depicts the direction of applied force in this instance

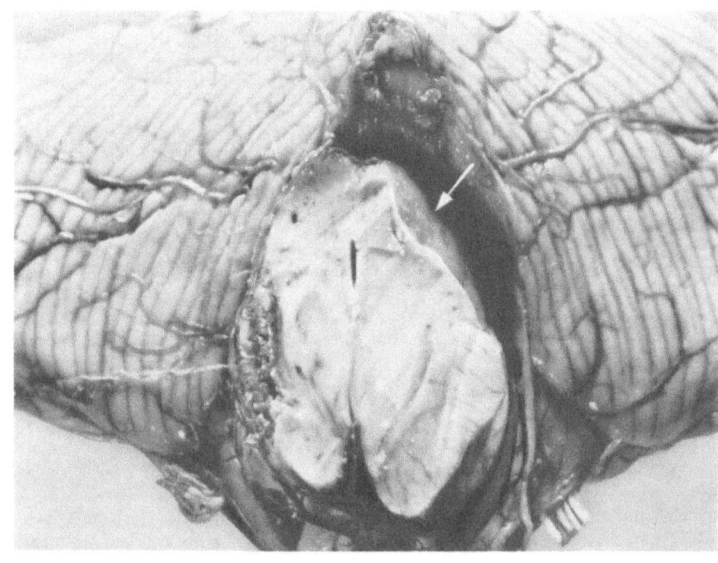

21

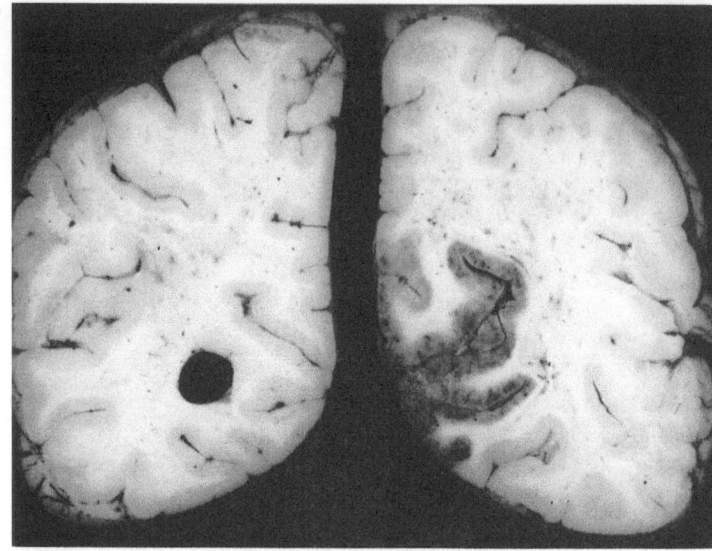

Fig. 33. Compromise of posterior cerebral artery in posterior transtentorial herniation resulting in hemorrhagic infarction of the medio-basal occipital lobe. Only the cortex is involved

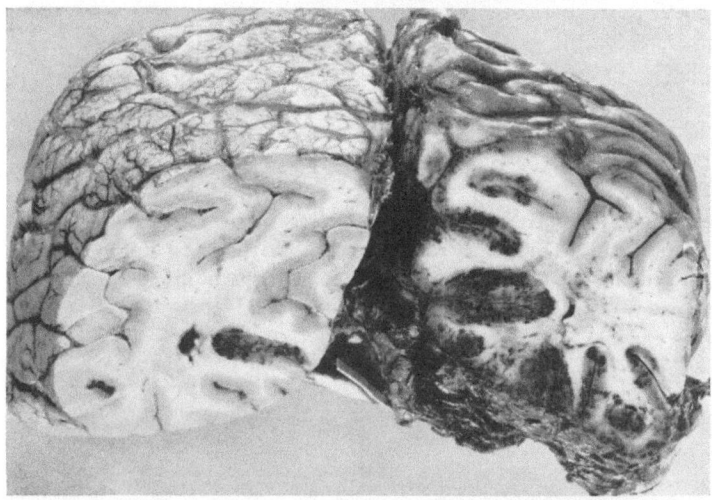

Fig. 34. A complete hemorrhagic infarction of the area of supply of the right posterior cerebral artery consequent to a massive subdural hematoma with bilateral temporal pressure cones (right more than left). Note the minor infarction in its typical location which has occurred contralaterally from similar involvement of the opposite posterior cerebral artery

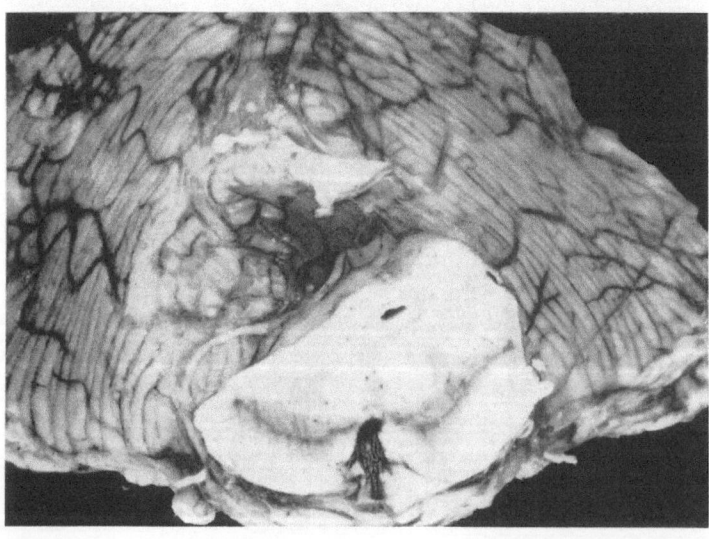

Fig. 35. Marked deformation of the midbrain by a tentorial pressure cone. Also note the indentation in the anterior lobe of the cerebellum

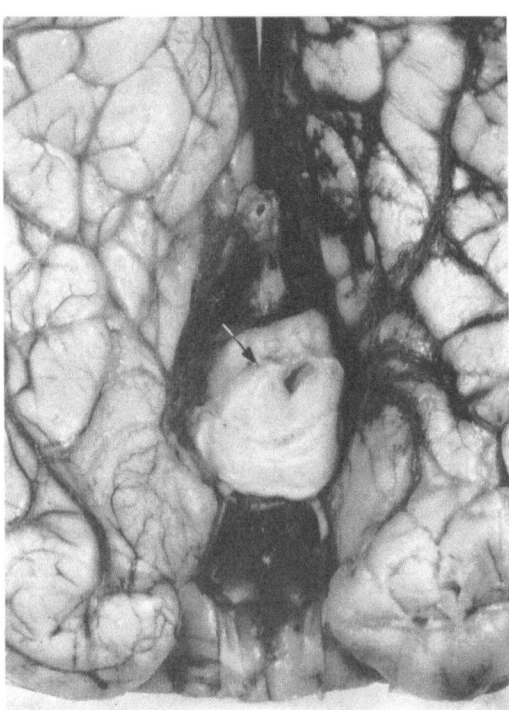

Fig. 36. Upward herniation of the anterior lobe of cerebellum with compression of the midbrain (arrow!) resulting in decerebration (clinically patient demonstrated so-called "cerebellar fits"). Primary lesion was a spongioblastoma of the cerebellum with a unilateral cystic component (see Fig. 41)

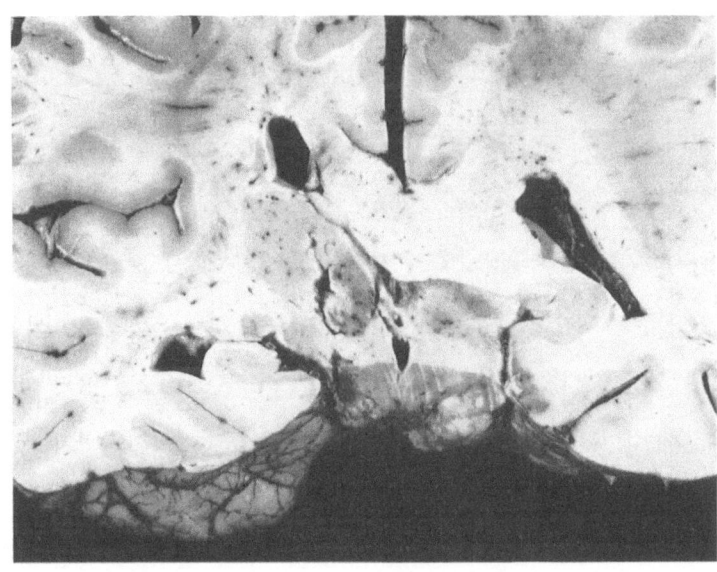

Fig. 37. Compromise of thalamic arteries of the opposite side in transtentorial herniation with shift of the midbrain and prominent secondary "notching" (note impression in the peduncle and hemorrhagic infarction in the thalamus)

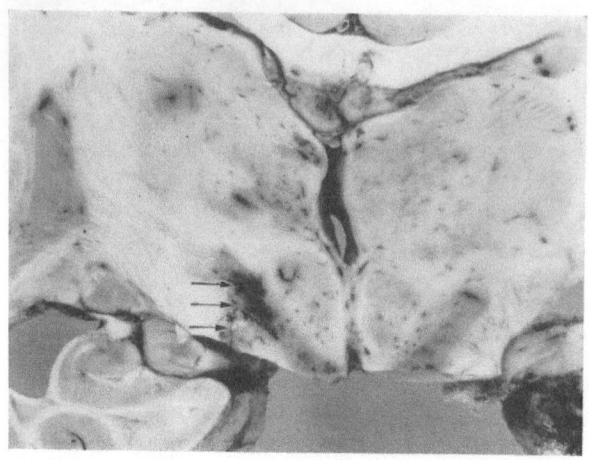

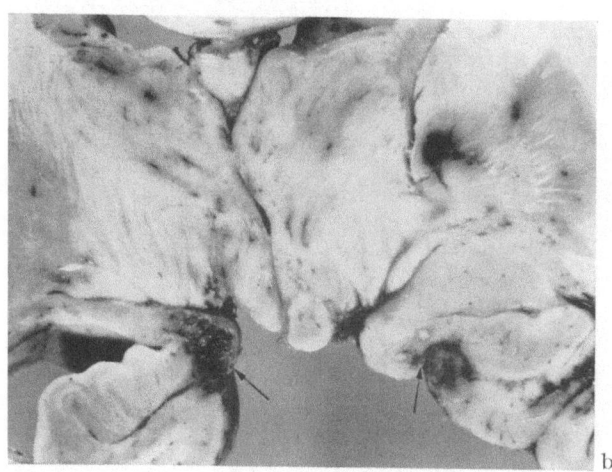

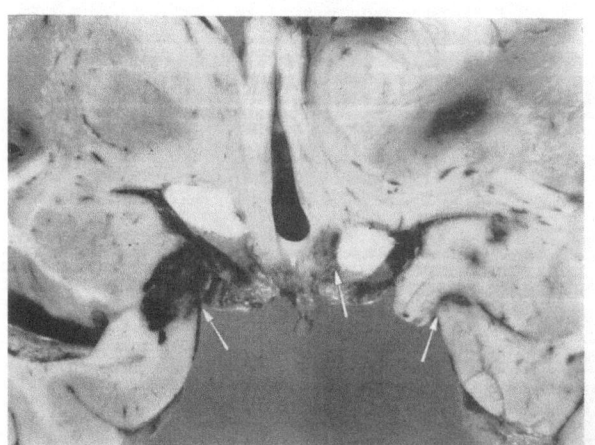

Fig. 38a—c. A rare case of a massive bilateral subdural hematoma which gave rise to some exceptionally rare mass movements. Note: a) that the sharp edge of the tentorial incisura has cut into the brain stem up to the level of the substantia nigra (arrows!) with resultant small hemorrhages; b) that the tentorial incisura has lacerated both hippocampal gyri (arrows!) with subsequent hemorrhage; and c) arrows demonstrating compromised basal structures of the brain secondary to their downward herniation

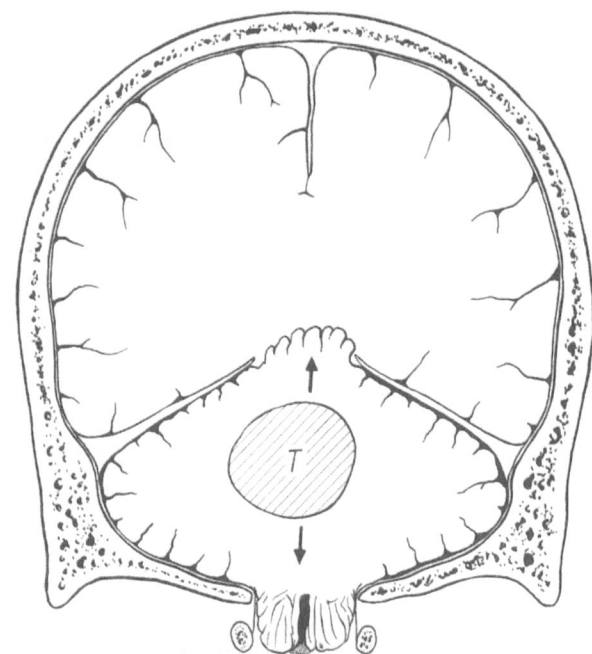

Fig. 39. Schematic diagram of the mechanisms of "upward" and "downward" herniation in the case of a space-occupying lesion of the posterior fossa

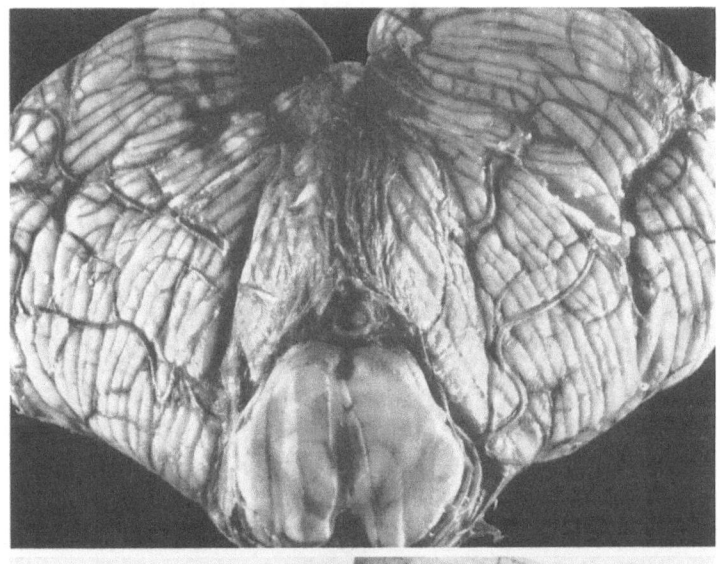

Fig. 40. View from above of upward herniation of the cerebellum through the incisura by a midline posterior fossa tumor. Note the sharp grooves!

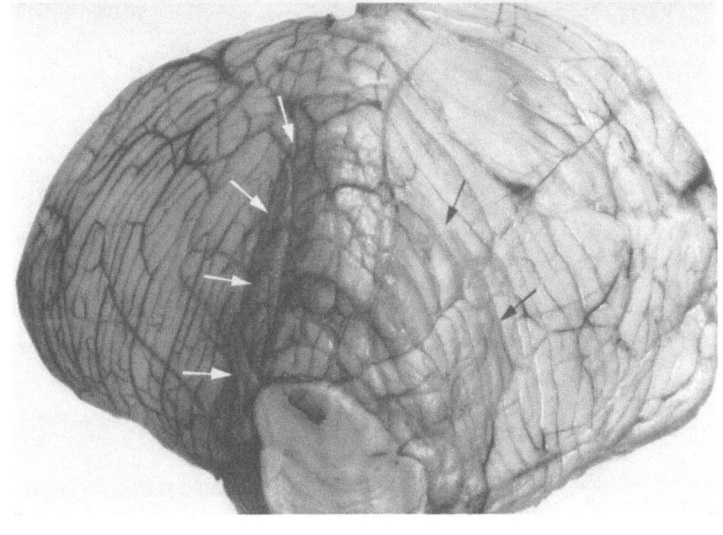

Fig. 41. Upward herniation (arrows!) of the anterior lobe of the cerebellum in a case of a left sided cerebellar spongioblastoma. The brain-stem is markedly displaced and the aqueduct distorted. There was clinical decerebration ("cerebellar fits") (see Figs. 36, 39)

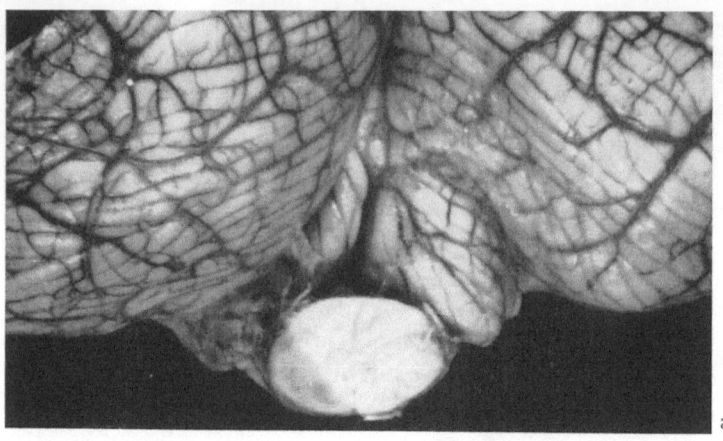

a

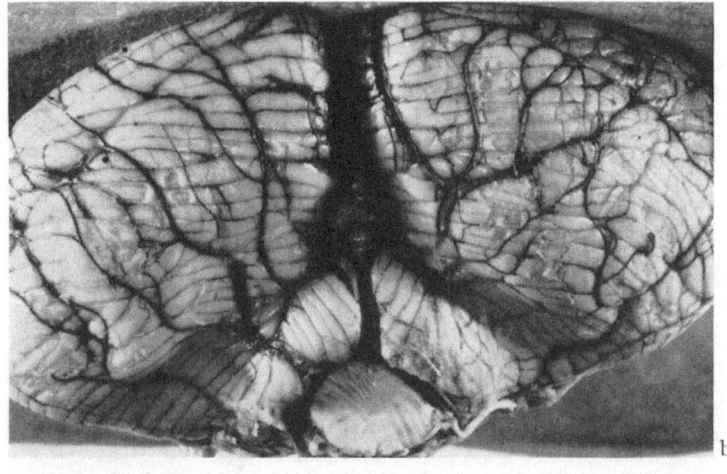

b

c

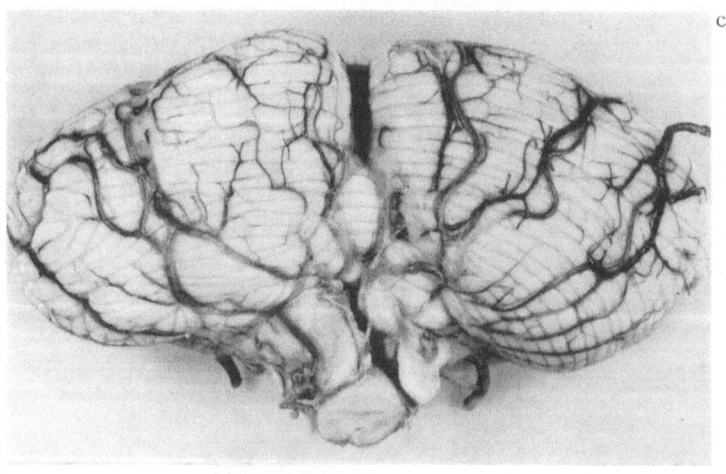

Fig. 42. Various configurations
of the cerebellar pressure cone

Fig. 43. Particularly prominent cerebellar pressure cone (III degree)

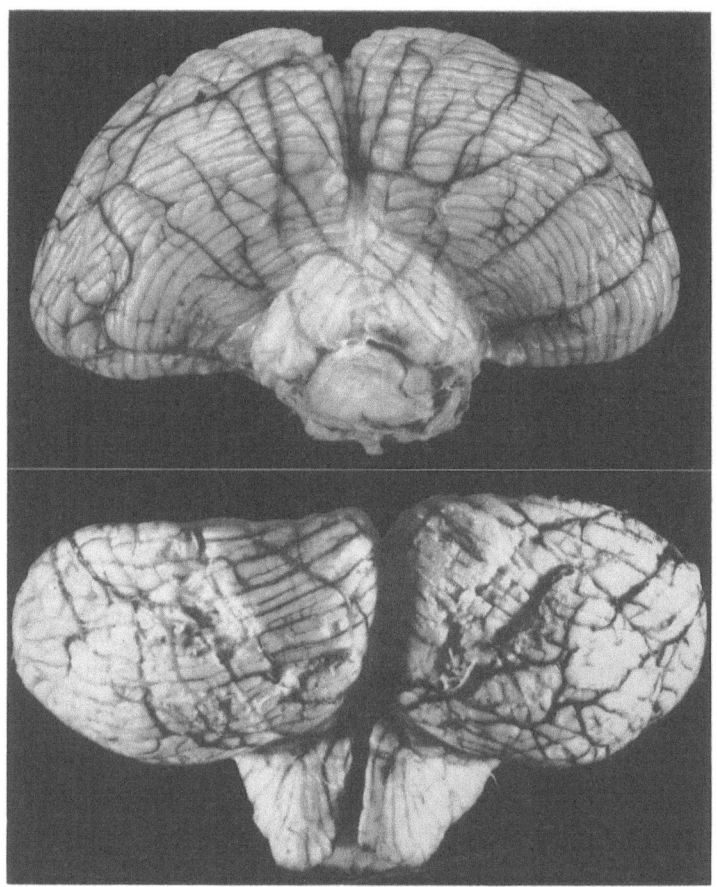

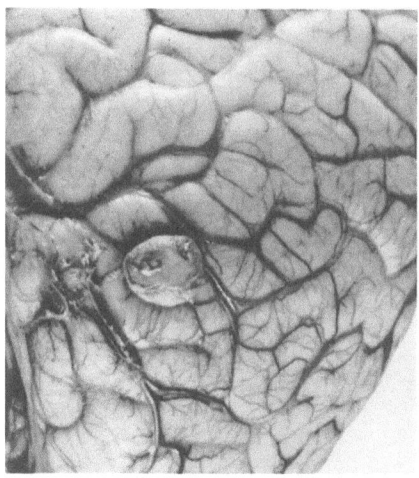

Fig. 44. Pea-sized herniation of adjacent brain substance into the burrhole for ventricular puncture in a case of increased intracranial pressure

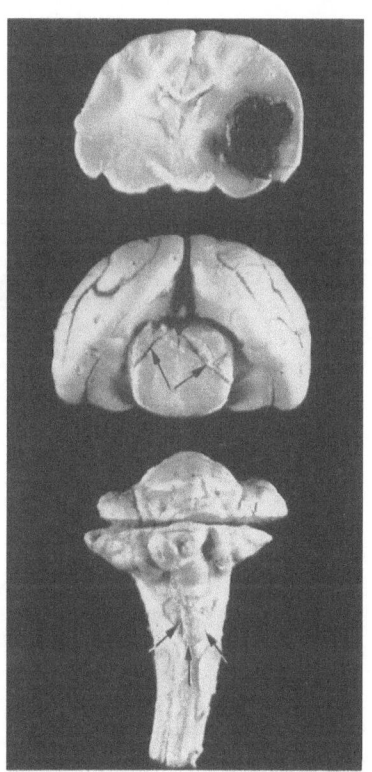

Fig. 45. Case of a simulated brain tumor in cat employing a paraffin injection. Both tonsillar and tentorial pressure cones are observed (see arrows!). Note the absence of edema

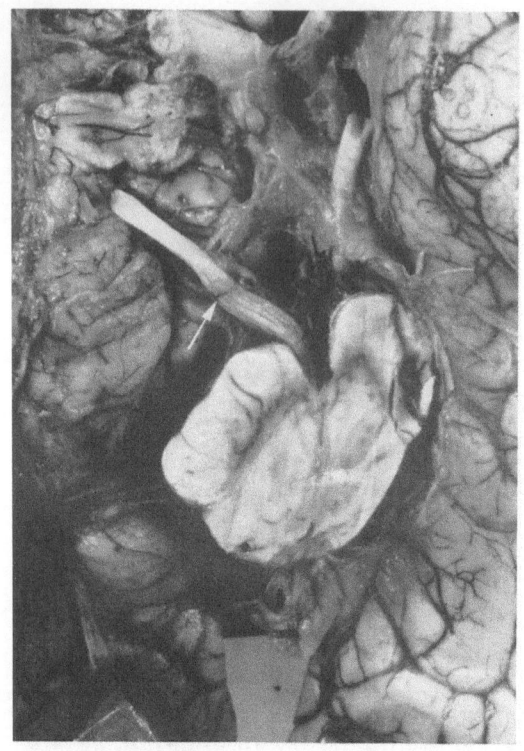

Fig. 46. Cross sectional view of the midbrain in a case with a space-occupying lesion in the right temporal lobe. Tentorial herniation resulted, producing a deep hemorrhagic notch in the third nerve ("distal" notch, see arrow) due to a downward displacement of the brain stem ("axial shift") and a compression of the nerve against the medial petroclinoid ligament (see Fig. 47)

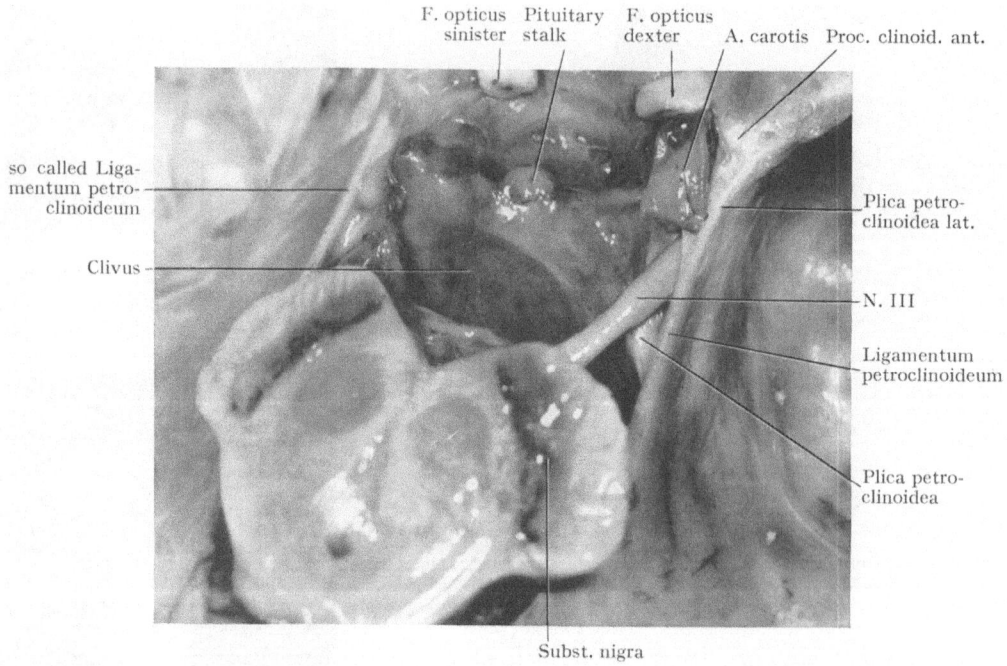

Fig. 47. A dissection illustrating the topographical relationships to the petroclinoid ligament

A. cerebri post.   N. III with proximal notching

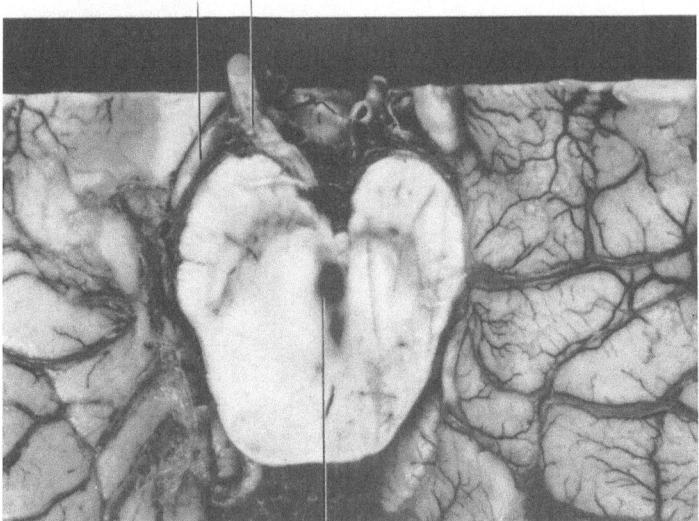

Fig. 48. "Proximal" notching of the third nerve occurring in midline shifts because of fixation of the nerve between the posterior cerebral and superior cerebellar arteries (see Fig. 5)

Small mesencephalic hemorrhage

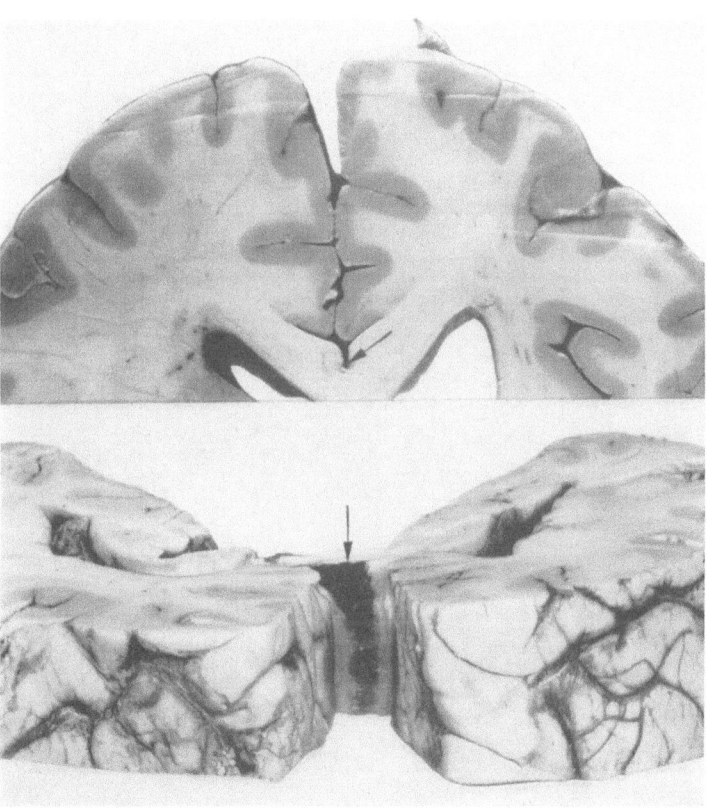

Fig. 49. Above: Beginning transection of corpus callosum by falx (note arrow!) in increased intracranial pressure. Below: Similar notching with fresh hemorrhages consequent to the cutting action of the falx on the splenium

29

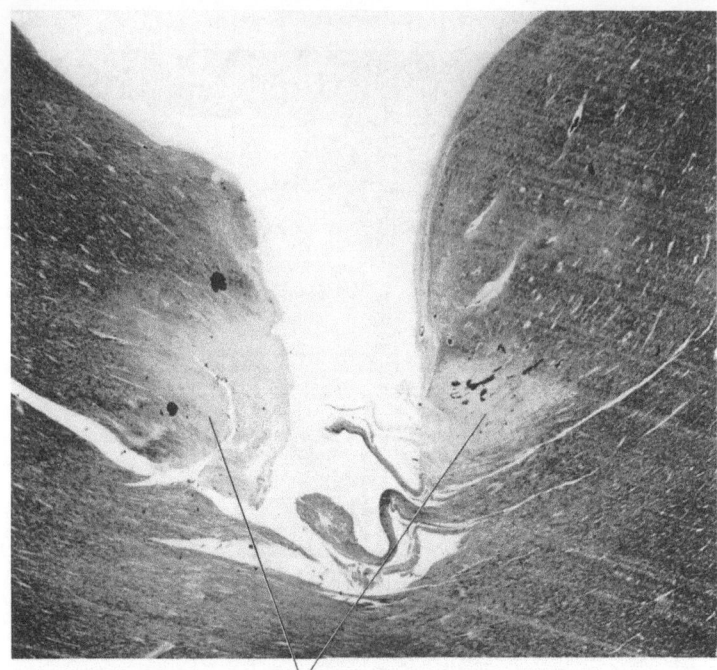

Demyelination and
small hemorrhages

Fig. 50. Myelin stain of a corpus callosum documenting its "in vivo" sectioning by the lower edge of the falx. This is demonstrated by bilateral demyelination on either side of the transection

1.1 Tumors and Related Processes

Classification and "Grading"

Most modern classifications are based upon principles adopted by BAILEY and CUSHING (1926), who proposed a classification of tumors of the glioma group on a histogenetic basis with a correlated study of prognosis. Whereas in general pathology tumors are usually grouped according to the *tissue* from which they are derived, the classification of most "brain tumors", on the other hand, is predominantly a *cytological* one. The original scheme was, however, very complicated and has been modified and condensed by other contributors from laboratories likewise working in close contact with neurosurgical clinics. Thus, most modern classifications group the tumors of neurosurgical importance into approximately 25 types of intracranial tumors. Every tumor classification must achieve two goals: a grouping of tumor types, first, according to the general principles of morphology, and second, according to a clinical and biological estimate of tumor growth—i.e., according to prognosis.

We must emphasize at this point that there is no general consensus of opinion regarding terminology. On the contrary, despite efforts to achieve this goal—in particular, at the Cologne International Tumor Symposium in 1961 (see ZÜLCH and WOOLF, 1964)—individual schools concerned with this matter have not been able to agree upon a common terminology for intracranial tumors. These schools include those of BAILEY and CUSHING (1926, 1930), of PENFIELD (1931, 1932), of KERNOHAN *et al.* (1949, 1952), of HENSCHEN (1955), of DEL RIO HORTEGA (1932, 1945), of RUSSELL and RUBINSTEIN (1971), RUBINSTEIN (1972) and others. Thus, there is still "verbal confusion" regarding terminology in this field, which impedes the statistical studies of those clinicians who wish to investigate the value of a specific mode of therapy (operation, radiation, cytotoxic drugs).

Consequently, we have chosen to adopt the compromise classification of the "Unio Internationalis Contra Cancrum" (UICC).

Since the ultimate classification has not yet been agreed upon, I have chosen to use the classification of our *Atlas of Histology* to facilitate comparison of the histologic and gross aspects of tumor morphology. However, we shall try to give recognition to other classifications by listing common synonyms (see Subject Index and individual Chapts, see also p. 12).

Our *Atlas of the Histology of Brain Tumors* was also based on the UICC classification in the hope of promoting international clarification and unification of the nomenclature (for details see ZÜLCH and WECHSLER, 1968). Subsequently, the World Health Organization established a system of "reference" and "collaboration" centers with the aim of continuing communication between the diverging factions and, ultimately, of recommending a more pragmatic classification which will probably be available in 1978 (see also p. 208).

Prognosis. A morphological classification is of little value to the clinician if it does not include an estimate of clinical prognosis based on morphology. This is an old task of pathology. The work of BAILEY and CUSHING (1926, 1930) might even be regarded as the precursor of a system of malignancy gradings, which they expressed in terms of post-operative survival time. However, one fundamental failing of such an abstract evaluation of biological behavior based solely on morphology is immediately apparent—it fails to account either for the effects of a space-occupying lesion within the closed confines of the intracranial cavity or for its vital position within the substance of the brain. This so-called "clinical" malignancy is often of much greater consequence than the morphologic picture indicates (see Table 2).

Table 2. "Clinical" malignancy of intracranial tumors = biological (histological) malignancy plus

1. Increased volume

2. Mass movements with herniations
$\left\{ \begin{array}{l} \text{temporal} \\ \text{cerebellar} \end{array} \right\}$ pressure cone

3. Action on CSF pathways: hydrocephalus

4. Action on arteries (infarcts!)

5. Action on vital centers: hypothalamus, mesencephalon, medulla oblongata etc.

Thus, tumors may invade a functionally sensitive structure like the diencephalon and even a pea-sized "benign" astrocytoma or spongioblastoma may block the pathway of the cerebrospinal fluid in the aqueduct. A tumor can strangulate a vessel of vital importance, which is occasionally seen with pituitary adenomas or basal meningiomas with respect to the carotid. Still other tumors, by virtue of their space-occupying effects, may be considered clinically "malignant" since the skull in adolescence and in adulthood is practically a closed box. Volume increases, including brain edema and even local obstructive hydrocephalus, can be expected to cause distortion and displacement of the adjacent brain tissue with increased intracranial pressure and with corresponding pressure zones ("herniations"). Thus, a morphologically benign frontal meningioma may prove to be fatal simply because of its location within the inelastic intracranial cavity, whereas most of the other body cavities are elastic. Therefore, both the site and the inherent growth potential of a brain tumor are of the utmost importance for the definition of its final overall malignancy.

The surgeon, however, seeks both precision and clarity of data in any tumor classification. This was the reason for the success of KERNOHAN's proposal of a classification based on 4 grades of malignancy for use in the routine collaboration between neuropathologist and neurosurgeon (KERNOHAN et al., 1949, 1952). Despite its popularity and its more obvious advantages, we feel KERNOHAN's classification has several basic flaws which prevent our endorsing it.

To arrive at an acceptable and meaningful malignancy grading system of a rather pleo-morphic group of neoplasms—compared to tumors of a more uniform organ such as the liver—one has to consider various problems inherent in any grading system. What criteria should be used? Should there be 2, 3, 4 or more grades? Considering these problems, we adopted a 4-scale grading system (ZÜLCH, 1962). Supporting this decision was a well-accepted four grade system in general pathology (BRODERS, 1926), the relatively widely recognized grading system of KERNOHAN et al. (1949, 1952), and the easy interpolation of four behavioral grades into descriptive designations—as "benign", "semibenign", "semimalignant" and "malignant". We are aware that in any grading system sharp borderlines cannot always be drawn and intermediate gradations exist. Also, varying growth rates within a tumor group and even within an individual tumor cannot be predetermined. The surgeon should bear in mind that the tissue he takes for biopsy may not be representative of all grades of activity in the particular tumor with which he is dealing. On the other hand, this system provides a valuable working hypothesis and applies reasonably well to all tumors of the nervous system.

Of these four different malignancy gradations, usually only one or two (and rarely three) are encountered in any one tumor group. Herein lies the basic difference from KERNOHAN's 4 grades for *every* tumor entity (KERNOHAN et al., 1949, 1952). The discussion of the International Cologne Symposium on Classification with respect to this matter revealed a fundamental difference in the definition of tumor malignancy between the Kernohan school (SAYRE, 1964) and our own rather pragmatic way which attempts to follow the example of BAILEY and CUSHING (1926, 1930) by utilizing postoperative results from an analysis of the great neurosurgical clinics of OLIVECRONA (1967), KRAYENBÜHL (1959), and TÖNNIS (1962)—all of whom employed similar classifications—to estimate malignant potential.

As SAYRE (1956, 1964) pointed out, in KERNOHAN's classification one must ideally analyze a multitude of cells, for his system of grading is based on degrees of de-differentiation or cellular anaplasia, in the fashion of BRODERS (1926). In fact, this latter author developed a system of grading based on the character of cells and the frequency of mitoses, choosing four grade categories to express his classification because of the mathematical simplicity of transposing 25th percentile groups into such a scheme. Thus, BRODERS (1926) originally stated that if three-fourths of a tumor were differentiated and one-fourth undifferentiated, it was to be graded I; if equally differentiated and undifferentiated, grade II; if three-fourths undifferentiated, grade III; and if there was no tendency for the cells to differentiate at all, grade IV. Analysis of tumors according to such a scheme and subsequent correlation with clinical course revealed that 90% good results were obtained with grade I tumors, 62 per cent good results with grade II tumors, while only 24 per cent of patients with grade III tumors had good results and this was reduced to 10% in those with grade IV tumors.

The transposition of such a grading system to the intracranial tumors, however, has not been simple, for one must take into consideration every manifestation of the tumor in its entirety—a difficult task. Subtle but significant areas of undifferentiated cells may be missed in the specimens submitted or may not have been included in the biopsy at all.

On the other hand, we have found that in the classification of brain tumors there are usually sufficient morphologic criteria present to decide whether a tumor previously grouped into one of the common categories is a more benign or a more malignant variant—a far simpler task. However, we do so only when such differences in malignant potential actually occur and have been proven to occur in correlated clinico-morphological studies. In this respect, our classification differs significantly from KERNOHAN's system; however, it is of some significance that the KERNOHAN group has admitted that "not all tumors (medulloblastomas) are classifiable according to grades". A good definition of what exactly constitutes "de-differentiation" in tumor cells is not available. What are "abnormal" or "malignant" cells of the astroglia, oligodendroglia or the ependymal lining? Our attempt to define the malignancy of tumors follows then a fundamentally different concept from that of KERNOHAN (1949, 1952), as follows:

step one: the general classification of the tumor;

step two (if indicated) : the determination of whether this particular tumor possesses an "isomorphous", uniform morphology and is amitotic or whether it shows signs indicative of a rapid, unrestricted growth pattern: "anaplasia" (presence of mitoses or increased number of mitoses or atypical forms of mitoses, pleomorphism of cells, disorganized arrangement of the stroma and its vasculature, reactive proliferation of vessels, presence of necroses, etc.), a variant which we designate by the term "polymorphous" or "polymitotic". Thus, even the manner of determining and defining "malignancy" differs significantly from one group to the other. We decide whether a given tumor is "isomorphous" or "polymorphous" or "anaplastic" only if previous clinico-pathological studies have indicated that such a division is warranted.

Initially it was necessary for us to establish with morphological/clinical correlations (the latter expressed by postoperative survival times) what general biological behavior was to be expected. Subsequently, we have learned that there are more rapidly growing variants of astrocytomas, oligodendrogliomas, ependymomas, plexuspapillomas, etc. Only careful clinical follow-up could teach us what to expect in the way of postoperative survival for these variants and such studies are now fortunately available.

The question then arises as to how to transmit the necessary histological prognosis to the clinician (Tables 3 and 4).

This could be done by applying time-honored pathological terms such as "benign" and "malignant", and this would suffice for some 50% of the tumors. However, a truly effective terminology must include the "transitional" or "intermediate" variants between these two poles. We decided to add two additional terms—semibenign and semimalignant—to include these marginal cases. This particular system is preferred to that of BRODERS (1926) or KERNOHAN (1949, 1952) because of the genuine differences which separate us, yet we feel that a 4-stage system has a certain acceptable flavor. Based on the published experiences of the great neurosurgical centers, we have attempted to fit each of the various tumor entities into whichever one of the four categories seemed indicated, and then to correlate this with corresponding morphological features, based on our extensive experience with tumor histology. In this manner we were able to characterize which features were unique to which tumor variants and thus could serve as morphologic criteria for predicting a member of a particular group

Table 3. Modified grading for tumors of the brain and related structures

Tumors	Grade I benign	Grade II semibenign	Grade III semimalignant	Grade IV malignant
Gangliocytoma				
isomorphous	+	+		
polymorphous			+	
Ependymoma				
isomorphous	+	+		
polymorphous			+	
Plexuspapilloma				
isomorphous	+			
polymorphous			+	
Astrocytoma				
isomorphous		+		
polymorphous			+	
Oligodendroglioma				
isomorphous		+		
polymorphous			+	
Glioblastoma				+
Spongioblastoma				
isomorphous	+			
polymorphous			+	
Medulloblastoma				+
Pinealoma				
isomorphous	+			
anisomorphous		+		
polymorphous			+	
Neurinoma				
amitotic	+			
polymitotic			+	
Meningioma				
amitotic/oligomitotic	+			
polymitotic			+	
Angioblastoma (LINDAU)	+			
Sarcoma				+
Pituitary adenoma				
isomorphous	+			
polymorphous		+		
Craniopharyngioma	+			

beforehand. Our concept of relative malignancy, however, is gained solely from a consideration of postoperative survival statistics, admittedly a rather arbitrary and often variable, yet effective method of estimating malignancy. From these efforts, we have fashioned a malignancy grading system for the neurosurgical tumors which we hope will provide the clinician with a basis for estimating prognosis, in so far as this can be implied from morphology. It must, however, be emphasized that this presentation should not be considered to reflect the absolute, invariable quality of each tumor, but rather should serve as a guide, an informed estimate of malignant potential. To expect more from such an inexact science—even in this age of computer technology—is to expect too much (Tables 3 and 4).

Table 4. Classification of brain tumors and their different degrees of malignancy

Degree of malignancy	Prognosis after "total" removal	Tumors	
		extracerebral	intracerebral
Grade I benign	Cure or survival of 5 and more years	Neurinomas Meningiomas Pituitary adenomas Craniopharyn-goimas	Gangliocytomas (temporobasal) Ependymomas of the ventricles Plexuspapillomas Spongioblastomas Angioblastomas (LINDAU)
Grade II semi-benign	Postoperative survival time: 3–5 years	Pituitary adenomas, polymorphous	Gangliocytomas of other locations Ependymomas, extraventricular Astrocytomas, isomorphous Oligodendrogliomas, isomorphous Pinealomas, isomorphous and anisomorphous
Grade III semi-malignant	Postoperative survival time: 2–3 years	Meningiomas, polymitotic Neurinomas, polymitotic	Gangliocytomas Ependymomas Plexuspapillomas Astrocytomas Oligodendrogliomas Pinealomas } polymorphous
Grade IV malignant	Postoperative survival time: 6–15 month	Sarcomas	Glioblastomas Medulloblastomas Primary sarcomas

The Preferential Sites of Brain Tumors

Brain tumors may occur singly or in multiple sites, are well-circumscribed but may be diffuse, and are usually restricted to the CNS. Most brain tumors, however, are single growths.

It is a matter of long experience (and easily understandable from what we know of embryology) that pituitary adenomas, pinealomas, and craniopharyngiomas occur only at one site, and that the neurinomas (of the cerebellopontine angle) prefer the eighth nerve. Meningiomas and cerebellar tumors also show a regularity in their distribution (CUSHING, 1930, 1931; CUSHING and EISENHARDT, 1938). OSTERTAG (1932, 1936) and SCHWARTZ (1932, 1936) are credited for having demonstrated similar relationships for the other types of glioma. Unfortunately, though, in their classification both authors paid little attention to the characteristic that is most decisive for the neurosurgeon: the tissue type of the tumor. Thus, tumors of the same location but of a different type were occasionally grouped together, an

understandable oversight since the idea of dysontogenetic origin was uppermost in the minds of the authors. I have reversed the former procedure by starting with the tumor types and then establishing their site of predilection. On the basis of considerable experience, I can confirm the concept of preferential sites for brain tumors in the overwhelming majority of instances and have found it especially pronounced in glioblastomas.

The following diagrams (Tables 5, 6) present the results in a schematic form; detailed description of these sites can be found in the chapters dealing with these specific tumors.

Table 5

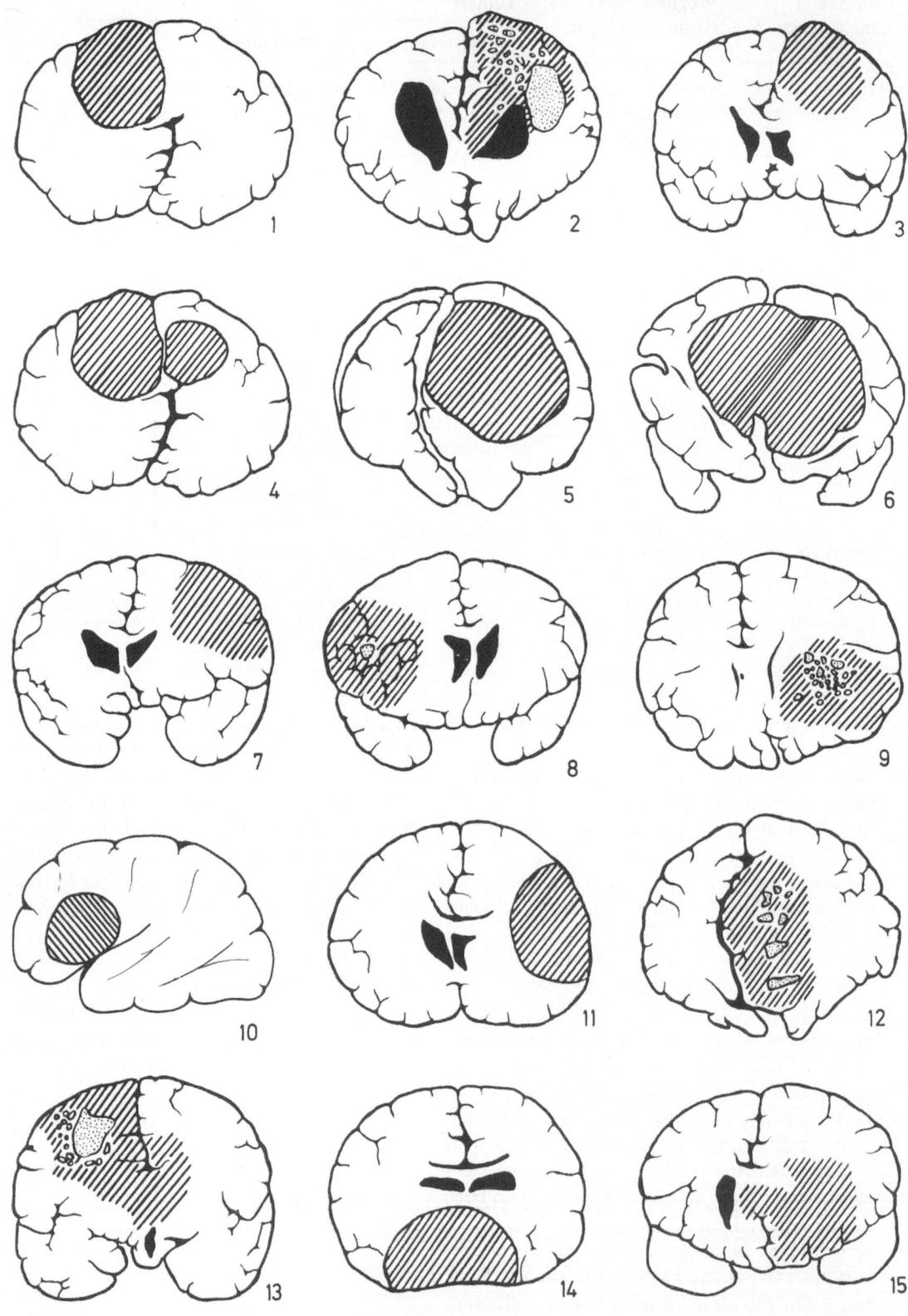

Table 5 (cont.)

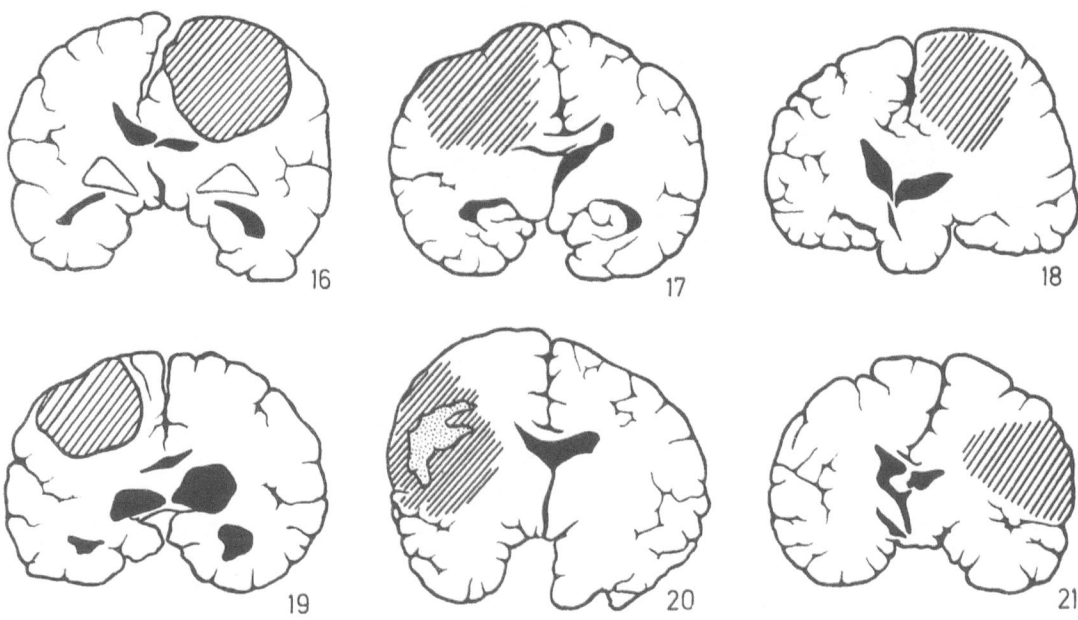

Parietal Tumors

16 Parietodorsal meningioma (meningioma of the middle third of the sagittal sinus). *17* Parietodorsal oligodendroglioma. *18* Parietodorsal glioblastoma. *19* Meningioma of the convexity. *20* Parietolateral astrocytoma. *21* Parietolateral glioblastoma

◁ Frontal Tumors

1 Meningioma of the anterior third of the sagittal sinus—frontodorsal meningioma. *2* Frontodorsal astrocytoma. *3* Frontodorsal glioblastoma. *4* Meningioma of the anterior third of the sagittal sinus (bilateral). *5* Meningioma of the falx (frontomedial meningioma). *6* Bilateral meningioma of the falx. *7* Frontolateral glioblastoma. *8* Frontolateral oligodendroglioma. *9* Frontolateral astrocytoma.

10 Frontolateral (F 3) meningioma. *11* Frontolateral meningioma (alsomeningioma of the convexity). *12* Frontomedial astrocytoma. *13* Frontomedial oligodendroglioma (parasagittal oligodendroglioma). *14* Olfactory groove meningioma (frontobasal meningioma). *15* Frontobasal glioblastoma

Table 5 (cont.)

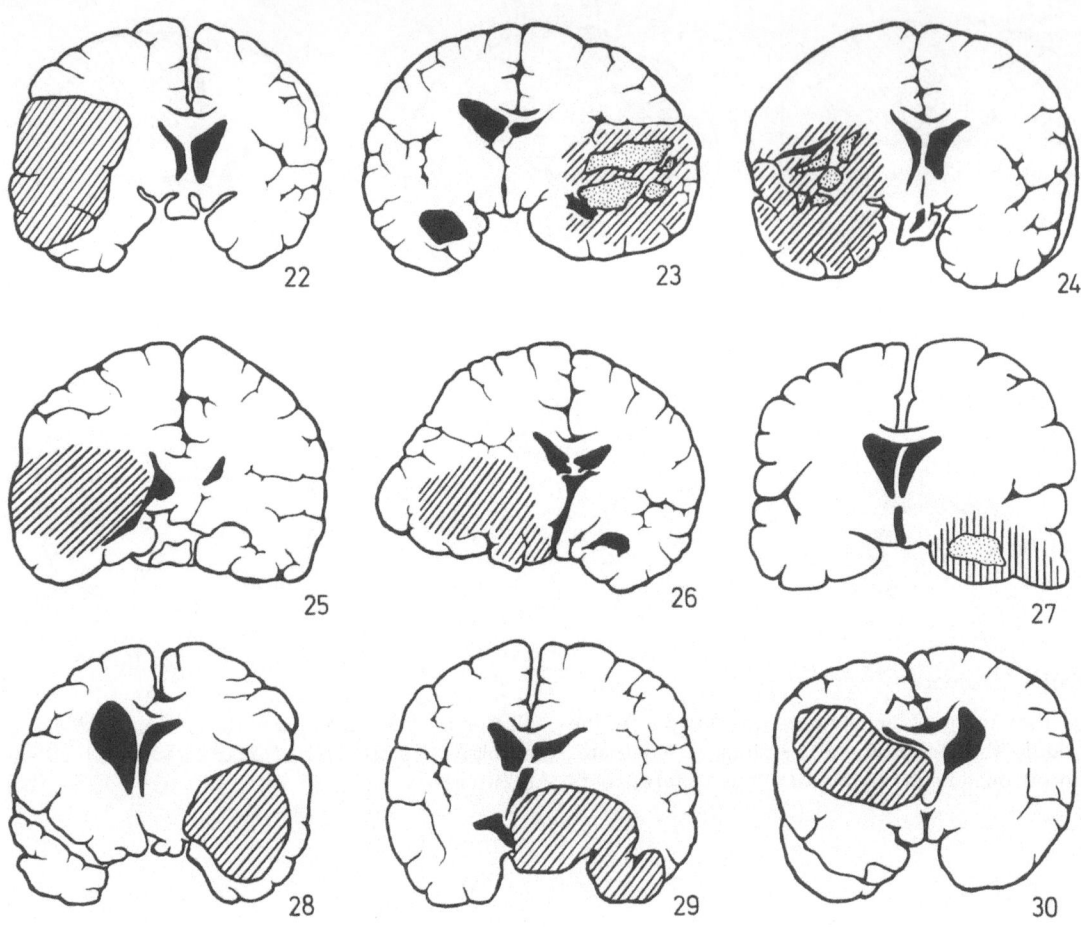

Temporal Tumors

22 Meningioma of the Sylvian fissure. *23* Temporal astrocytoma. *24* Temporal oligodendroglioma. *25* Temporolateral glioblastoma. *26* Temporomedial glioblastoma. *27* Temporobasal gangliocytoma. *28* Meningioma of the sphenoid ridge, round. *29* Meningioma of the sphenoid, en plaque. *30* Ependymoma of the cerebral hemisphere

Midline Tumors ▷

31 Meningioma of the olfactory groove. *32* Meningioma of the tuberculum sellae. *33* Craniopharyngioma. *34* Craniopharyngioma. *35* Meningioma of the tuberculum sellae. *36* Craniopharyngioma. *37* Pituitary adenoma. *38* Pituitary adenoma. *39* Spongioblastoma of the chiasm. *40* Ependymal (colloid) cyst of foramen of Monro. *41* Glioblastoma of the rostral corpus callosum. *42* Glioblastoma of the caudal corpus callosum. *43* Oligodendroglioma of corpus callosum. *44* Lipoma, supracallosal

Table 5 (cont.)

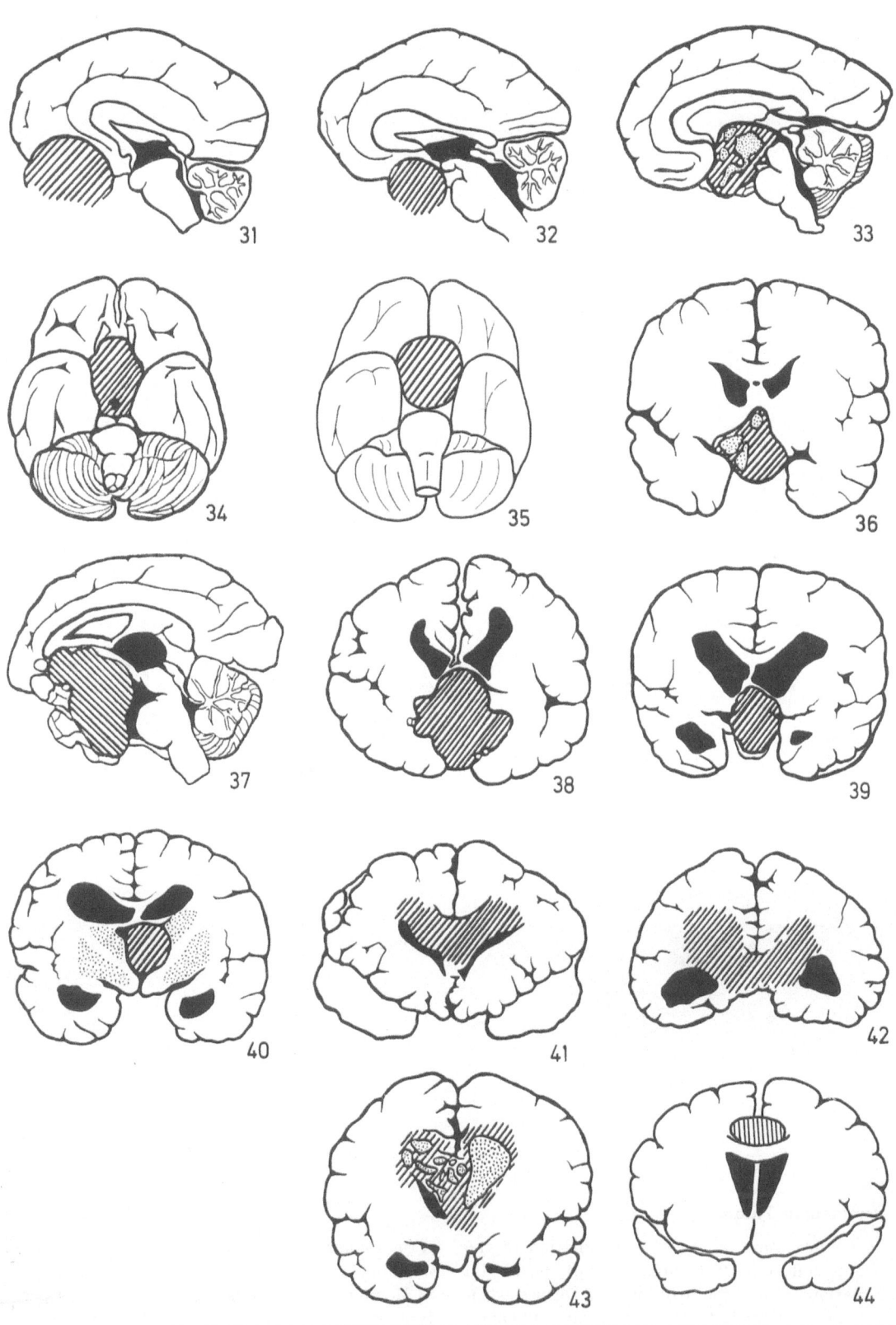

Table 5 (cont.)

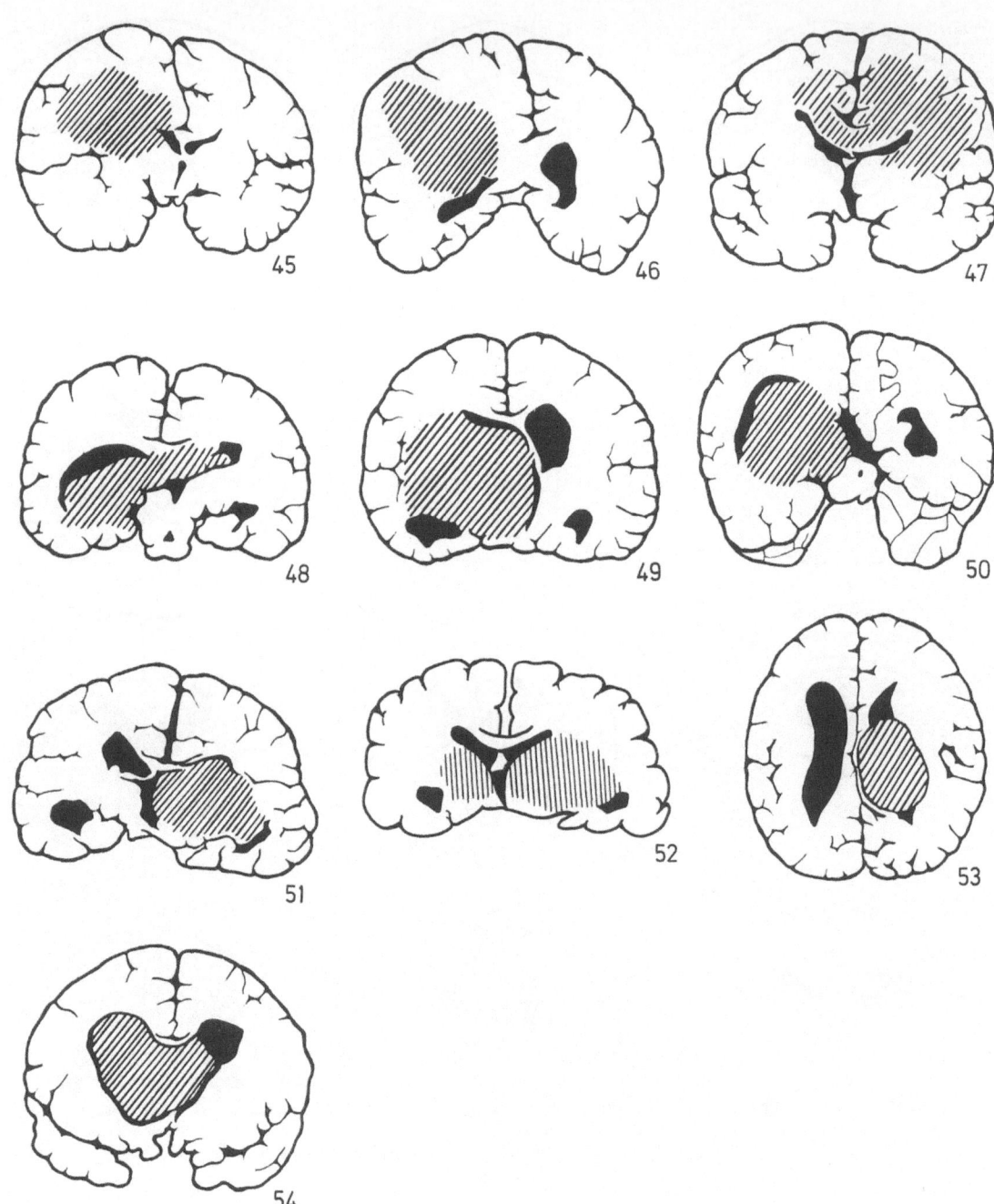

Paramedian Tumors

45 Glioblastoma of the rostral radiation of the corpus callosum. *46* Glioblastoma of the caudal radiation of the corpus callosum. *47* Diffuse astrocytoma. *48* Glioblastoma of the fornix. *49* Oligodendroglioma of the thalamus. *50* Glioblastoma of the thalamus. *51* Astrocytoma of the thalamus. *52* Glioblastoma of the thalamus (bilateral). *53* Meningioma of the lateral ventricle. *54* Ependymoma of the lateral ventricle (foramen of Monro).

Table 5 (cont.)

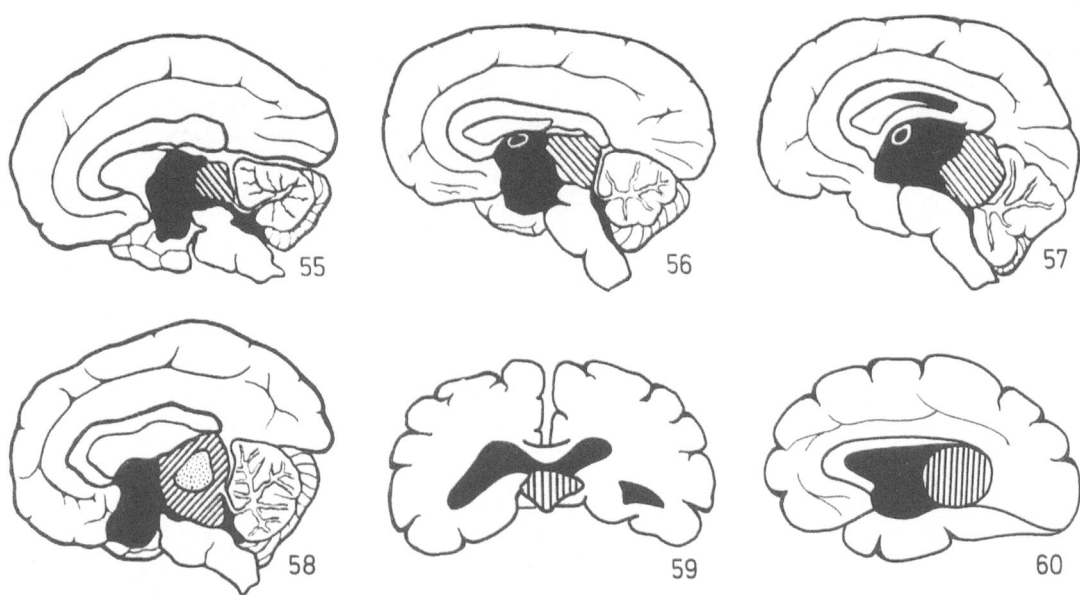

Midline Tumors (mesencephalic)

55 Pinealoma. *56* Ependymoma of the third ventricle (region of the quadrigeminal plate). *57* Glioblastoma of the midbrain. *58* Spongioblastoma of the midbrain. *59* Pinealoma. *60* Meningioma of the tentorial hiatus

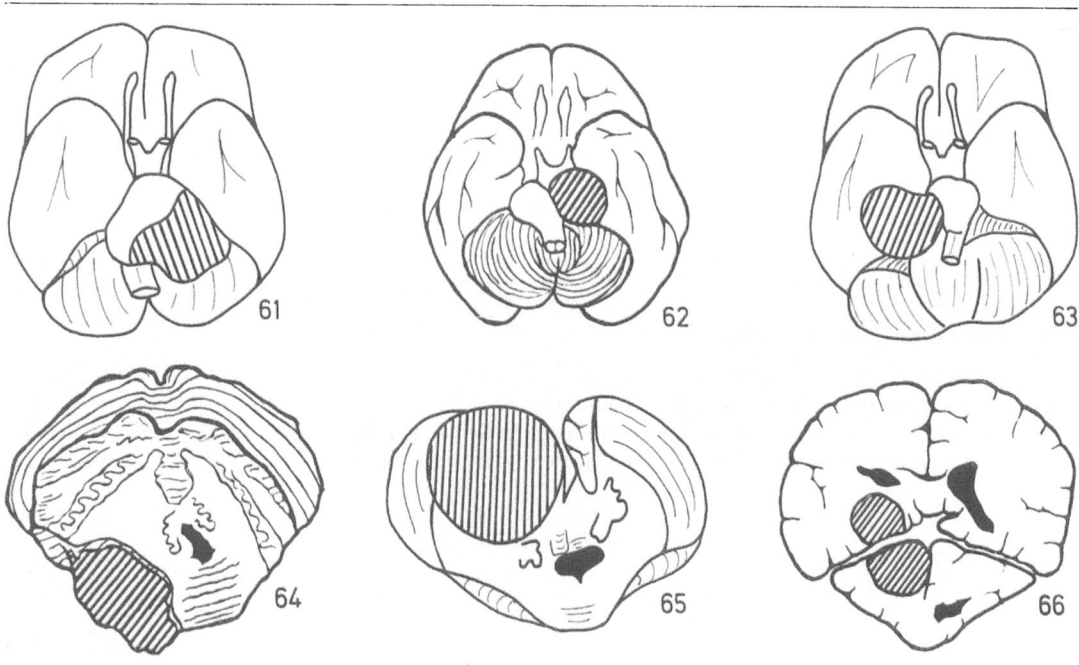

Posterior Fossa Tumors (paramedian)

61 Epidermoid of cerebellopontine angle. *62* Meningioma of the petrous pyramid (cerebellopontine angle). *63* Neurinoma of the cerebellopontine angle. *64* Neurinoma of the cerebellopontine angle. *65* Meningioma, peritorcular. *66* Meningioma of the tentorium

Table 5 (cont.)

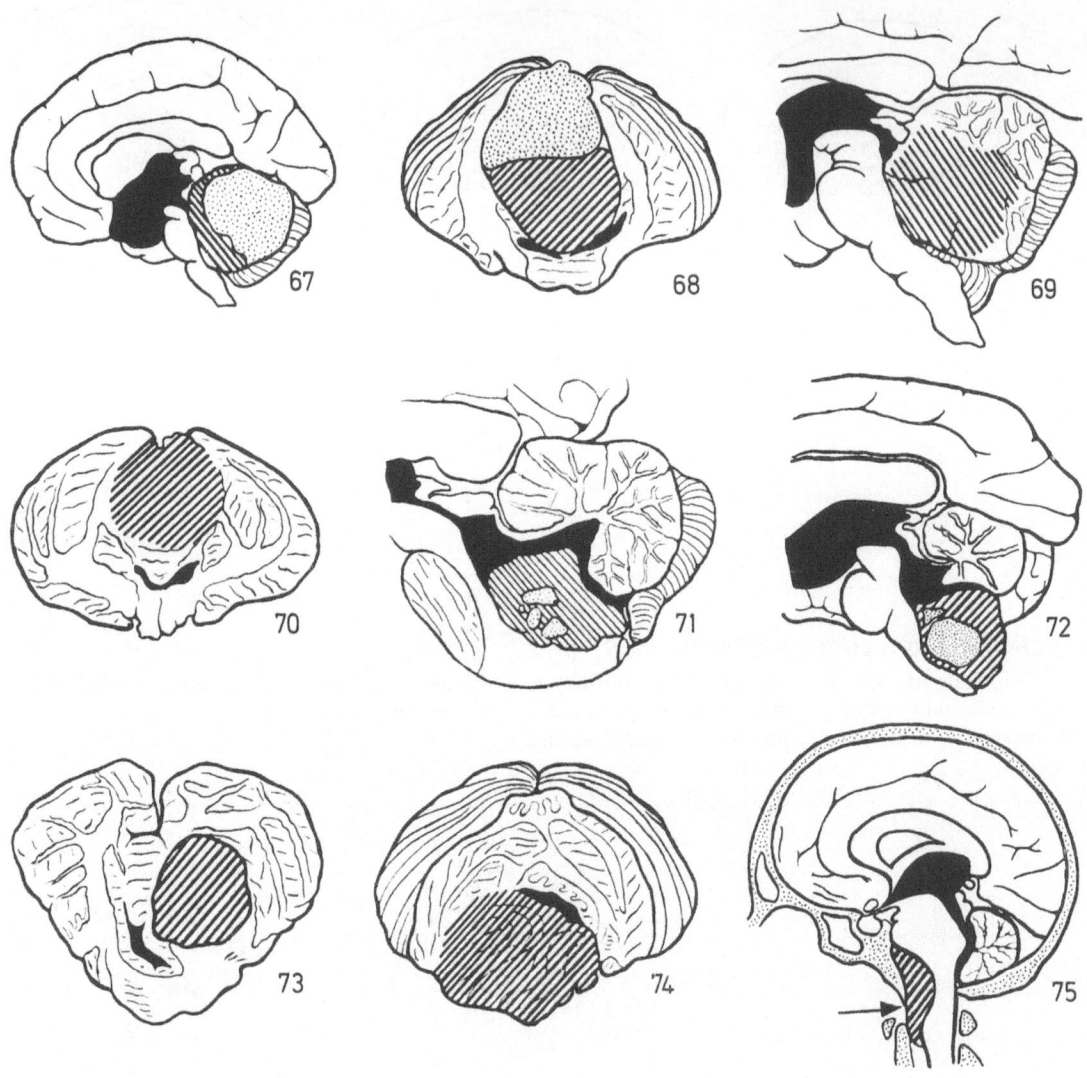

Posterior Fossa Tumors (midline)

67 Spongioblastoma of the cerebellum. 68 Spongioblastoma of the cerebellum. 69 Medulloblastoma of the cerebellum. 70 Medulloblastoma of the cerebellum. 71 Ependymoma of the fourth ventricle. 72 Angioblastoma in the fourth ventricle. 73 Angioblastoma of the cerebellar hemisphere. 74 Astrocytoma of the pons. 75 Meningioma of the clivus (cranio-spinal)

Table 5 (cont.)

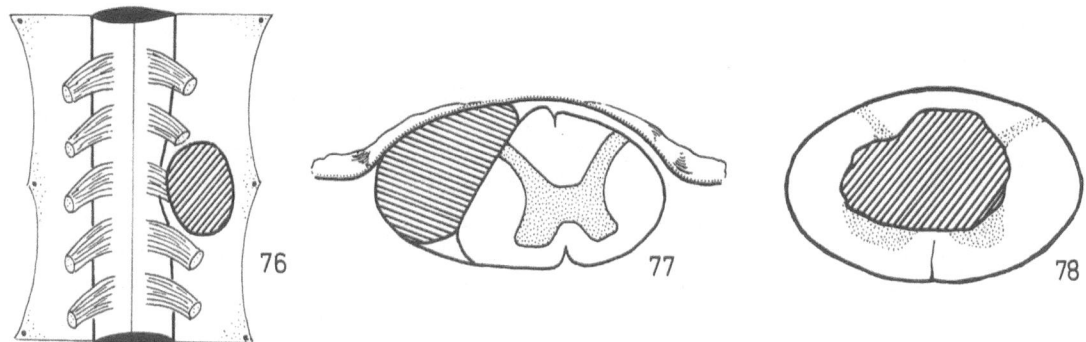

Spinal Tumors

76 Neurinoma, spinal. *77* Meningioma, spinal.
78 Ependymoma of the spinal cord

Table 6. Schematic representation of the site of the common tumors of the base of the skull

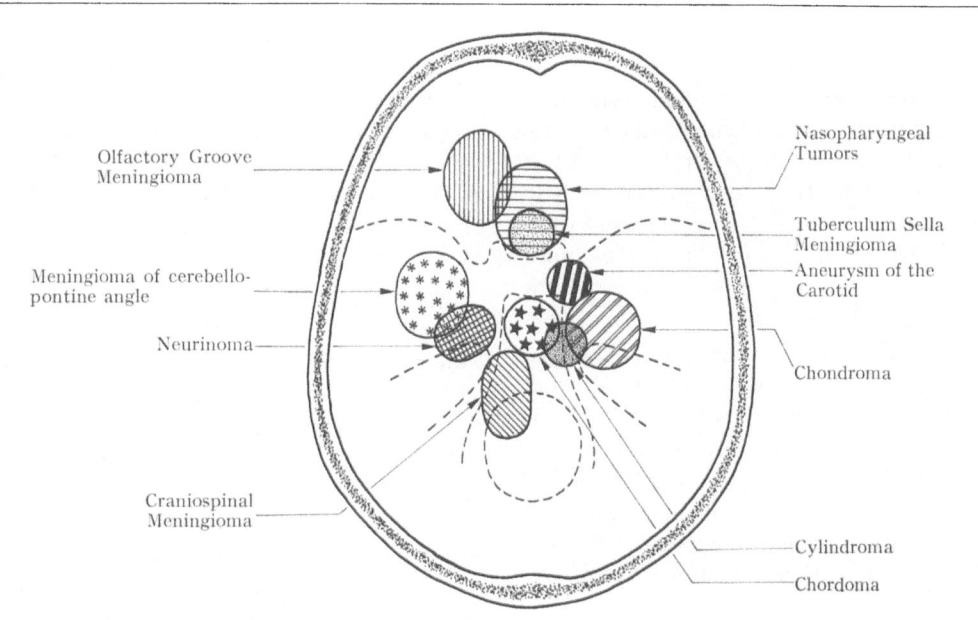

Sex Distribution of Patients with Brain Tumors

Sex distribution and the discovery of a clear sex predilection for of certain tumor types has proven to be particularly noteworthy.

An analysis of our series has resulted in the general conclusion that there is a slight preponderance of males over females (52.8 to 47.2%, or approximately 11:9), which corresponds to results previously mentioned in the literature. Moreover, certain brain tumors showed a particularly pronounced sex predilection. The preponderance of males over females in a selected group of cases was as follows:

Ependymomas	6:4
Astrocytomas	7:5
Oligodendrogliomas	5:4
Glioblastomas	6:4
Medulloblastomas	7:3
Angioblastomas	2:1
Angiomas and aneurysms	4:3
Pinealomas	2:1
Metastases	7:4
Craniopharyngiomas	2:1
Teratomas	4:3

A preponderance of females over males was found in:

Neurinomas	2:1
Meningiomas	9:5

It was of special interest that this general sex preponderance of patients with a given tumor was even more pronounced in a particular decade of life or at a particular site. Thus the male preponderance of craniopharyngiomas attained a ratio of 4:1 when restricted to the first two decades of life. After the age of 40 females were four times more often affected by neurinomas than males, and even eight times more at the age of 55. In the meningiomas, females up to the age of 50 were more frequently affected than males (at a ratio of 3:2), whereas at the age of 60 matters became reversed and twice as many men were affected.

While females with meningiomas, in general, outnumbered males by only 9:5, they were affected with chiasmal (tuberculum sellae) meningiomas twice as often as males and with cerebellopontine angle meningiomas and spinal meningiomas four times as often as men.

Age Incidence

Determination of the age incidence of individual tumor types was one of the most important achievements in the biology of brain tumors. We owe the precise definition of tumor groups—i.e., entities with similar location, age incidence, and tissue type—to CUSHING (1930, 1931) and BAILEY (1936, 1951) in their description of the cerebellar tumors (medulloblastomas and the so-called cerebellar astrocytomas and many other groups). If age incidence is plotted against frequency for all tumor groups, the resulting curves show characteristic age peaks (Table 7a–n). But since the actual time of onset of tumor growth cannot be determined, we use the age at the time of admission to the hospital or, where there has been no hospital treatment, at the time of death. The discrepancies in such an arbitrary system between onset of tumor growth and hospital admission or death are obvious, particularly in the case of slow-growing tumors, such as astrocytomas, oligodendrogliomas, some gangliocytomas, meningiomas, craniopharyngiomas, epidermoids, etc.

With all the age curves plotted together on a single ordinate, we would notice a crossing of many of the curves at around age 20—i.e., the ascending and descending limbs of a number of curves cross one another. This indicates the biological significance of this age period which represents the end of childhood and adolescence.

We also see that certain tumor types show a predilection for the third and fourth decades and that the fifth and sixth decades, too, are preferred by certain kinds of tumors. We define childhood and adolescence as the ages between 1–20 years, middle age from 21 to 45, the age of involution from 46–65, and old age from 65 on.

If we evaluate a large number of patients from the point of view of age incidence, we come to the following conclusions: in childhood and adolescence the most common tumors in the cerebral hemispheres are ependymomas, with the other gliomas and ganglion cell tumors appearing less frequently. Monstrocellular sarcomas are also encountered. On the other hand, we see only a few of the meningiomas, which form the single largest group in the older age groups. In the chiasmal region craniopharyngiomas and spongioblastomas are frequent, while pituitary adenomas are nearly absent. The complete absence of neurinomas is very impressive, while in the cerebellum itself the bulk of all tumors occurring in the younger age groups consists of medulloblastomas and spongioblastomas (so-called cerebellar astrocytomas of the juvenile type).

The angioblastomas of the fourth ventricle are not very evident as yet, but in the region of the quadrigeminal plate teratomas and pinealomas do occur in this age group; nearly all spongioblastomas and astrocytomas around the aqueduct occur under the age of 20. Other tumors occurring in childhood and in adolescence are the oligodendrogliomas of the thalamus, and astrocytomas and spongioblastomas of the pons.

The middle decades of life (third and fourth decades) are characterized by the frequent occurrence of gliomas in the cerebral hemispheres (astrocytomas and oligodendroglio-

mas), meningiomas at various sites, pituitary adenomas, the neurinomas of the cerebello-pontine angle, and the angioblastomas of the cerebellum. The two cerebellar groups of tumors of the younger age groups are found only rarely.

The latter decades of life (fifth and sixth decades) show more frequent occurrence of malignant glioblastomas and of metastatic tumors. Oligodendrogliomas and astrocytomas, meningiomas, angioblastomas, and neurinomas are also encountered.

In the sixth and seventh decades glioblastomas, meningiomas and neurinomas comprise 82% of the brain tumors and, together with the metastatic lesions, clearly predominate. We have little information about comparable data on tumors in the very aged, since autopsy is seldom performed on those who die of old age. Also, in the very youngest age groups the distribution of brain tumors may vary and contains many uncommon types of tumors.

Table 7a—n. Incidence of individual tumor types according to age groups

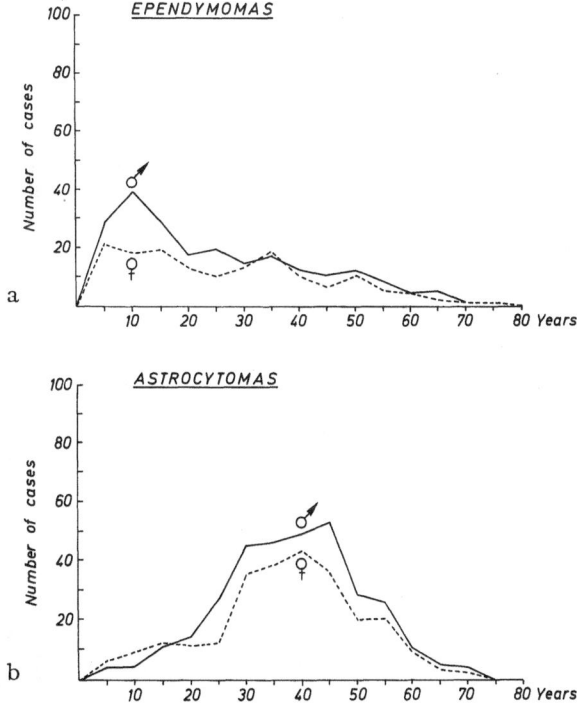

Table 7 (cont.)

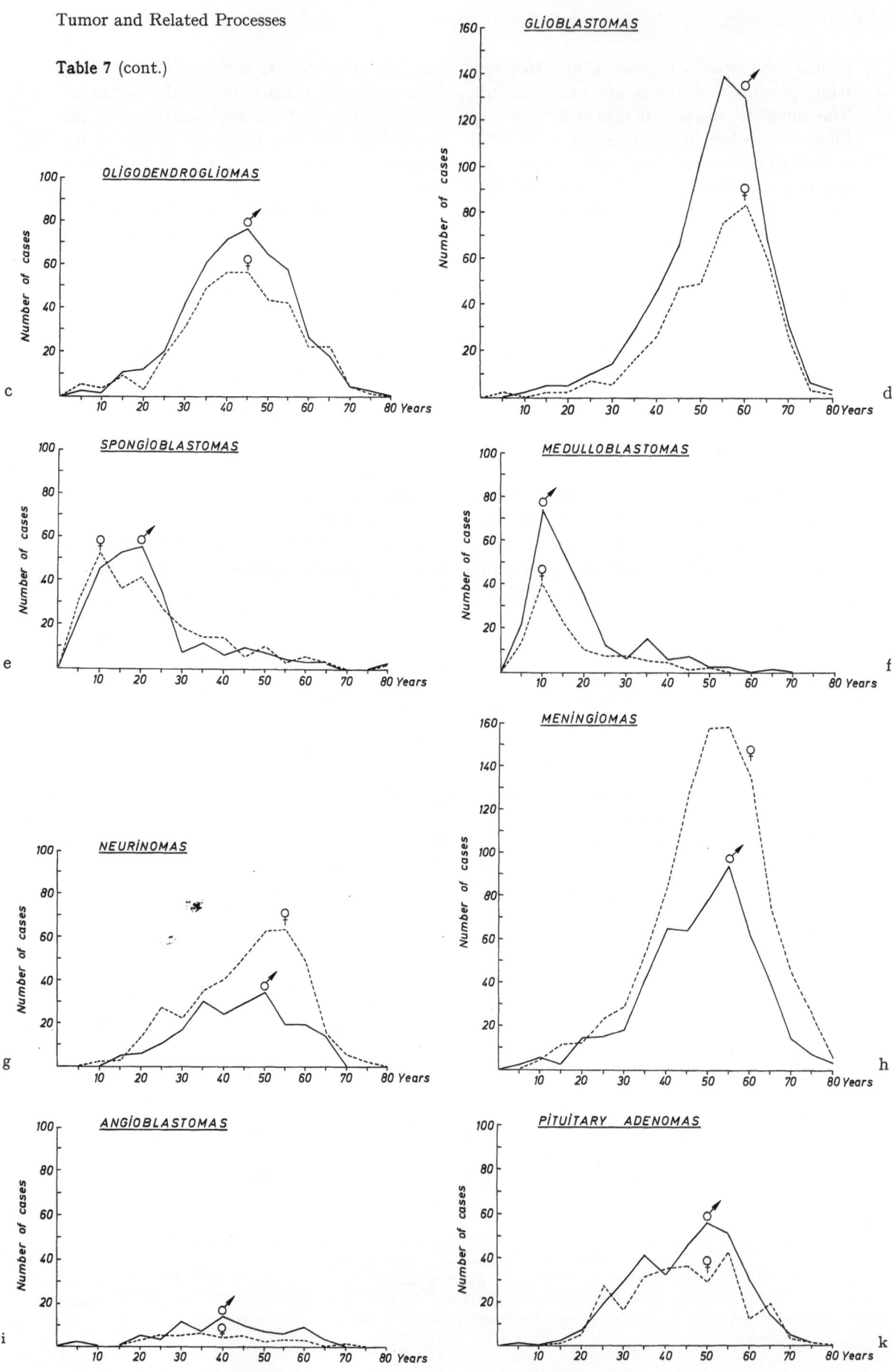

Table 7 (cont.)

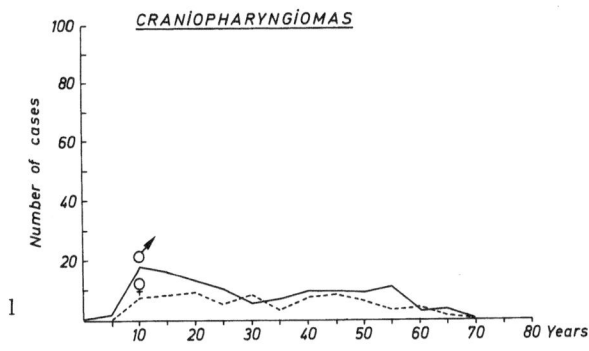

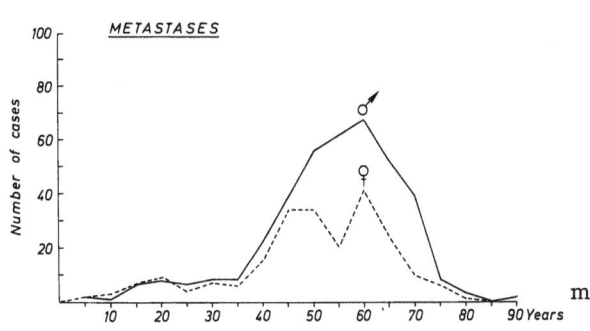

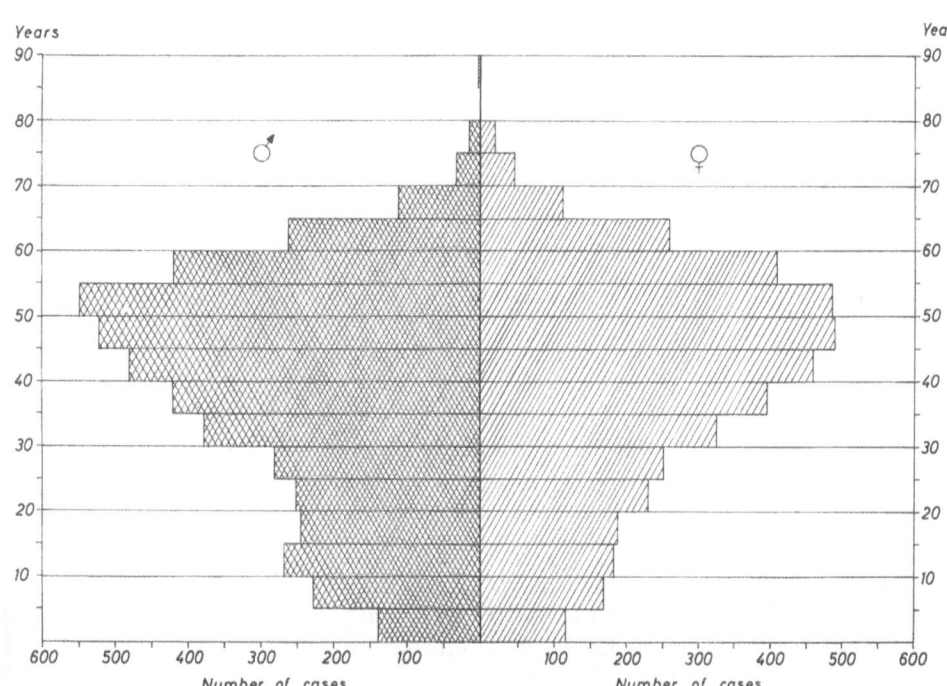

Review of the Classification of 4000, 6000 and 9000 brain tumors, compared with Cushing's (1932) and Olivecrona's (1958) series

	Personal series of 4000		Personal series of 6000		Personal series of 9000[a]		Cushing's series	Olivecrona's series	
	cases	% of total	cases	% of total	cases	% of total	% of total	cases	%
Gangliocytomas	15	0.4	27	0.4	38	0.4	0.2 ⎫		
Ependymomas	184	4.6	259	4.3	384	4.3	1.3 ⎪		
Plexus papillomas	20	0.5	30	0.5	52	0.6	0.6 ⎪	21	0.3
Astrocytomas	283	7.1	381	6.4	591	6.6	9.8 ⎪		
Oligodendrogliomas	312	7.8	490	8.2	859	9.6	1.3 ⎬	2816[b]	45.6[b]
Glioblastomas	530	13.3	738	12.3	1093	12.2	10.3 ⎪		
Spongioblastomas (including the socalled cerebellar astrocytomas)	292	7.1	419	7.0	538	6.0	6.1 ⎪		
Medulloblastomas	161	4.0	230	3.8	373	4.2	4.3 ⎭		
Neurinomas	297	7.5	451	7.6	614	6.8	8.7	469	7.6
Meningiomas	723	18.1	1079	18.0	1492	16.6	13.4	1125	18.2
Angioblastomas	60	1.5	78	1.3	119	1.3	1.2	140	2.3
Angiomas and aneurysms[a]	83	2.1	151	2.5	337	3.8	1.0	528	8.5
Sarcomas	74	1.9	162	2.7	372	4.3	0.7		
Pinealomas	16	0.4	25	0.4	48	0.5	0.7		
Pituitary adenomas	282	7.1	478	8.0	596	6.6	17.8	528	8.6
Craniopharyngiomas	107	2.7	150	2.5	185	2.1	4.6	116	1.9
Epidermoids ⎫ Dermoids[a] ⎬ Teratomas ⎭	78	1.8	128	2.1	166	1.8	0.9 ⎫ ⎬	22	0.4
Chordomas	9	0.2	14	0.2	75	0.8	0.1 ⎭		
Chondromas ⎫ Osteomas[a] ⎬ Lipomas ⎭	28	0.7	53	0.9	—	—	0.8		
Cylindromatous epitheliomas	8	0.2	12	0.2	—	—			
Fibromas	5	0.1	7	0.1	—	—			
Metastases	163	4.1	242	4.0	636	7.1	3.2	232	3.8
Unclassified tumors	151	3.8	221	3.7	286	3.2	9.6		
Parasites[a]	6	0.2	9	0.1	—	—	0.1		
Granulomas	32	0.8	45	0.7	—	—	2.2	56	0.9
Arachnoiditis and ependymitis[a]	53	1.3	92	1.5	—	—	1.1		
Miscellaneous (myelomas, Schüller-Christian disease etc.)	28	0.8	39	0.6	146	1.6		116	1.9

[a] This last classification comprises the earlier series of 4000 and 6000; the recent series of 9000 however was compiled according the scheme proposed by the UICC. Therefore some alterations between the earlier and the last series were necessary: dermoids and epidermoids were put into one rubric. Some entities which were not contained in the UICC classification, were deleted and the tumors summarized under the heading "miscellaneous".

[b] Including pinealomas, excluding plexus papillomas.

1.2 Tumors of Nervous and Supporting Tissue Origin

1.2.1 Nerve Cells

The Gangliocytomas (Gangliogliomas, Neuroblastomas, Neuroastrocytomas)

The gangliocytomas are theoretically of more importance to the neuropathologist than to the neurosurgeon. However, there is a particular gangliocytoma of the temporal lobe in adolescence (Table 5/27) which is readily amenable to surgery. These tumors have long histories and usually develop toward the end of the adolescent period. Gangliocytomas occur in the medial part of the temporal lobe, where they form large cysts (Fig. 51) and show a marked tendency to nodular growth in the leptomeninges; they are, however, very benign and the patients may be "cured" in cases of total removal of the tumor. Similar tumors occur rarely in the tuberal region, the thalamus, the mesencephalon, and in the medulla oblongata (Figs. 52, 53). They are also quite rare in the cerebellum and form a well-defined group, characterized by the hyperplastic-looking infiltrated cerebellar folia.

The peripheral tumors in the sympathetic nerves are tough but partly necrotic inside, they grow mainly by expansion, and vary in size from that of a chestnut to that of a child's head. The order of frequency is lumbar, thoracic and cervical.

Metastases in the cerebral form are an exception to the rule; postoperative recurrences in all forms are known. In general, only the two groups of the temporobasal cerebral and the thoraco-lumbar gangliocytomas are of importance to the neurosurgeon. Immature gangliocytomas of the sympathetics can freely metastasize.

In rare cases, gangliocytomas of the cerebral hemispheres may dedifferentiate (Fig. 52) and become polymorphous, assuming the malignant character of a glioblastoma multiforme. Of our series of 9000 tumors 38 are gangliocytomas; 23 were from male and 15 from female patients.

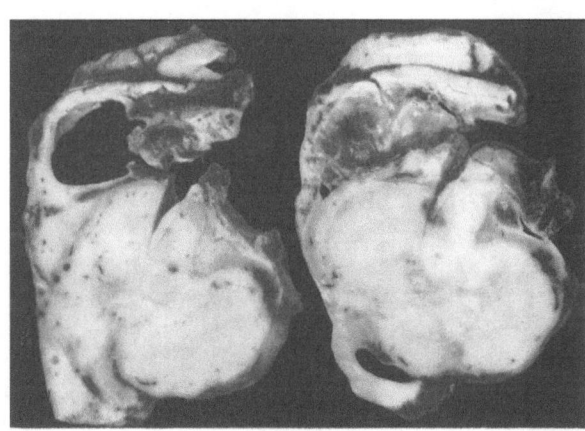

Fig. 51. Section through a surgical specimen of a temporobasal gangliocytoma with a large cyst in its upper half

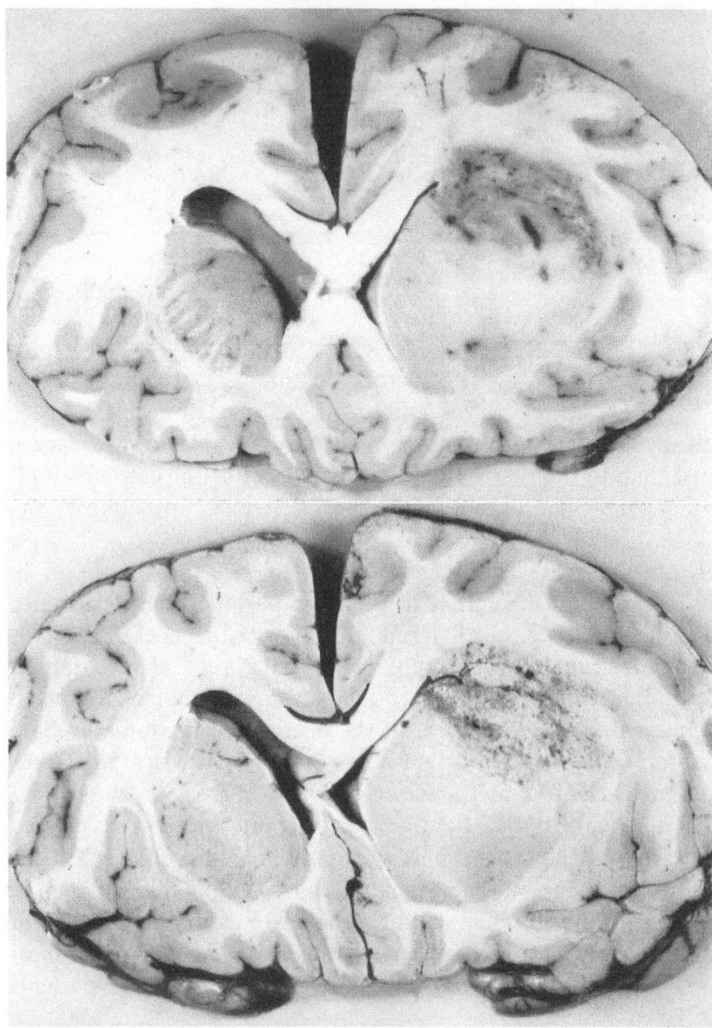

Fig. 52. Malignant form of gangliocytoma simulating a glioblastoma multiforme

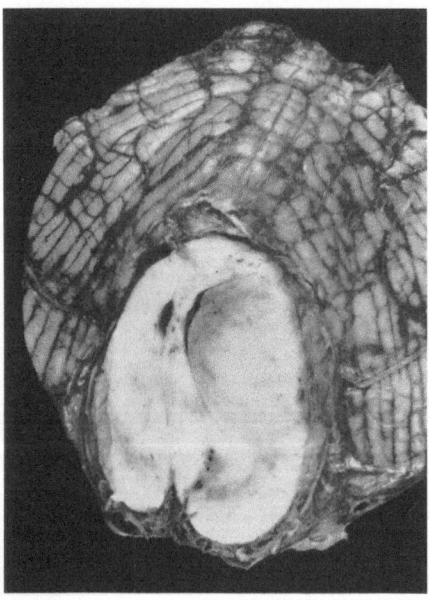

Fig. 53. Circumscribed gangliocytoma of the midbrain displacing and occluding the aqueduct

1.2.2 Neuroepithelium

The Ependymomas (Ependymoblastoma, Glioependymoma, "Neuroepithelioma")

Ependymomas occur predominantly in the vicinity of the ependyma, and may have an intraventricular or extraventricular site of origin. The order of frequency of the "intraventricular" ependymomas is as follows: fourth ventricle (Figs. 59–63), lateral ventricles (Figs. 54, 55), third ventricle (Fig. 56), aqueduct. However, none of these is more prevalent than the "extraventricular" ependymoma of the cerebral hemisphere, which abuts against the lateral ventricle (particularly the trigone) (Figs. 64–72). From there it can expand into and displace the adjacent cortex (particularly the angular and supramarginal gyri), and may occasionally even break through the cortex (Figs. 64, 65). The surface of most ependymomas is lobulated and tufted (Figs. 68, 69); the danger of tearing off these tufts during operation is considerable. The cerebral extraventricular forms may be calcified and usually have a large rostrally-placed cyst (Fig. 64). They have been known to reach the size of a tennis ball. On the other hand, the ependymomas of the fourth ventricle are usually the size of a plum (Figs. 59–63) and are attached firmly to the floor of the ventricle (Figs. 62, 63). A portion of the tumor often extends into the cisterna magna or the lateral recess (Figs. 59, 60), occasionally reaching down to the mid-cervical cord (down to C 5 in one of our cases) (Fig. 60). Less frequently, ependymomas lie within the lateral ventricle at the foramen of Monro (Figs. 54, 55), in the third ventricle rostral and dorsal to the quadrigeminal plate (Fig. 56), and finally—though rarely—in the cerebellopontine angle (Fig. 58) and actually in the aqueduct. In the spinal cord they may assume the shape of a pencil, extending over several segments in the region of the posterior columns, or they may appear as large white gelatinous tumors in the region of the cauda and on the filum terminale. Here they may reach a length of 7–10 cm.

In the spinal cord there is often a cavity both above and below the tumor, resembling syringomyelia, but more closely corresponding to the cyst of the cerebral form; the elongated shape conforms to the longitudinal orientation of the spinal cord tracts.

Generally, ependymomas grow by expansion, but in the marginal zone growth occasionally occurs by means of advancing papillae. Metastases occasionally occur spontaneously, but are not uncommon after operation on those of the cerebral hemisphere, in fact, the entire CSF circuit may be diffusely involved with nodules and plaques (Figs. 70–72). Another characteristic of the ependymoma of the cerebral hemisphere is a tendency to recur even after "total" removal. The other ependymomas, fortunately, do not share these traits.

In some recurrences, particularly of the cerebral forms, malignant "anaplastic" de-differentiation may take place, in which case the ependymoma assumes a more "polymorphous" histological character and is of greater malignant potential.

Ependymomas make up around 5 % of intracranial tumors (in our series of 9000 cases, 4.3 %). The comparable figure in BAILEY's and CUSHING's (1926, 1930) material was 1.3 %, in OLIVECRONA's series (RINGERTZ and REYMOND, 1949) 6.3 %. The number of male and female patients in our series showed a slight male preponderance (226 males, 158 females). The ependymomas of the spinal canal, according to KERNOHAN and SAYRE (1952), form 60% of the gliomas of the spinal cord (117 of 200 cases).

The "extraventricular" cerebral ependymomas occur almost exclusively in childhood and adolescence (see p. 45; Table 7a–n) and are the most common gliomas of the cerebral hemisphere in this age group. The other age groups show a predilection for the "intraventricular" ependymomas.

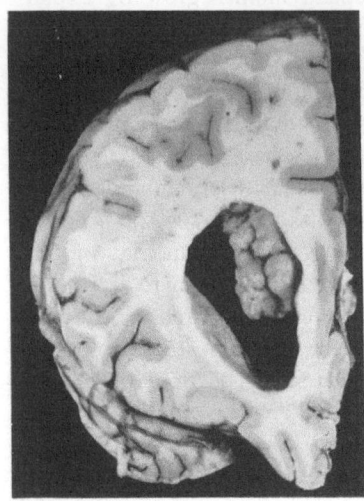

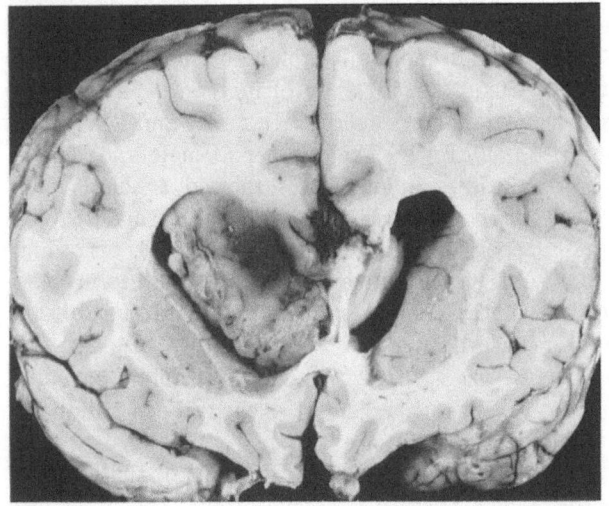

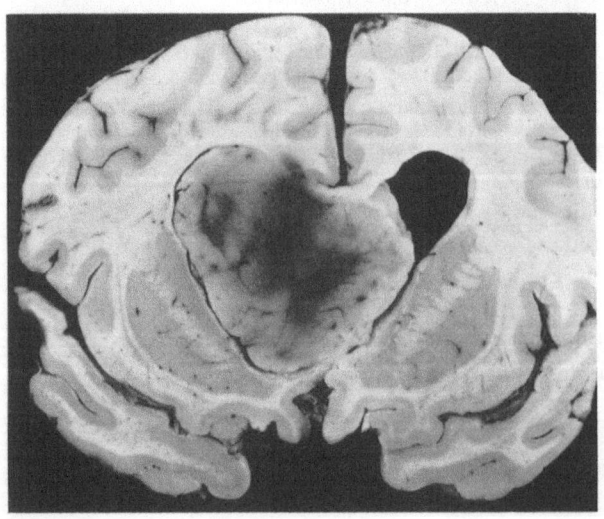

Fig. 54. Ependymoma of the foramen of Monro with hemorrhages into the tumor. The septum is markedly shifted to the opposite side with ipsilateral occlusion of the foramen of Monro and contralateral stenosis

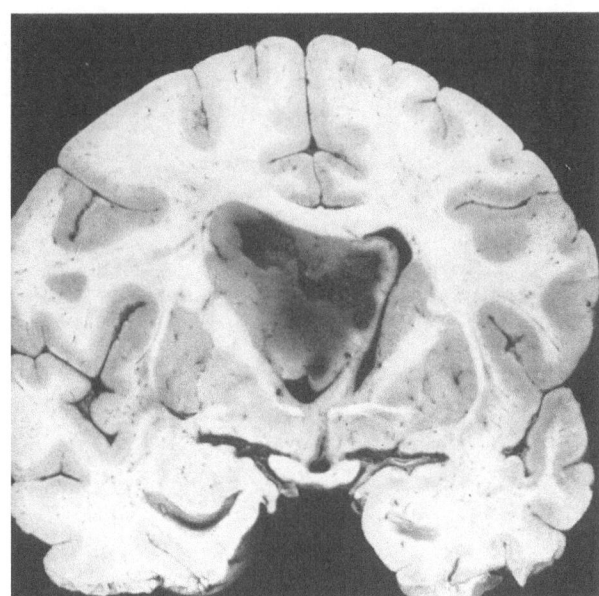

Fig. 55. Ependymoma in the left anterior horn originating from the region of the foramen of Monro. Note the shift of the septum pellucidum towards the right which has produced a secondary occlusion of the opposite foramen of Monro

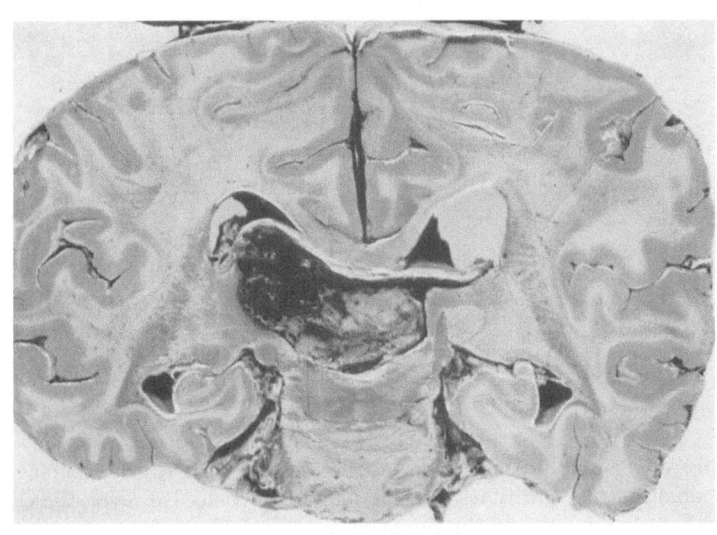

Fig. 56. Acorn-sized ependymoma filling the posterior part of the third ventricle and depressing the quadrigeminal plate

53

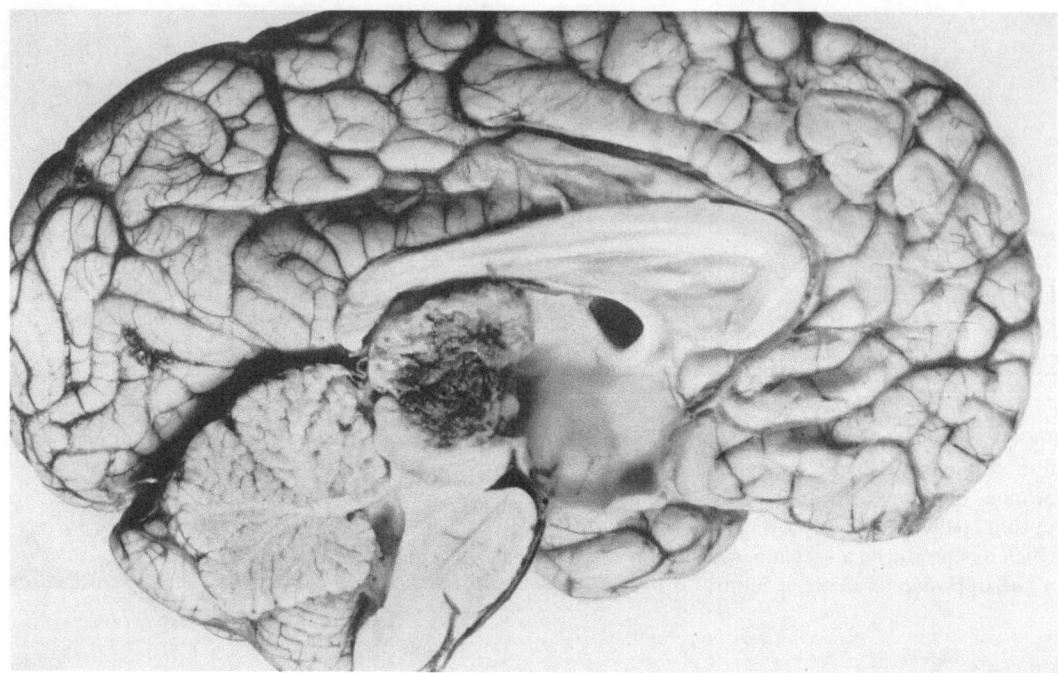

Fig. 57. Typical ependymoma in the posterior portion of the third ventricle compromising the quadrigeminal plate. Obstructive hydrocephalus of the 3rd ventricle has occurred

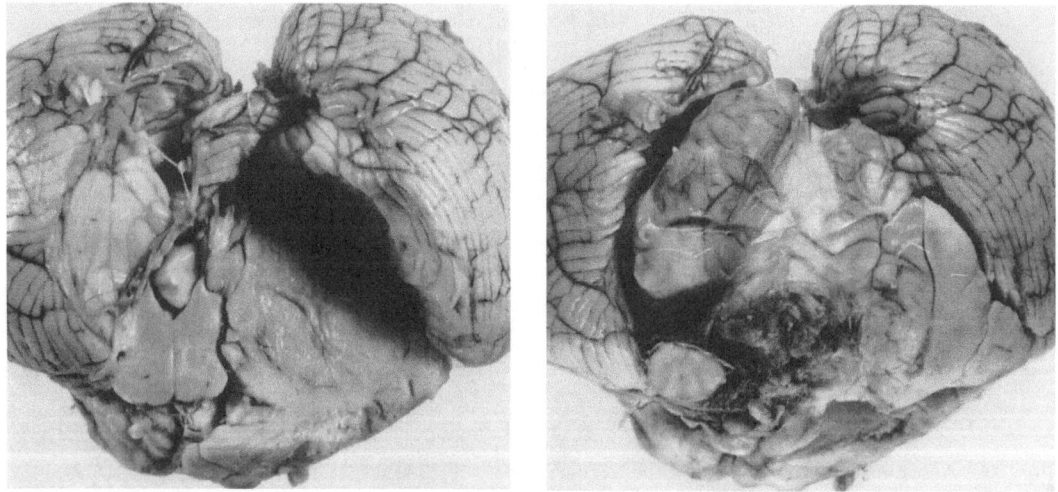

Fig. 58. Primary ependymoma of the lateral recess which occupies the cerebellopontine angle. Only a small portion protrudes into the fourth ventricle. However, the cisterna magna is completely filled with and expanded by the tumor mass

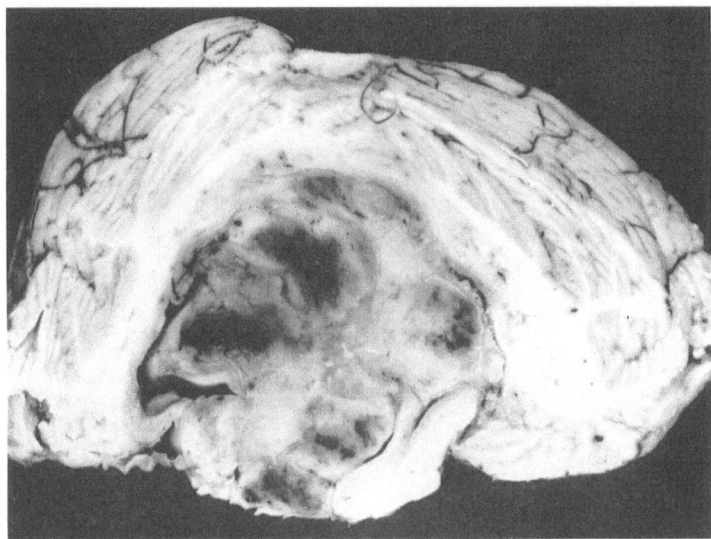

Fig. 59. Large ependymoma of the fourth ventricle expanding into the cerebellopontine angle via the foramen of Luschka

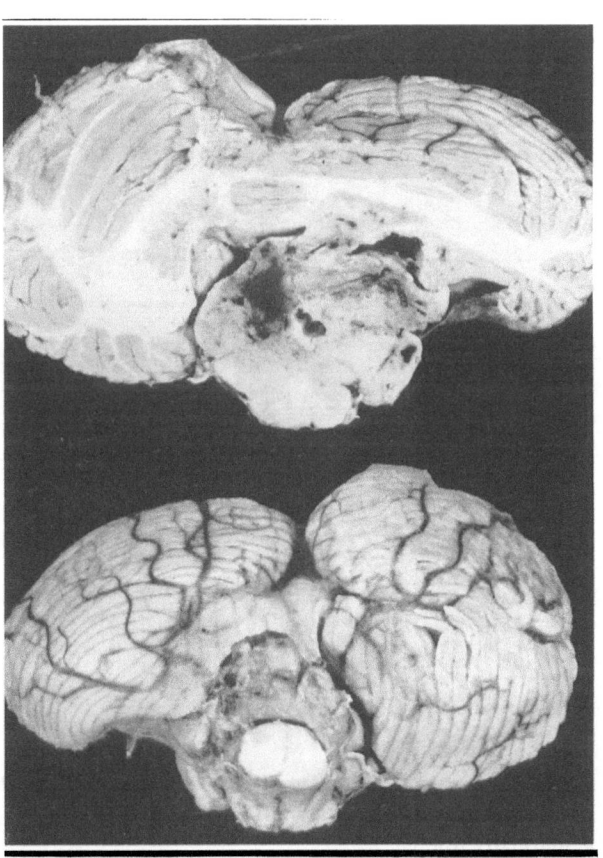

Fig. 60. Typical ependymoma of the fourth ventricle extending through the lateral recess. Note the tumor expansion in the cisterna magna

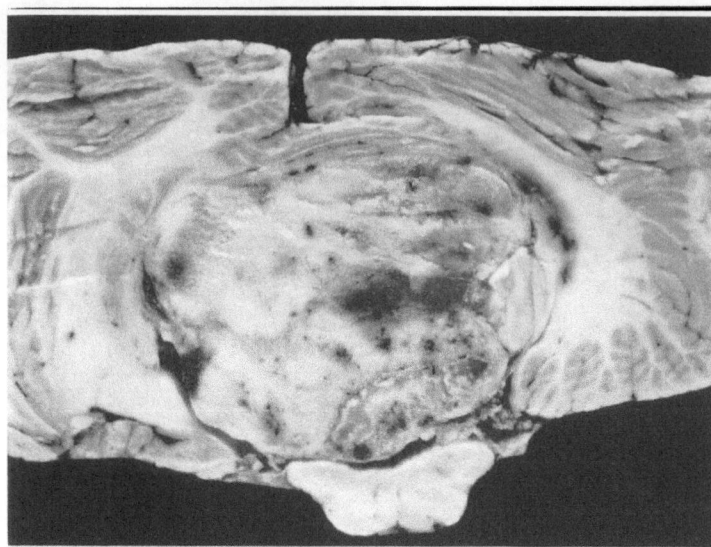

Fig. 61. Large ependymoma of the fourth ventricle which has massively expanded its lumen

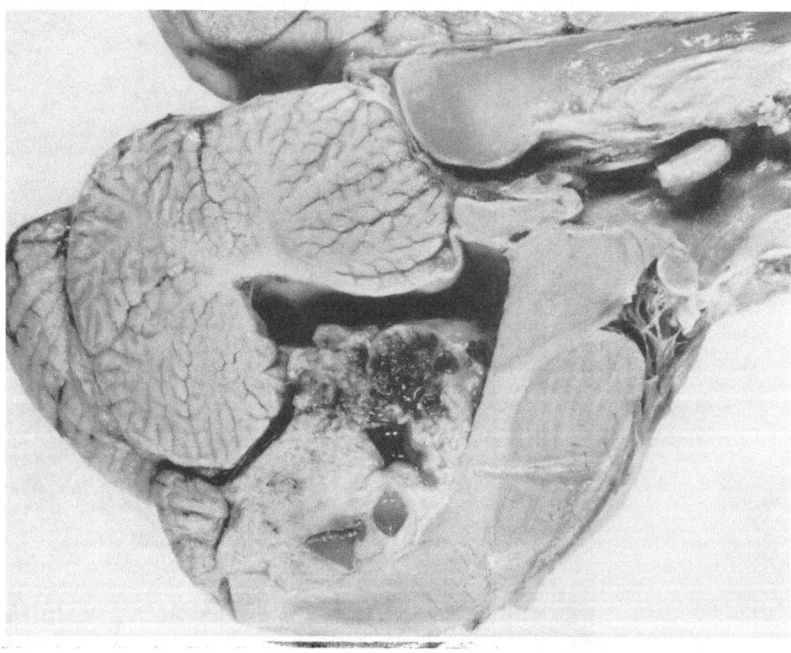

Fig. 62. Typical ependymoma of the fourth ventricle with a small process extending into the cisterna magna. Small cysts and hemorrhages have occurred. The anterior portion of the fourth ventricle is markedly dilated

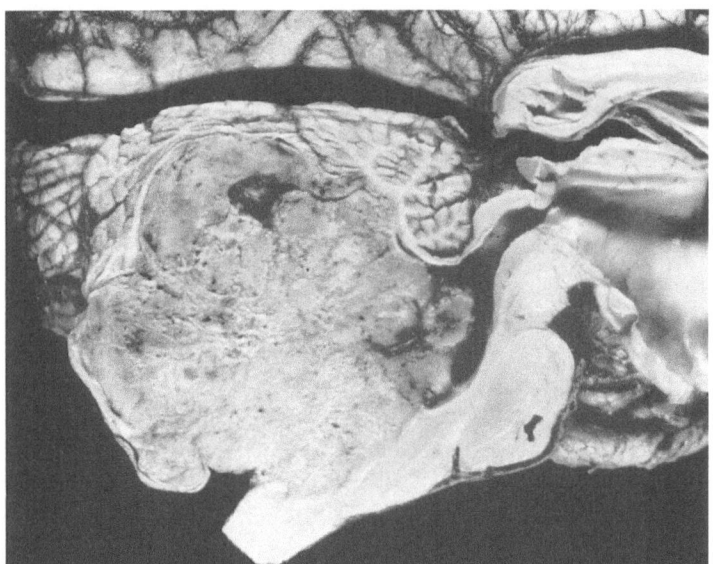

Fig. 63. Enormous ependymoma-like tumor of the fourth ventricle which is firmly attached to the floor and has broken through the ependyma at many points

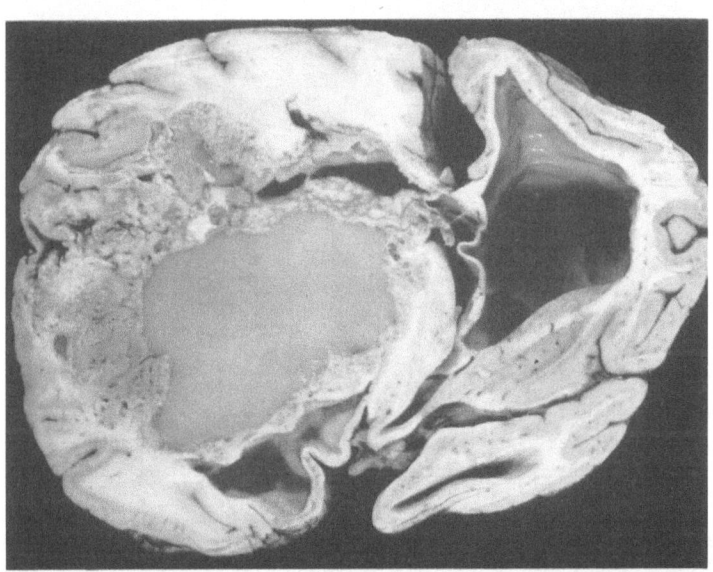

Fig. 64. Large cerebral ependymoma which is attached to the outer wall of the trigone. Large cysts within the tumor and a lobulated outer surface are apparent, as is the secondary hydrocephalus on the opposite side

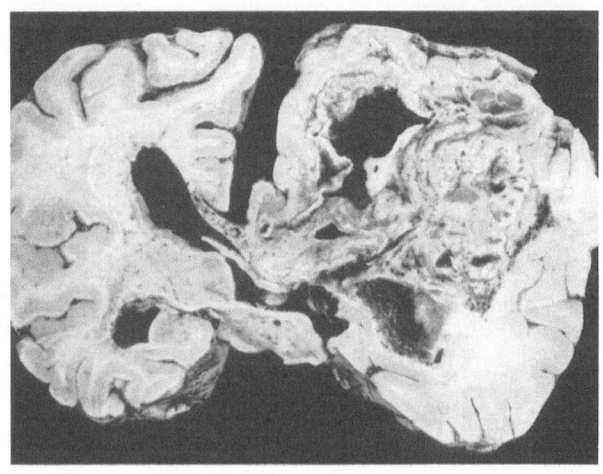

Fig. 65. Cerebral ependymoma with large cysts. The tumor probably originated in the outer wall of the cella media of the ventricle and extended to the surface of the convexity in the parieto-temporo-occipital region

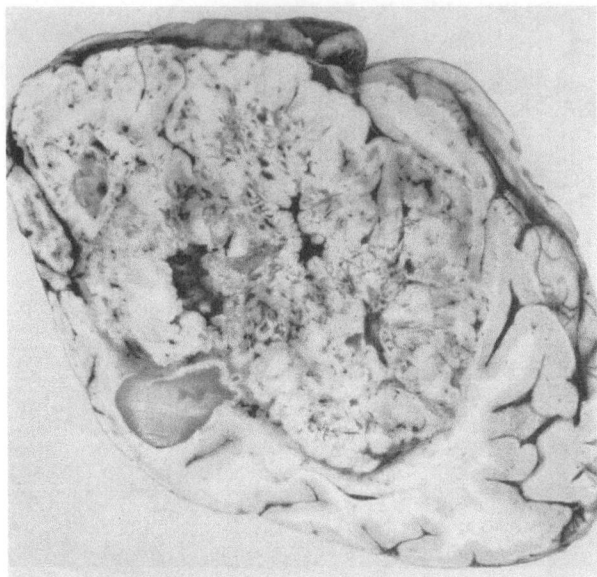

Fig. 66. Large cerebral ependymoma which has expanded within the parietal lobe (see Fig. 65) and then extended through the occipital lobe to reach the surface

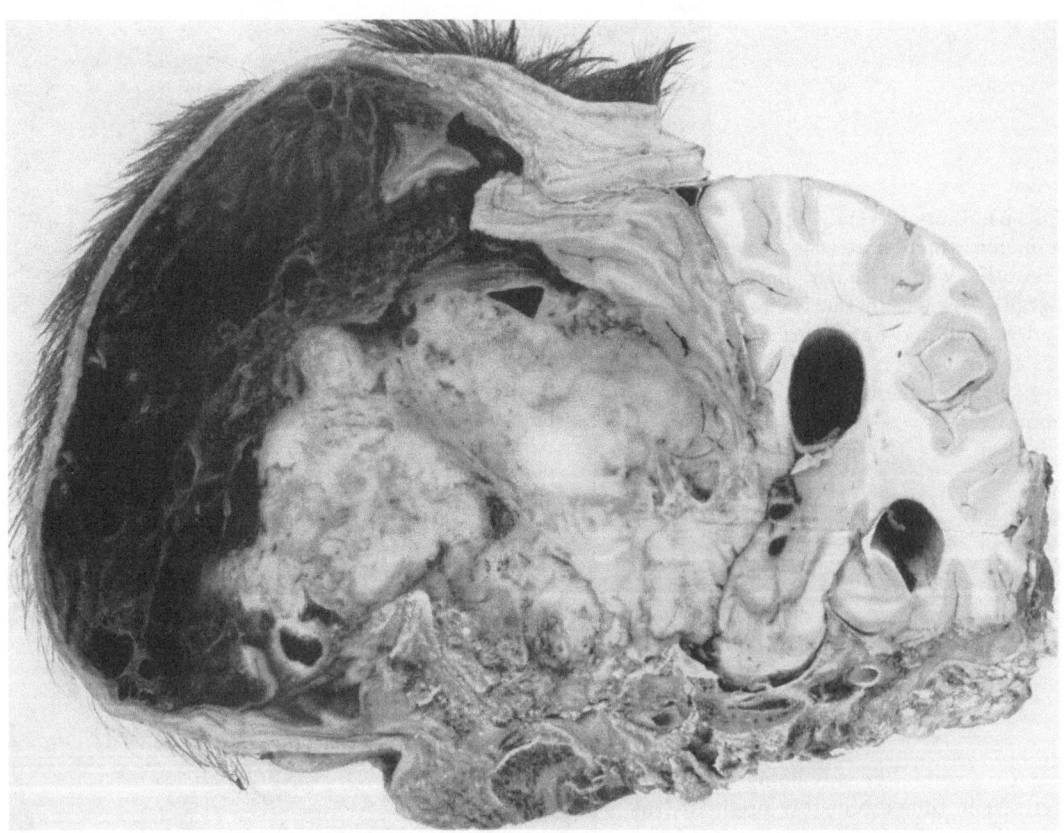

Fig. 67. Giant cerebral extraventricular ependymoma in its typical location with a grotesque postoperative prolapse

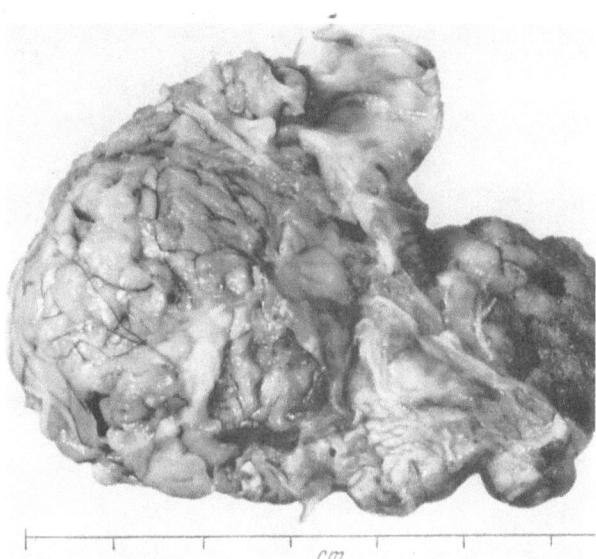

Fig. 68. Large recurrent cerebral ependymoma which was surgically removed

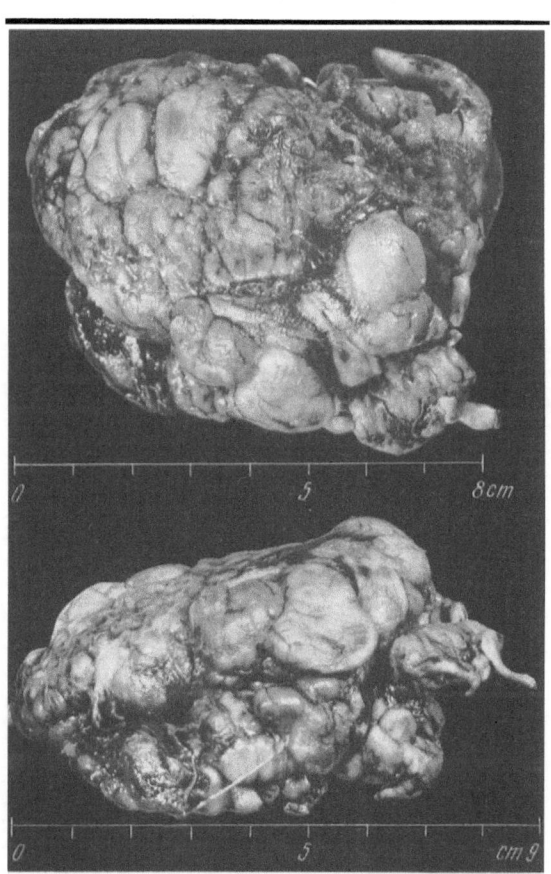

Fig. 69. Surgically removed ependymoma. The surface is lobular and somewhat resembles the appearance of a placenta

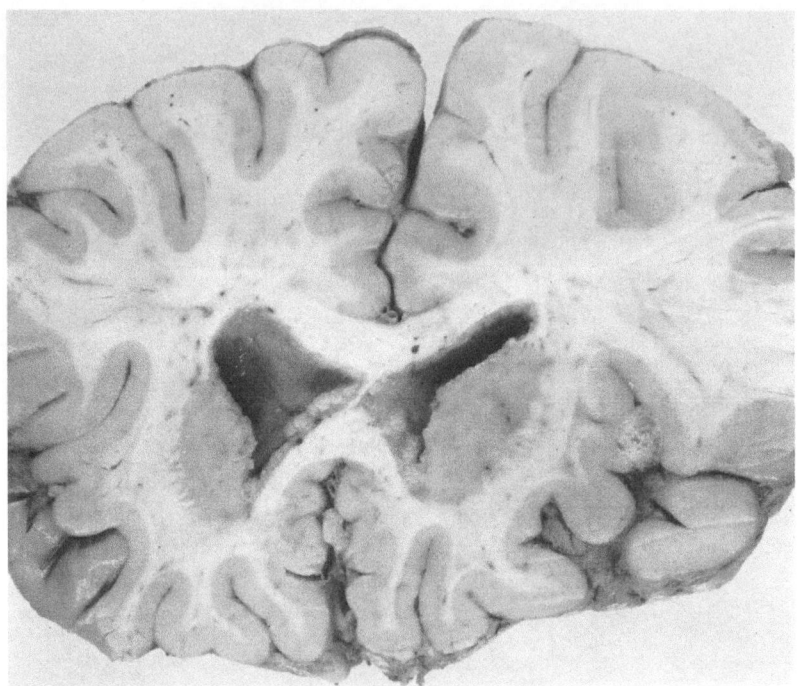

Fig. 70. Post-operative nodular seeding of an extra-ventricular cerebral ependymoma on the ventricular walls and throughout the subarachnoid spaces (see Fig. 71 and 72)

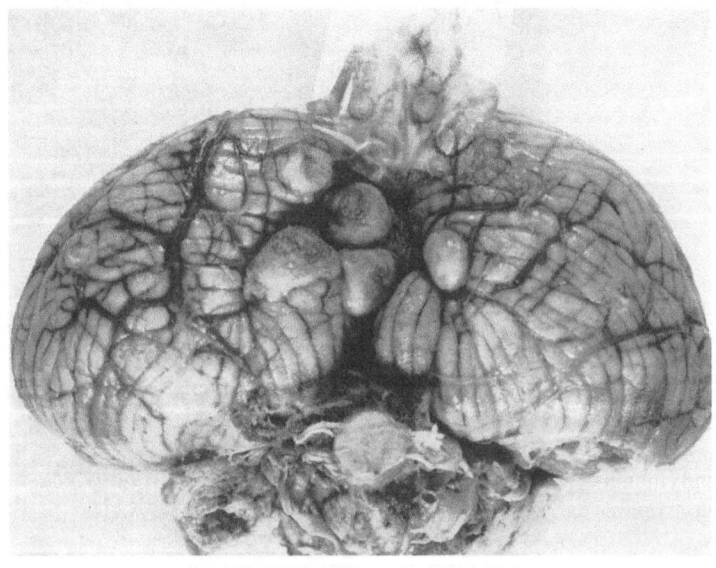

Fig. 71. Extensive (rare) nodular metastases into the basilar cisterns in the same case as Fig. 70 and 72

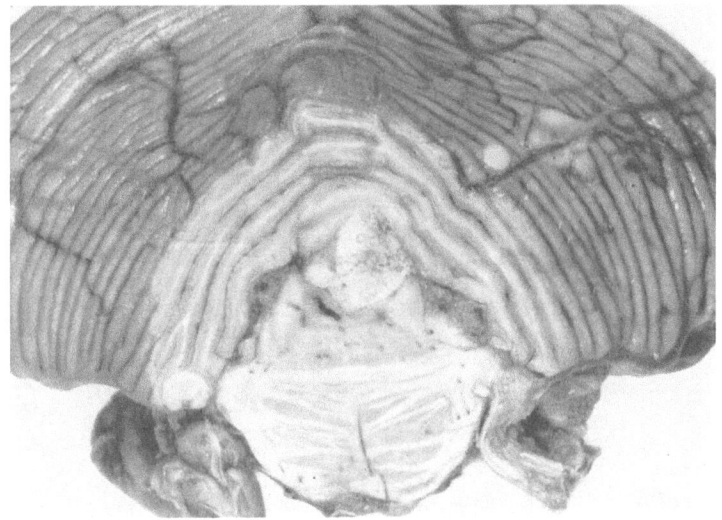

Fig. 72. Nodular cerebellar metastasis overlying the quadrigeminal plate following surgical removal of a cerebral ependymoma. Note the distorted aqueduct and the spotty superficial cortical metastases on the cerebellar surface (see Fig. 70 and 71)

The Ependymal Cysts (Colloid or Paraphysial Cysts). The so-called "colloid" or ependymal cyst of the foramen of Monro may have the size of a pea when encountered as an incidental finding (Fig. 74), or that of a cherry (Fig. 73) when they make their presence known to the neurosurgeon by blocking the foramina of Monro and producing an obstructive hydrocephalus. They are filled with greenish colloid-like fluid which subsequently coagulates.

They probably represent malformations of a pinched-off remnant of the embryonic paraphysis. They lie under the fornix between the foramina of Monro, are lined with a single layer of ependyma which is often ciliated, and tend to bulge through the foramina of Monro with the choroid plexus attached.

Other ependymal cysts are noted as malformations in the mesencephalon (Figs. 75, 76).

Cysts of the Cavum Septi Pellucidi and Cavum Vergae. These cavities have no embryological relation to the ventricular system, although they have been named the fifth and sixth ventricles. They can, however, communicate secondarily with the lateral ventricles. In rare cases they undergo dilatation and cause hydrocephalus by blocking the foramina of Monro (Fig. 77 a, b).

Ventricular Tumors in Tuberous Sclerosis (Subependymal Glomerate Astrocytomas). They are distantly related to the ependymomas. Those of potential surgical importance (Fig. 78) are especially apt to occur in the lateral ventricles around the foramen of Monro where they range in size from a cherry to a tangerine, are medium hard, often calcified, nodular and produce a block at the foramen of Monro (Figs. 78, 79 a–c). They may be "forme fruste", i.e., without the typical clinical triad.

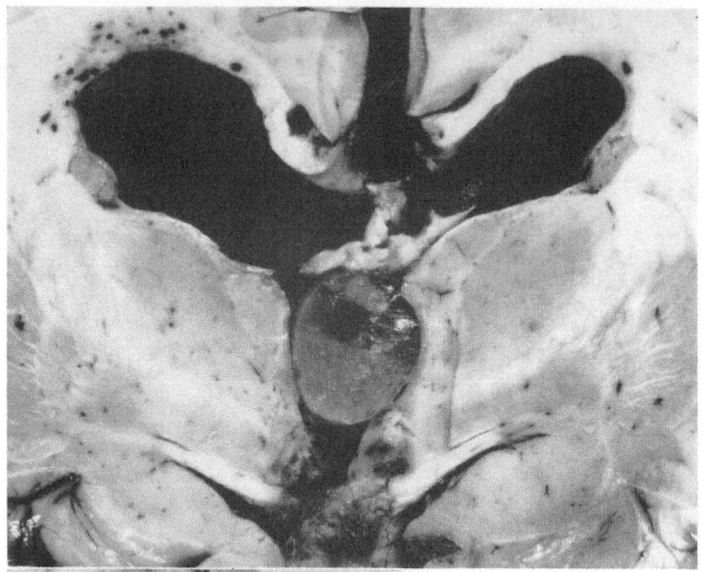

Fig. 73. Cherry-sized colloid cyst (ependymal cyst) of the foramina of Monro "in situ". The lesion had been approached surgically by a transcallosal route

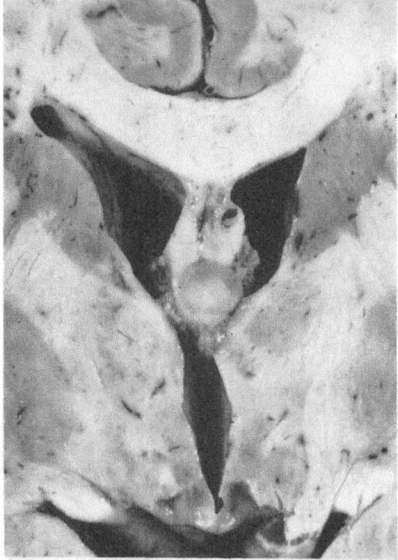

Fig. 74. Colloid cyst of the foramina of Monro (incidental finding)

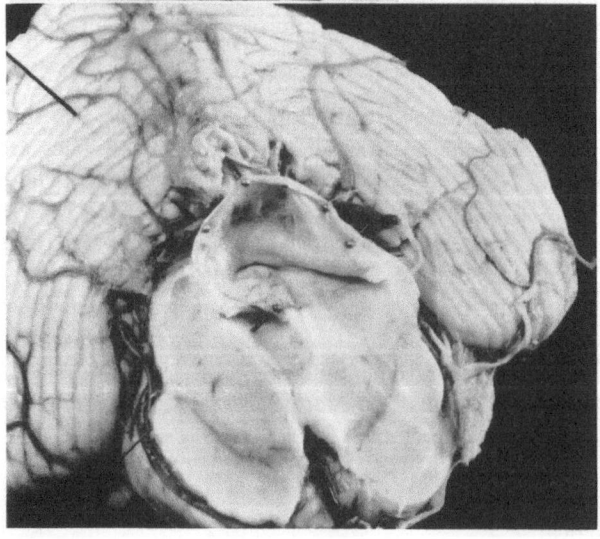

Fig. 75. Ependymal cyst of the quadrigeminal plate with resultant aqueductal occlusion (c.f. Fig. 332)

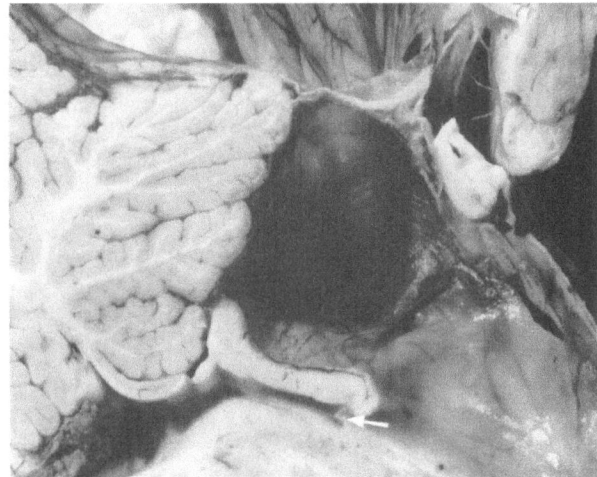

Fig. 76. Occlusion of the aqueduct by a membraneous ependymal malformation (arrow!). The suprapineal recess has been enormously expanded, impinging on the upper vermis and compromising the quadrigeminal plate. Atrophic changes in this latter structure are apparent

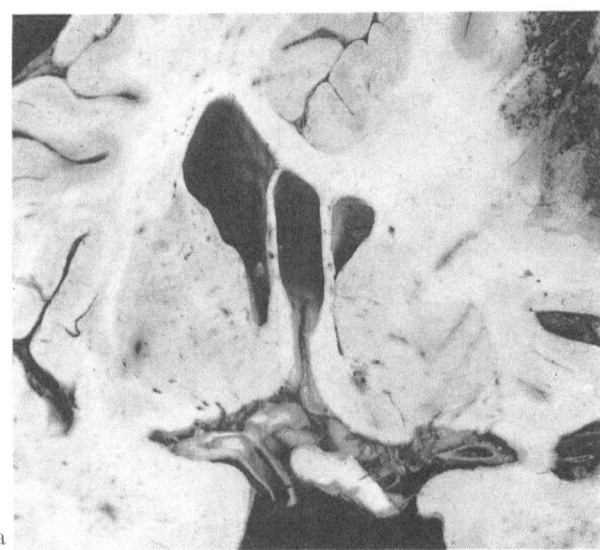

a

b

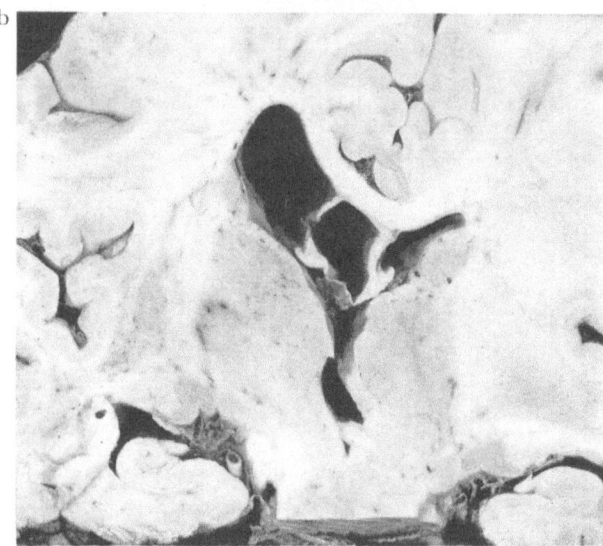

Fig. 77. Cyst of the septum pellucidum and cavum vergae

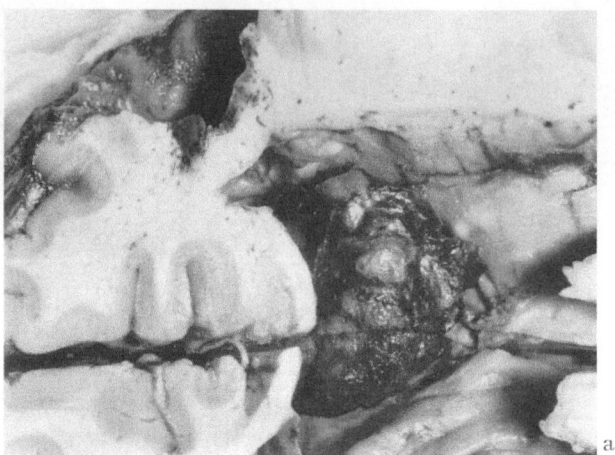

a

b

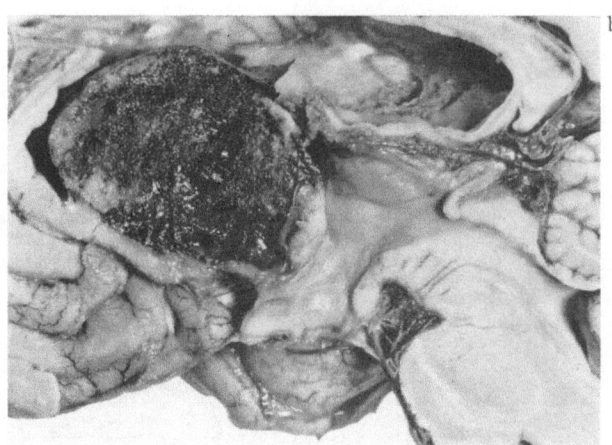

Fig. 78. Ventricular tumor in tuberous sclerosis in the lateral ventricle around the foramen of Monro

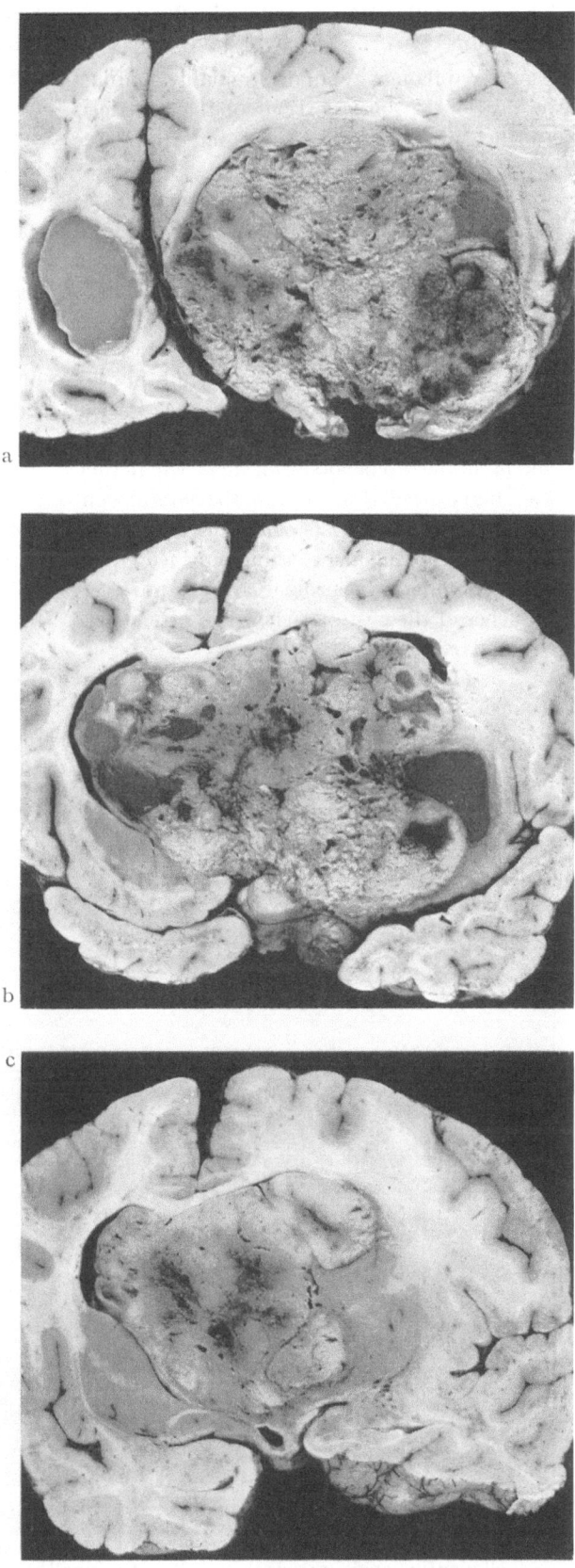

Fig. 79. Enormous ependymoma-like tumor of the right lateral ventricle with cystic degeneration in a case of tuberous sclerosis

The Plexus Papillomas (Choroid Plexus Papilloma)

Plexus papillomas are understandably confined in location to those portions of the ventricles which contain choroid plexus, but they have certain preferential localizations.

The preferential site of these tumors is (1) in the fourth ventricle (the size of a plum) where they expand the lumen (Fig. 82); (2) in the lateral ventricles (reaching the size of a fist), particularly in the trigonum at the junction of the temporal horn, where they completely obliterate the lumen and may expand all the way out to the cortex; (3) in the third ventricle, where they reach the size of a chestnut (Fig. 81); and (4) in the cerebellopontine angle where they are cherry-sized (Fig. 80). In the lateral ventricular type, large cysts can occur next to the tumor. The papilloma is commonly fed by an enlarged anterior choroidal artery; however, branches of the posterior choroidal artery may be involved.

The plexus papillomas are well-demarcated from the surrounding tissue, but tufts of tumor can be forced into the cerebral substance by pressure. Plexus papillomas are grayish-pink, have a fine or coarsely tufted surface, and even though they possess a certain general firmness, are tender, friable and tear easily. On occasion, they are highly calcified, particularly those encountered in the trigonum.

Metastases and Recurrence. Removal of plexus papillomas without recurrence is difficult since the tumor itself is so friable; small fragments, easily torn off, can be liberated and may lead to artificial seeding of tumor "transplants". The plexus papillomas are also very apt to metastasize spontaneously (Fig. 80). There exist (Fig. 82), therefore, a number of cases of multiple plexus papillomas with definite evidence of spread via the cerebrospinal fluid. Disregarding these implantation metastases, the tumor generally grows slowly and only by expansion. There are a few cases of polymorphous tumors with de-differentiation and a higher malignancy.

In our series of 9000 cases they comprised 0.58%, in CUSHING's 0.6% (CUSHING, 1932, 1935). Males and females were equally represented. The peak of incidence falls between 25 and 30 years.

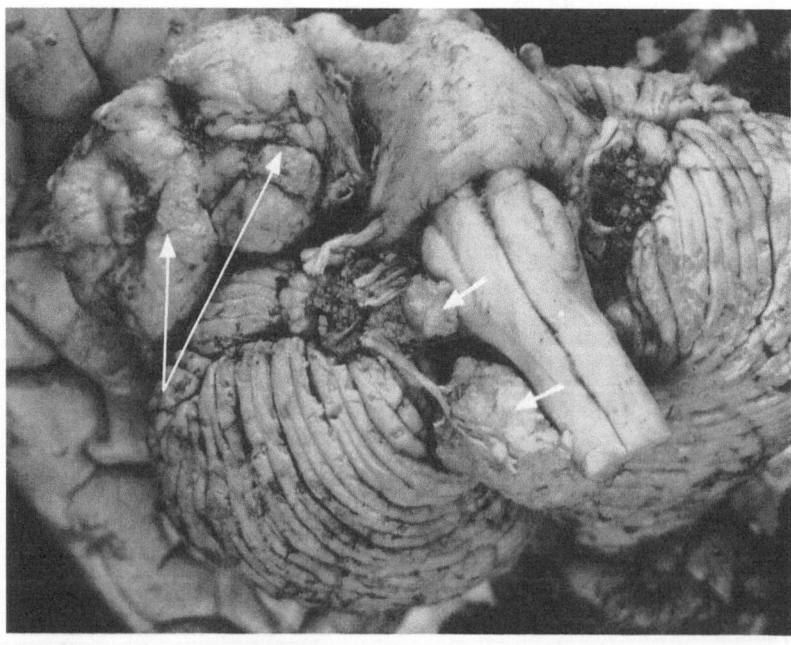

Fig. 80. Metastases from a plexus papilloma of the left trigone. Note the acorn-sized knot in the right cerebellopontine angle (arrows!) as well as the small two para-bulbar lesions (arrows!)

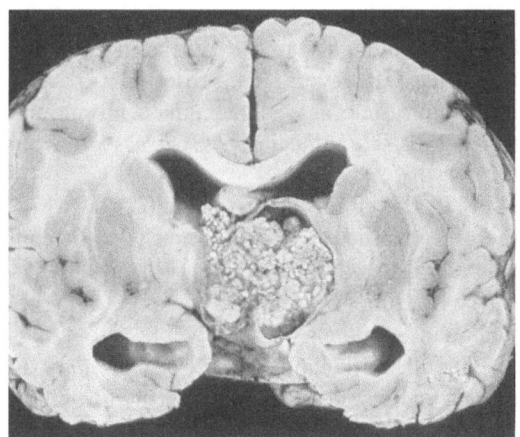

Fig. 81. Large plexus papilloma of the third ventricle. Secondary obstructive hydrocephalus

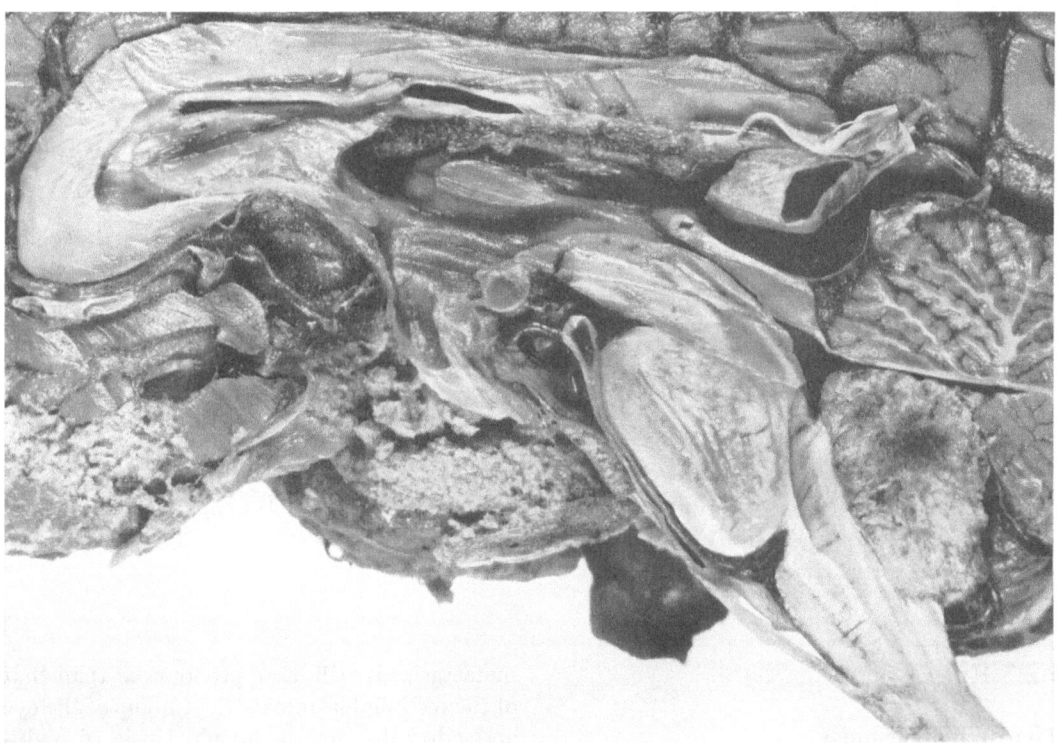

Fig. 82. Widespread diffuse involvement of the external CSF pathways from a fourth ventricular plexus papilloma

Neuroepitheliomas and Medulloepitheliomas

These two tumor entities, part of BAILEY and CUSHING's (1926, 1930) detailed classification of neuroepithelial tumors, are so extremely rare that for a long time there was much debate as to whether they ought to be kept in the classifications. However, they definitely do occur

(Fig. 83) and do play a certain role in experimental neurooncology, so that they will be mentioned briefly.

The neuroepitheliomas are characterized by the occurrence of a particular cellular architectural pattern, namely, the true rosette. These are radial arrangements of cells around a minute true lumen. They are frequently observed in retinoblastomas (neuroepitheliomas of the eye) and in highly undifferentiated medulloblastomas. However, "true rosettes" are seen in benign tumors as well—i.e., in ependymomas (for details see: *Atlas of the Histology of Brain Tumors*).

It is, therefore, the histologic picture which dictates whether a specific tumor is to be considered an ependymoma or a neuroepithelioma, the latter tumor belonging to the class of highly malignant tumors.

Medulloepitheliomas are also malignant tumors which are characterized by the formation of rows of tubules lined by high cylindrical cells resembling the embryological medullary epithelium. Again, similar ependymal tubules —even resembling the central canal of the spinal cord—may be observed in the more benign ependymomas caudad to the midbrain. However, the general histologic picture and the high cylindrical epithelium of the tubules usually allow the diagnosis of medulloepithelioma to be made with some degree of certainty.

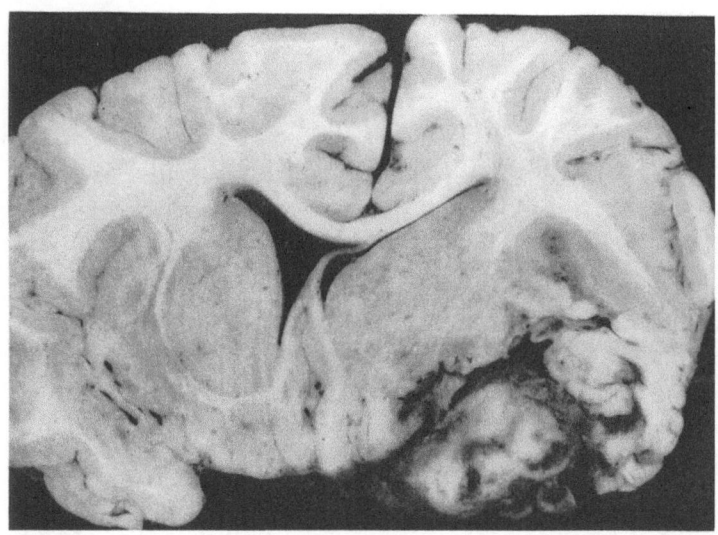

Fig. 83. Rare case of a true medulloepithelioma of the temporal lobe. (Courtesy of Dr. Ikuta/Niigata

1.2.3 Eye

The Retinoblastomas

We compare the tumors of the retina, together with the tumors of the pineal region, sympathetic trunk, and adrenals, occurring in early infancy and childhood, grossly with the medulloblastomas; they are histologically very similar to the cerebellar tumors and biologically also very malignant. Their tendency to metastasize is still more pronounced than that of the medulloblastomas; the tumors of the eye and adrenals directly invade tissue of a different embryonic origin (mesoderm) or metastasize to it—retinoblastoma particularly to the bones and lymph nodes, and sympathoblastoma to the bones, lymph nodes, and liver. The pineoblastoma does not metastasize except via the CSF. The histological character (with or without true rosettes) is of no biological significance.

1.2.4 Glia

The Astrocytomas

The astrocytomas consist of various subtypes, each with a somewhat different appearance to the naked eye. They may tend to be sharply circumscribed, firm, whitish, solid tumors (Figs. 93–96) with an almost cartilaginous consistency. Depending on the admixture of glial fibers present, however, some are tough and rubbery, while others are soft and "edematous" (Figs. 87, 92) and can be readily removed by the surgical sucker. Between these two extremes, "mixed" cases can occur which are tough in some parts and softer in others. The pattern of growth is a combination of infiltration at the margins and expansion from the center with infiltrated convolutions appearing broadened (Fig. 93), flattened, greyish-white and glossy. If circumscribed, these involved convolutions may even resemble a mushroom (Fig. 96). The cortical vessels, both large and small, seem to be spread apart from each other by the separating effect of these flattened and often distorted convolutions (Fig. 95). If cortical invasion is heavy, lobulation of the tumor tissue may even occur (Fig. 96).

Cysts of different sizes are seen regularly. In the most fibrous (tough) types, which tend to be only sparsely vascularized—for instance, those near the Rolandic area—the cysts may be large and unilocular (Fig. 85). Other types may have multiple small cysts (Figs. 86, 89) or even a network of cysts (Fig. 91). Apart from the "cortical" tumors, variants with a strictly subcortical localization occur which tend to show a more diffuse growth pattern (Fig. 98). Astrocytomas almost never calcify, become necrotic, or undergo fatty degeneration, the predominant regressive change being liquefaction with cystic degeneration. In some rare cases the end result is a great cyst with a small, hard, solid tumor nodule somewhere in the cyst wall (Fig. 85).

Astrocytomas commonly lie over the convexity of the brain and can be subdivided into many types. In the frontal lobe we find: frontodorsal astrocytomas of the first and second frontal convolutions growing deep (Figs. 84, 85) in the direction of the anterior horn and often containing a large cyst (Fig. 85); frontomedial astrocytomas extending into the white matter from the frontal pole along the first frontal convolution and along the medial gyri (Fig. 89), often infiltrating and expanding the septum pellucidum (Fig. 90); frontolateral astrocytomas in the laterobasal convolutions directly under the third frontal gyrus (Figs. 86–88) spreading into the frontal white matter and occasionally forming a large cyst (here, a finger-like extension usually reaches into the white matter of the insula) (Fig. 88); and diffuse frontal astrocytomas (Fig. 97) of the entire frontal white matter which may even extend through the corpus callosum to the opposite side. In the temporal lobe astrocytomas of the temporal poles (Fig. 91) are found growing in an occipital direction through the white matter, or penetrating into the basal region of the frontal lobes (Fig. 92) and medially into the basal ganglia, while in the parietal lobe parietolateral (Figs. 93, 94) astrocytomas (central or postcentral) are found spreading in the direction of the ventricular wall and frequently containing large cysts. Parietal parasagittal tumors (Fig. 95) often reach the mesial surface of the brain (parietomedial astrocytomas) (Fig. 96). There are, in addition, astrocytomas of the thalamus (Figs. 99, 100) (often bilateral), of the midbrain, of the pons (Fig. 101), and of the spinal cord. A carefully studied breakdown of 52 cases according to regions by large serial sections showed that frontal astrocytomas were most common, followed by temporal and centroparietal astrocytomas, with only sporadic occurrences in other regions.

Based on criteria of "growth" astrocytomas belong to the "semibenign" gliomas. However, survival statistics are not very encouraging since "complete" removal is rarely possible because of diffuse infiltration of the adjacent tissues. Recurrences are therefore common. Only small, well-circumscribed astrocytomas can be radically removed.

Around 10% of astrocytomas "totally" excised and examined by serial sections showed foci of malignant degeneration. These "polymorphous" variants show a higher mitotic rate, areas of necrosis, and disorganization of the vascular stroma—i.e., many characteristics of the glioblastoma multiforme. In one autopsy case we found a firm, circumscribed astrocytoma the size of a small fist (Figs. 95, 96) blending into an adjacent tumor (possessing the afore mentioned malignant features) which had diffusely permeated the entire hemisphere and had even spread via the corpus callosum to the opposite side. The more malignant portion in this case had quite obviously arisen at a later stage from its more benign mate.

Astrocytomas predominantly occur in middle age, where the peak of incidence falls rather precisely around 35–45 years (see p. 45). Of our series of 9000 cases, 56.2% were males and 43.8% were females. The astrocytomas comprised 9.8% in CUSHING's series (1932, 1935) and 6.6% in our material. However, comparable figures are difficult to obtain since in our series the "cerebellar astrocytomas" were excluded from the astrocytoma group and put in the same group as the spongioblastomas.

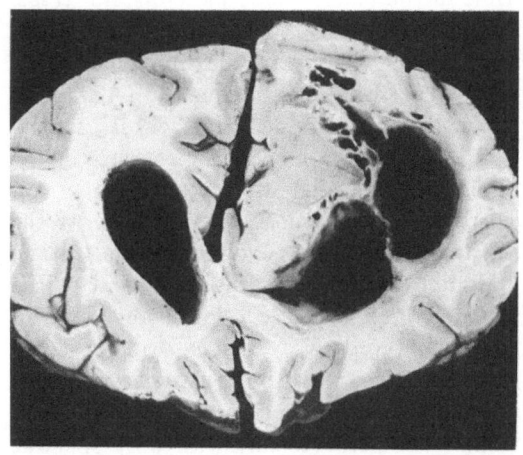

Fig. 84. Frontodorsal astrocytoma with a massive cyst dorsolateral to the anterior horn

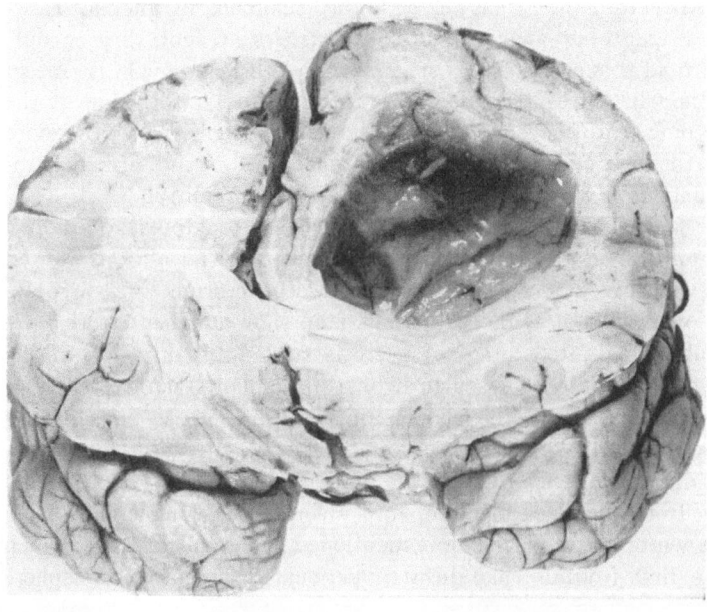

Fig. 85. Huge cyst in a frontodorsal gigantocellular astrocytoma. Considerable mass shifting has occurred

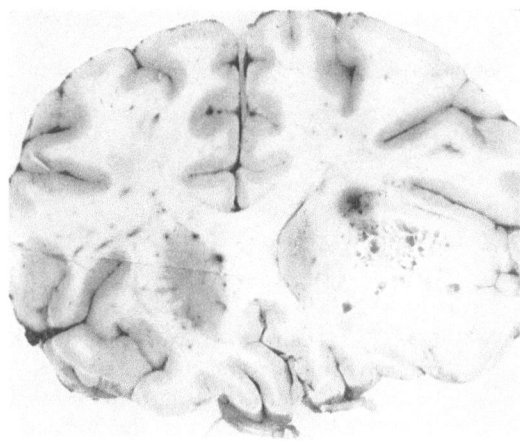

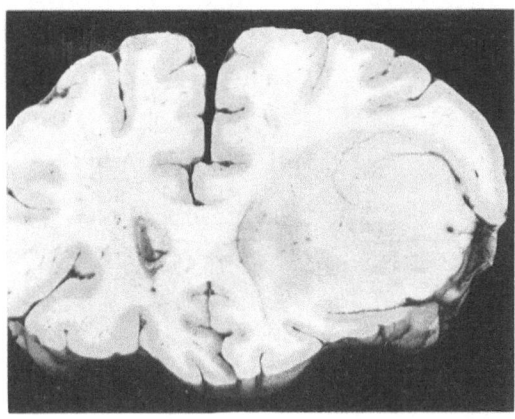

Fig. 86. Frontolateral astrocytoma with central cystic degeneration. In this case extension into the white matter of the insula typical for tumors in this location was seen

Fig. 87. Frontolateral astrocytoma which has infiltrated the third frontal convolution. Minimal shift of midline structures

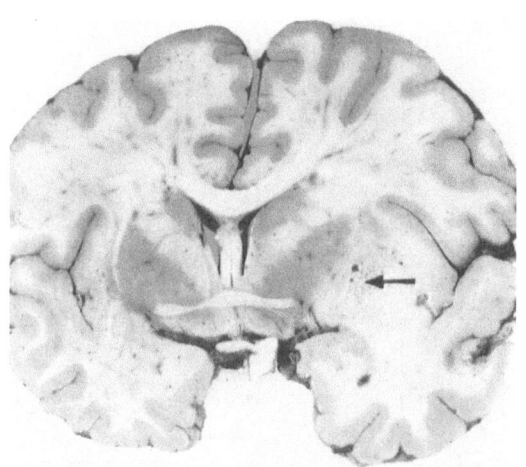

Fig. 88. Typical insular extension of a fronto-lateral astrocytoma (arrow!)

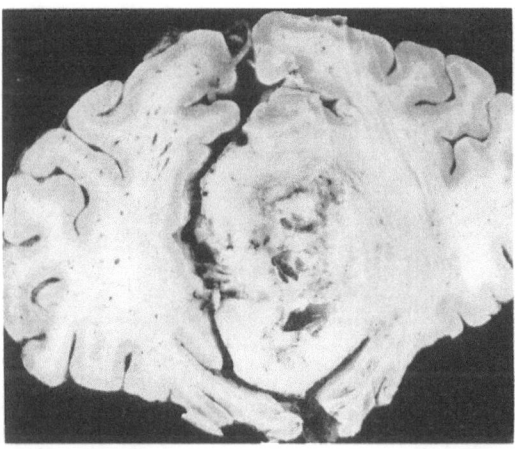

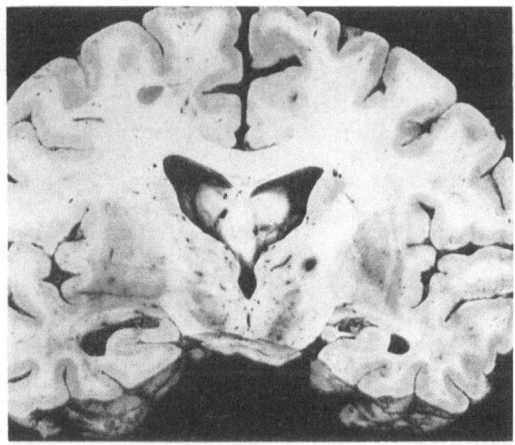

Fig. 89. Typical frontomedial astrocytoma. Note the multiple small cysts which are a frequent occurrence in such tumors

Fig. 90. Frontomedial astrocytoma which has invaded and expanded the septum pellucidum and which invaginates the anterior horn

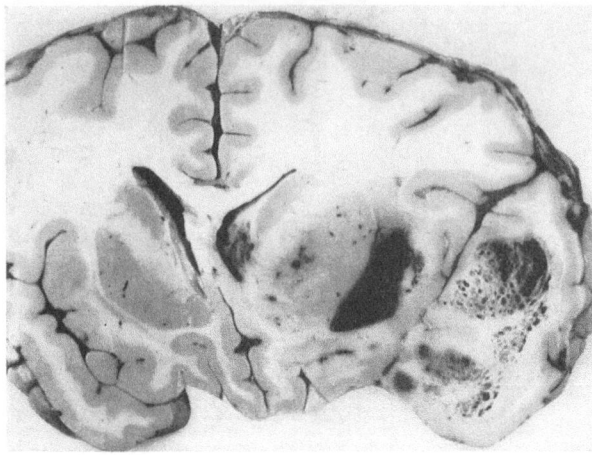

Fig. 91. Temporal astrocytoma with extensive microcystic degeneration and hemorrhage. Note extension into the basal frontal lobe, perhaps via the uncinate fasciculus

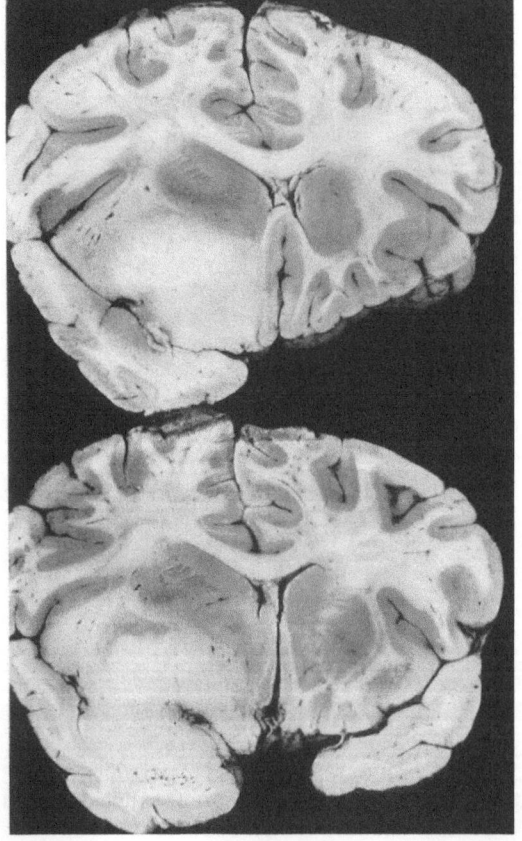

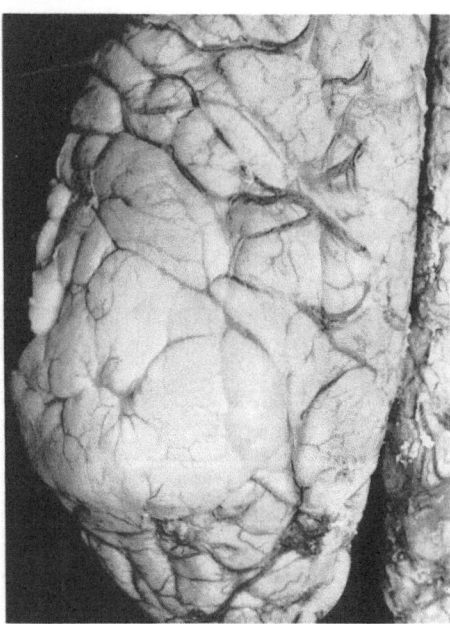

Fig. 93. Typical parietolateral astrocytoma in the left hemisphere. The gyri are expanded and hardened, only a few vessels are seen

Fig. 92. Frontobasal astrocytoma (rare) with extension into the temporal lobe

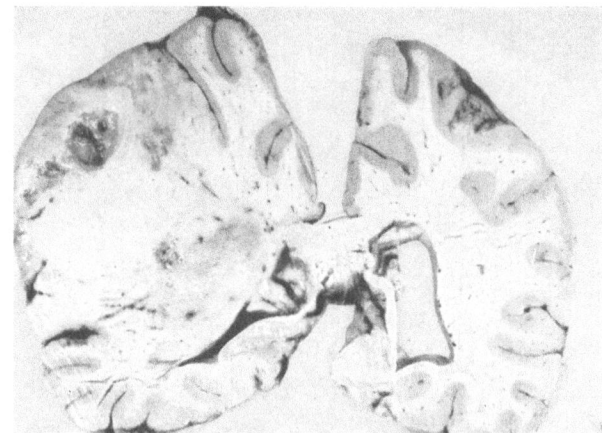

Fig. 94. Parietolateral astrocytoma which presented on the surface of the convexity as a mushroom-shaped mass and had extended to the wall of the ventricular trigone. Note the subcortical cystic degeneration

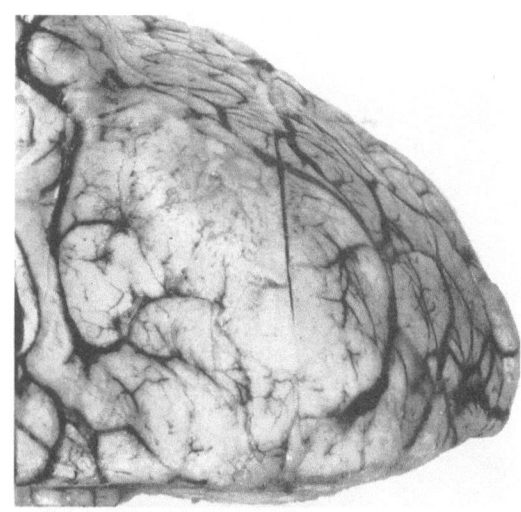

Fig. 95. View from above of a well-circumscribed parietal astrocytoma which had eroded the overlying skull (rare!) and which showed areas of malignant degeneration. Histologic picture was otherwise that of a typical fibrillary astrocytoma (see Fig. 96)

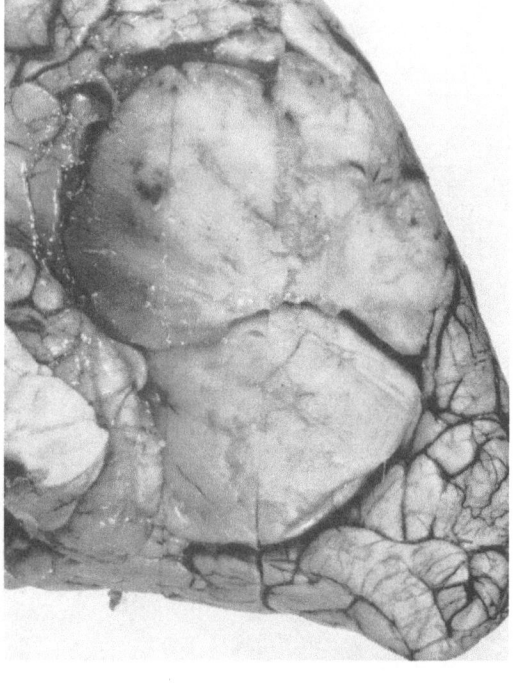

Fig. 96. Medial view of previous case. Note the knotty, hard appearance of this apparently well-circumscribed tumor. However, a more malignant portion was found to have traversed the corpus callosum to the opposite hemisphere. A tentorial pressure cone is readily apparent adjacent to the left inferolateral border of the tumor

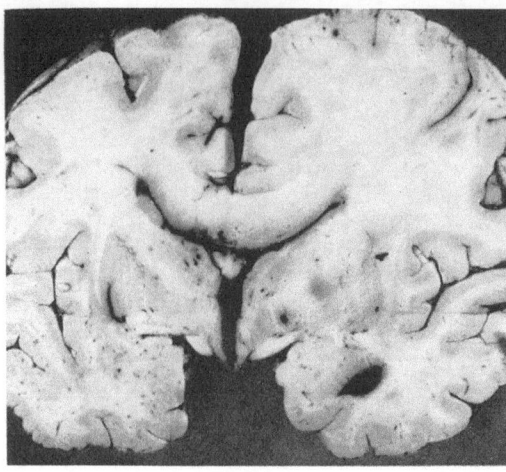

Fig. 97. Diffuse (protoplasmic) astrocytoma with extensive involvement of the corpus callosum

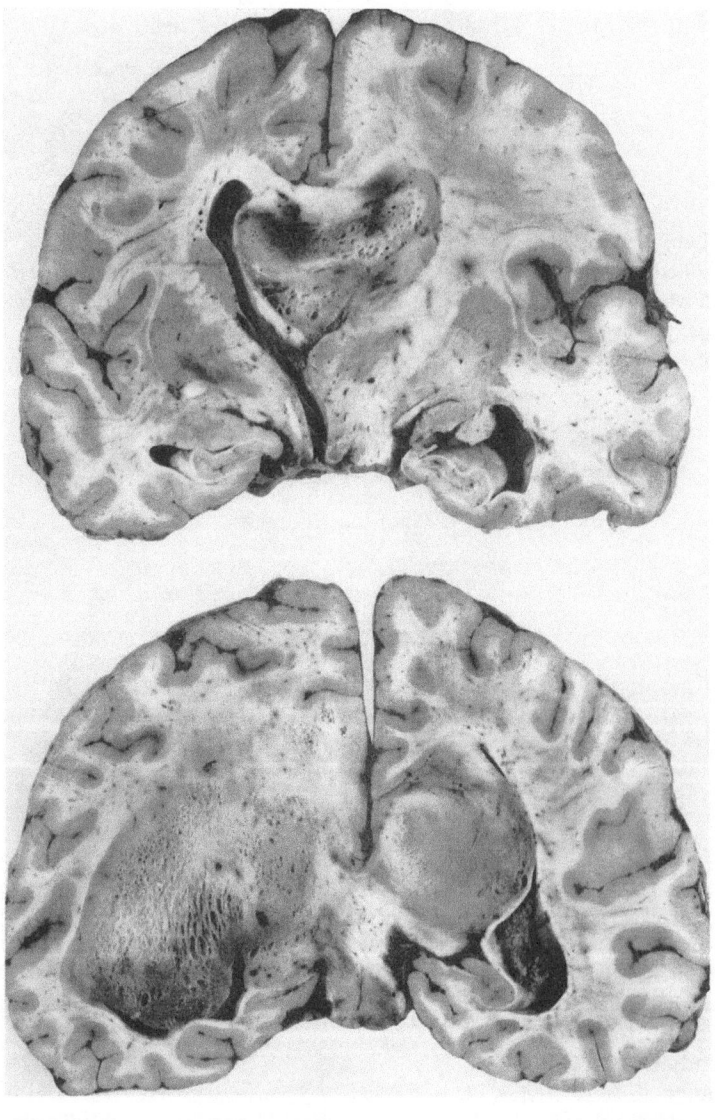

Fig. 98. Extension of a cystic astrocytoma along the fornices which are grossly distorted. The adjacent occipital lobe was also involved

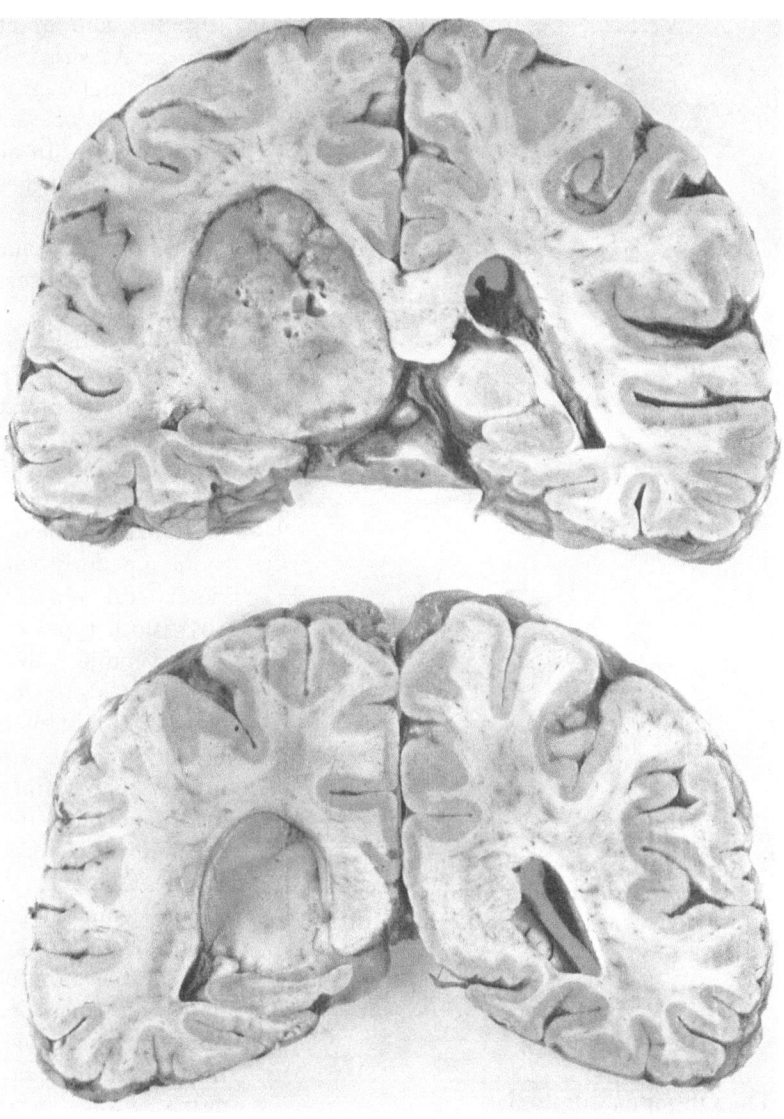

Fig. 99. Malignant astrocytoma of basal ganglia

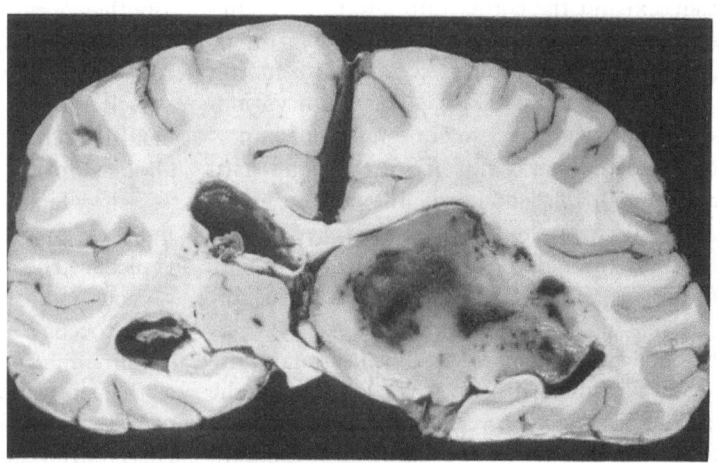

Fig. 100. A large glassy-appearing astrocytoma of the thalamus with hemorrhage

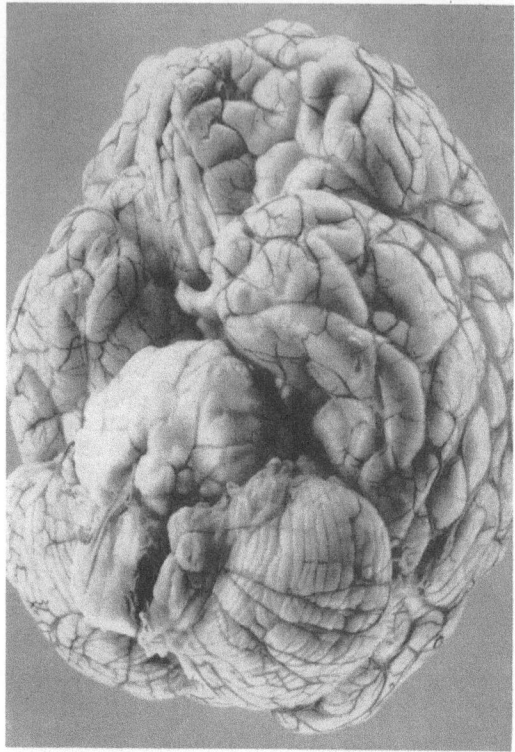

Fig. 101. Typical astrocytoma of the pons which has greatly expanded this structure. Note the tumor processes extending inferolaterally into the adjacent cisterns and the marked cerebellar pressure cone

The Oligodendrogliomas

The oligodendrogliomas are more frequently cortical than "deep seated" tumors. In general they expand the cortex diffusely in a circumscribed area making it appear hypertrophic (Fig. 103), while the underlying white matter shows mucoid cysts (Figs. 102, 105) of various sizes and sometimes small necroses. Of importance to the neurosurgeon are the small hard readily-palpable nodules in the cortex, which are also apparent to the naked eye. Upon breaking through the meninges, the tumor may form large lumps that project beyond the surface like bluish-red mushrooms (Fig. 104). This tendency is particularly marked frontolaterally near the Sylvian fissure (Fig. 102) and in the upper parietal regions. Such oligodendrogliomas tend to adhere (but not to infiltrate!) the dura

(Fig. 102) and are often first taken for meningiomas. At surgery, they appear either firm or moderately, gray-red or the colour of raw meat, friable or calcified and occasionally necrotic in parts. In addition, the extent of the necrosis often suggests the histological variant present; smaller areas of necrosis are more typical of the "isomorphic" type, while larger areas are more suggestive of the "polymorphic" type.

The oligodendrogliomas lie quite frequently at the base of the second or third frontal convolutions (frontolateral oligodendrogliomas) (Figs. 102, 103), where they may reach the size of an egg and invade the convolutions above the Sylvian fissure and the underlying white matter. The same subtype may lie caudally and more superiorly within the parietal gyri (parietolateral oligodendrogliomas) (Figs. 104, 105). Both types can simulate "mushrooms" as they project above the level of the cortex. There are also rarer parasagittal oligodendrogliomas (Fig. 106) located either in the gyri bordering the sagittal fissure, from where they invade the rostral corpus callosum (frontomedial oligodendrogliomas) (Fig. 106), or the splenium of the corpus callosum itself (Fig. 110). In the temporal lobe they infiltrate the gyri of the temporal pole (temporal oligodendrogliomas) (Fig. 107a, b) and from here they can invade the frontobasal or temporomedial (hippocampal) regions (Fig. 108). In the occipital region they lie medially or occupy all of the cortex. A favorite location—although nearly always in children—is the thalamus (Fig. 109) which may be blown up to the size of a tennis ball. Rare are oligodendrogliomas of the corpus callosum (Fig. 110). Exceptionally they occur in the spinal cord or cerebellum.

Oligodendrogliomas are rather vascular tumors, usually with an abundance of smaller vessels. However, only the polymorphous oligodendrogliomas approach the vascularity of glioblastomas, often containing "sinusoid" vessels which may be seen by angiography; but even here the arteriovenous "fistulae" so typical of the glioblastoma never occur. Spontaneous metastasis via the CSF pathway can rarely occur (Fig. 111), in which case the metastatic nodules continue growing at the same rate as the parent tumor. Sometimes diffuse seeding over the ventricular and arachnoidal systems is seen after surgery (Fig. 112).

The oligodendrogliomas occur in the middle decades with the peak of incidence falling between 30–55 years, only those of the thalamus showing a preference for the younger age groups (see p. 46). The figures on incidence vary between 1.3% of CUSHING's (1932, 1935), 5% of KERNOHAN's and SAYRE's (1952) and 9.6% of our own series. In our series of 9000 tumors 484 (56.3%) were males and 375 (43.7%) females. The oligodendrogliomas generally belong to the "semibenign" group; however, not infrequently tumors with "cellular" or "structural" polymorphy are encountered and these have a poorer prognosis ("semimalignant" tumors).

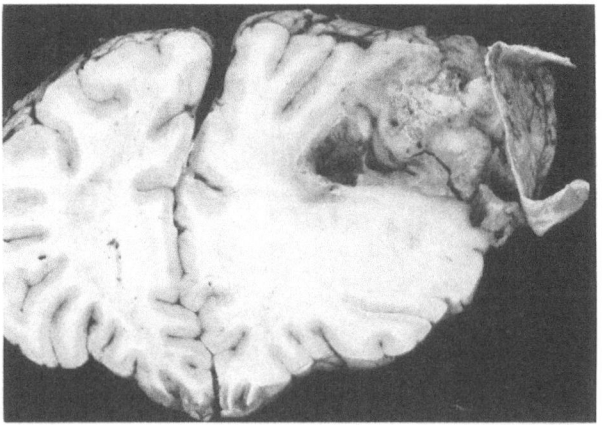

Fig. 102. Frontolateral oligodendroglioma which has broken through to the cortical surface, assuming the form of a mushroom, and widely infiltrating dura. A pigmented cyst is seen in the depths of the tumor, as well as some fresh hemorrhage

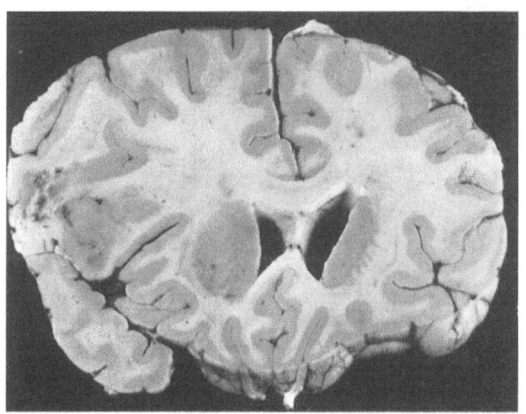

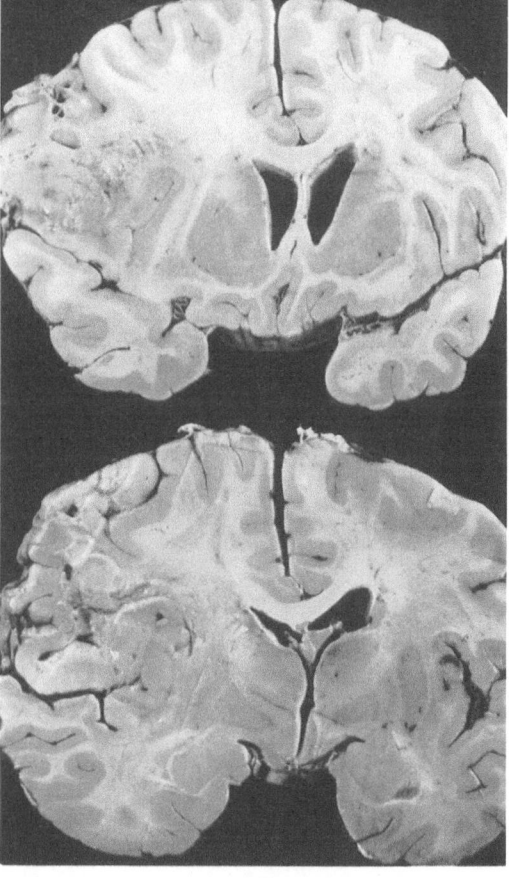

Fig. 103. Frontolateral oligodendroglioma which also invades the insular gyri. Moderate contralateral displacement is evident. Note the "hypertrophy" of the convolutions

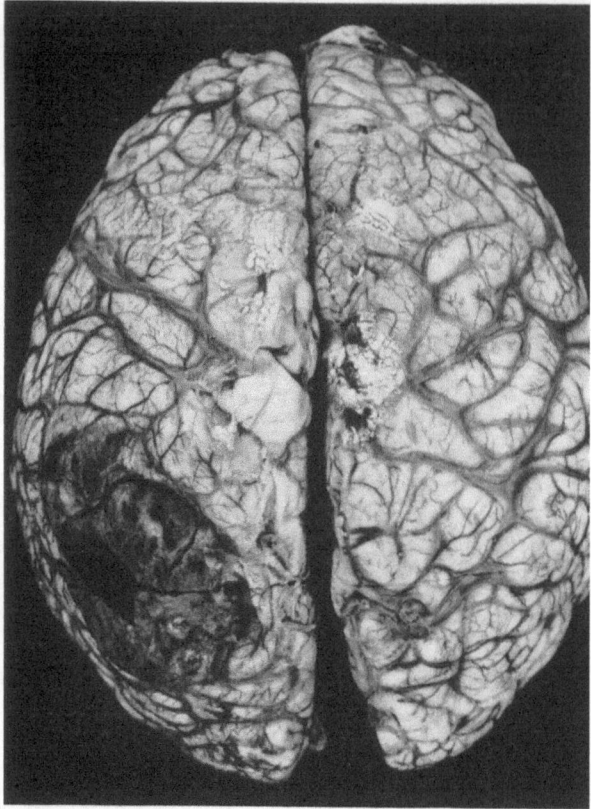

Fig. 104. Large mushroom-like parieto-lateral oligodendroglioma with fresh hemorrhage within the tumor

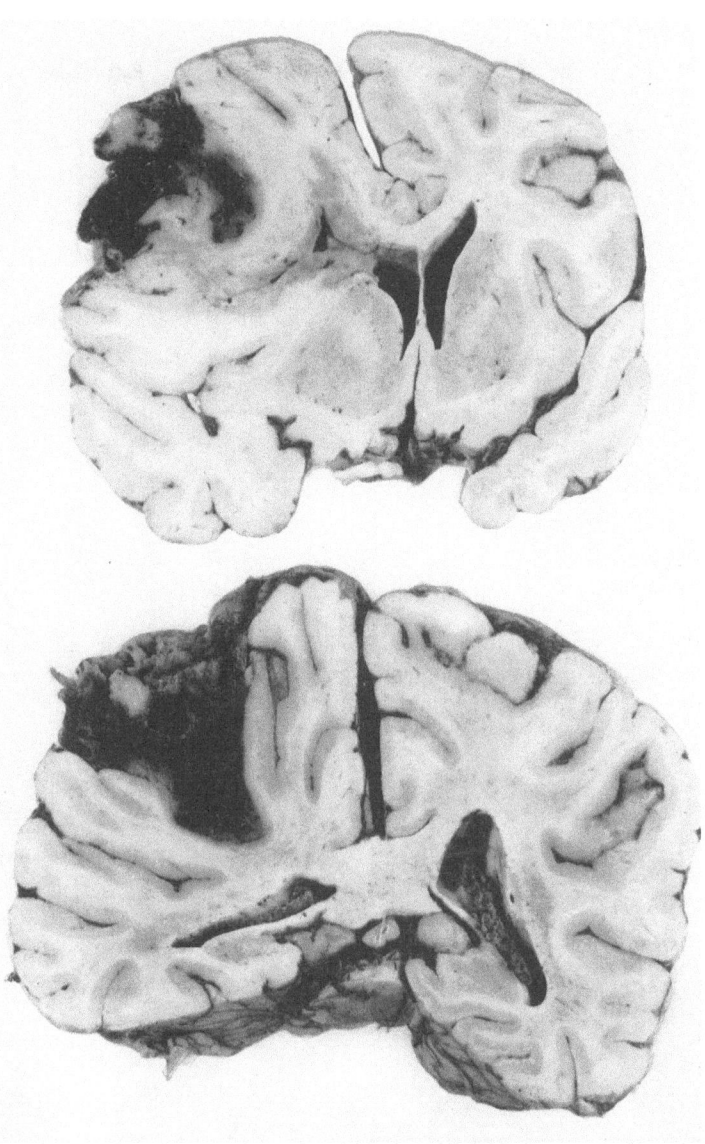

Fig. 105. Mushroom-shaped parietolateral oligodendroglioma. A large cyst is seen which communicates with the anterior horn of the lateral ventricle. Fresh hemorrhage into the tumor is also apparent

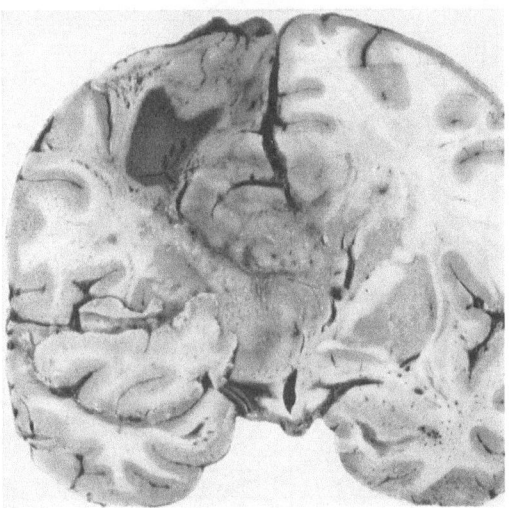

Fig. 106. Large frontomedial oligodendroglioma with subcortical cyst formation. The tumor has obliterated the anterior horn and has extended through the corpus callosum to the opposite hemisphere

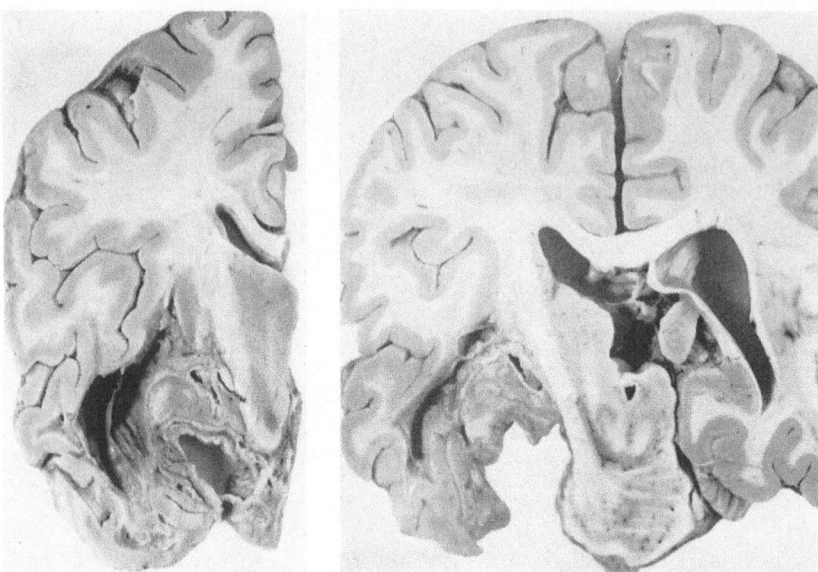

Fig. 107. Large temporomedial oligodendroglioma after intensive radiation therapy. The entire temporal white matter has undergone cystic degeneration secondary to the effect of the radiation, the cortical parts of the tumor being unaffected

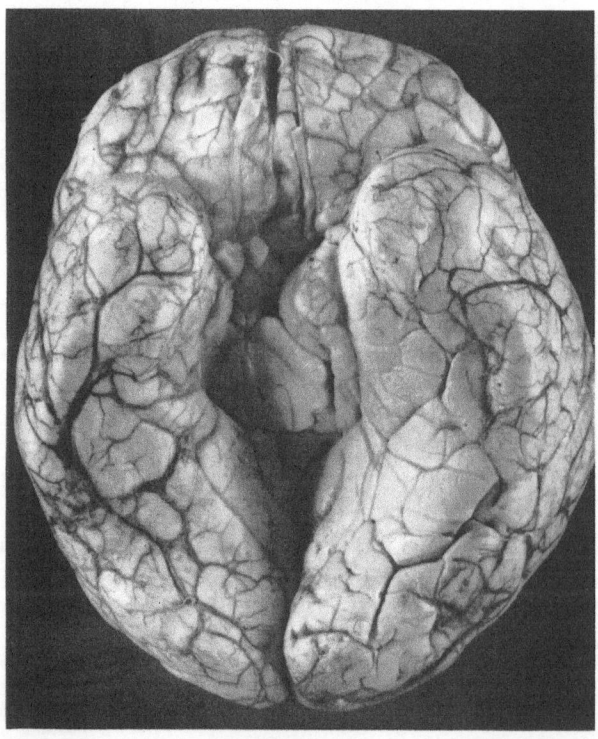

Fig. 108. Large left temporomedial oligo-dendroglioma with extensive herniation into the tentorial hiatus

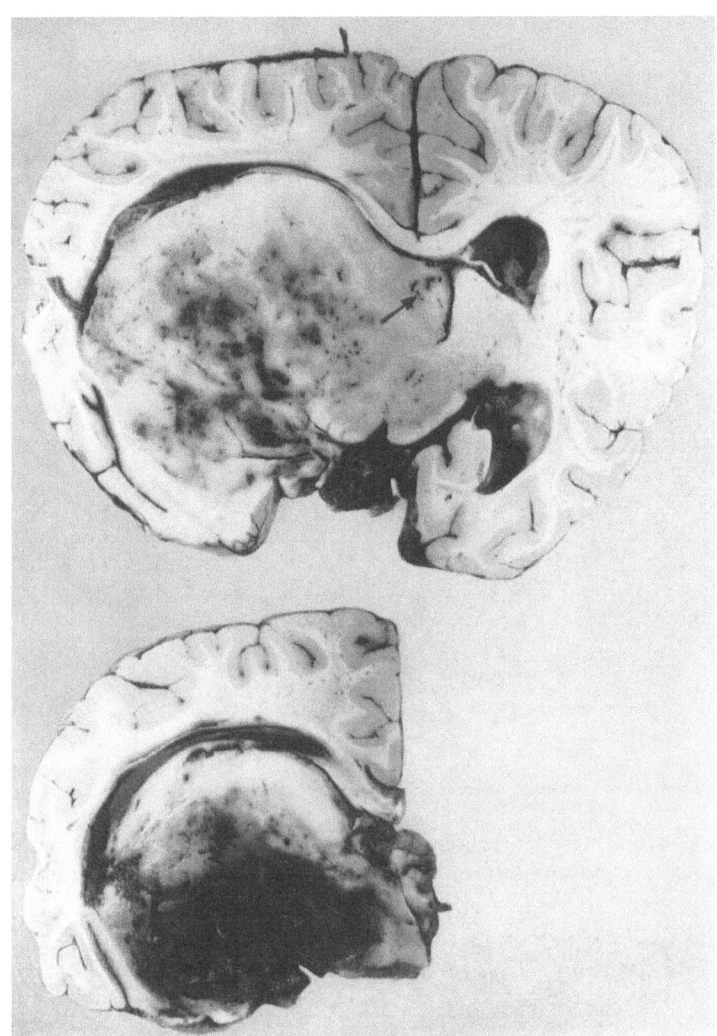

Fig. 109. Enormous thalamic oligodendroglioma with invasion of the midbrain. Apoplectic hemorrhage into the tumor has occurred, which can be seen to have extended into the ventricular system

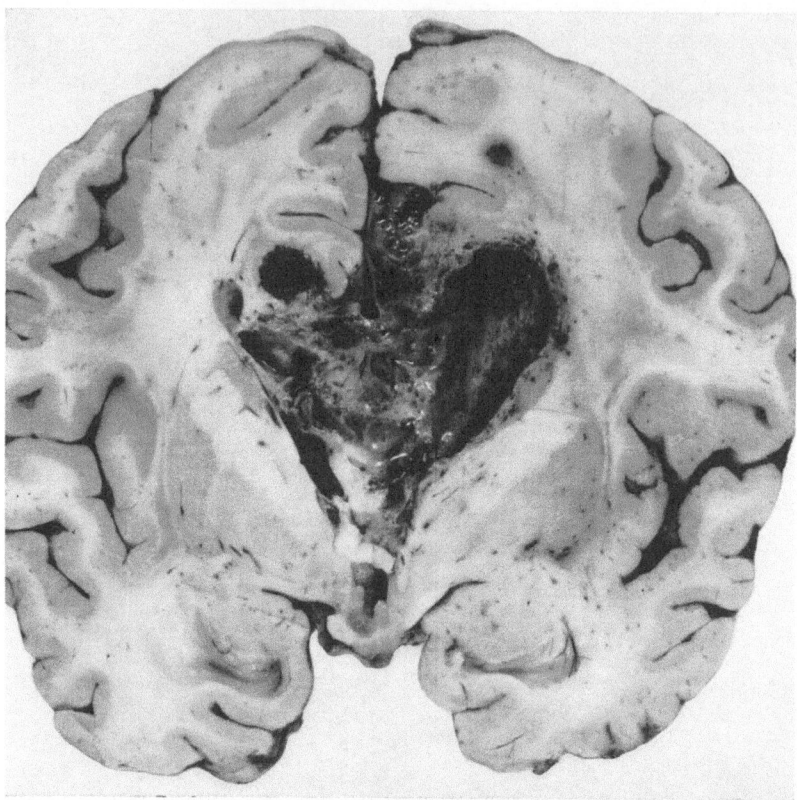

Fig. 110. Oligodendroglioma of the corpus callosum and of the septum pellucidum. The adjacent cingulate gyri are infiltrated. Cystic degeneration and numerous hemorrhages are apparent

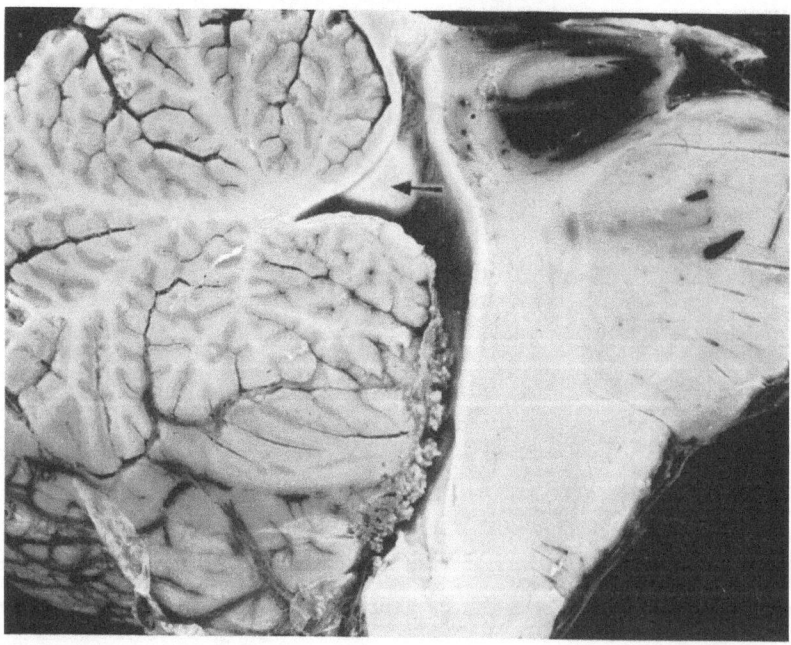

Fig. 111. Pea-sized, spontaneous metastasis (very rare) to wall of fourth ventricle (arrow!) in a cerebral oligodendroglioma. Midbrain hemorrhage was secondary to increased intracranial pressure and axial shift from the primary tumor

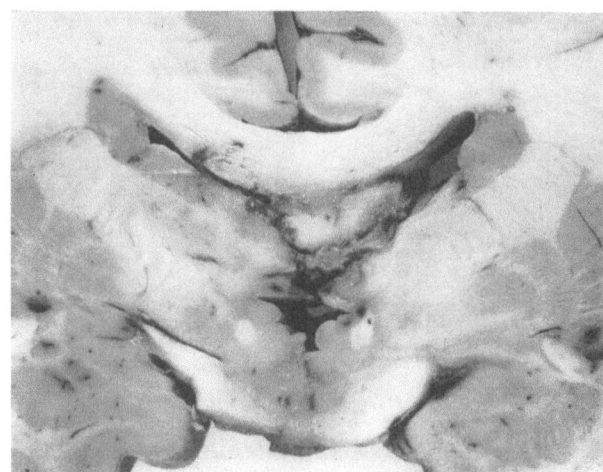

Fig. 112. Post-operative diffuse spread of an oligodendroglioma via the cerebro-spinal fluid into the ventricles and external CSF pathways

The Glioblastomas

The glioblastoma multiforme, when it invades the surface of the brain, is recognized by a flattening of the convolutions (Fig. 117) and by a brownish-red or yellowish and glassy discoloration. Sometimes—particularly if the convolutions are glassy and pale—it is apt to resemble an astrocytoma (Fig. 121, 130). However, in the depths of the tumor increased vascularity is found (Figs. 132, 135, 136) as well as a variegated color pattern—i.e., fatty degeneration: yellow to ochre-yellow; necroses: gray; hemorrhages of various stages: brown to red—all of which characterizes the glioblastoma (Fig. 116). In addition, softening of the adjacent brain as a result of the marked number of regressive changes induced is seen. Most cases of glioblastoma, however, do not reach the surface of the brain, but limit themselves to infiltration of the white matter.

Dilated blood vessels with lumens occasionally as large as a match (Fig. 136) may surround many of the tumors in their peripheral zones. Often, such vessels are visible on the cortical surface as large, hyperemic, engorged vessels with a bright red, "arterial" color corresponding to "early veins"). Larger vessels in the depths of the tumor adjacent to or within an area of necrosis may be thrombosed (Figs. 130, 141). Cysts are not common (Fig. 119), but do occasionally occur and contain a yellowish-brown fluid; necrosis, however, is a far more

common finding (Fig. 139, 141). Taken as a group, the glioblastomas are often unusually well-circumscribed for gliomas (Fig. 116). Occasionally, they are less well-demarcated and may resemble a "necrotizing inflammation" (Figs. 132, 138). Here, dilated blood vessels prevail (Figs. 133, 136), some resembling the lacunar and fistulous vessels which appear on angiography. Hemorrhages and thromboses are frequent and, if large (Figs. 116, 123, 137), may induce acute "apoplectiform" episodes. The surrounding brain edema and swelling are well known (Fig. 134) and are at least partly responsible for the early and very marked increase in intracranial pressure seen with these tumors. The consistency of the glioblastoma depends upon the amount of regressive change on the one hand, and on the amount of connective tissue stroma on the other. Stromal reaction may be so marked and so abundant that hard nodules consisting of "fibrosarcomatous" connective tissue—with many of the features of a malignant mesodermal tumor—are occasionally encountered within the glioblastoma.

For the glioblastomas, too, it is now possible to point to various sites of preferende (Table 5). They are found in a frontolateral location (Fig. 113; the size of a hen's egg), in particular in the third frontal convolution and subcortical white matter; in a frontodorsal location (Fig. 114) in the first and second convolutions, extending to the tip of the anterior horn; and in a frontobasal location (Fig. 115) within the

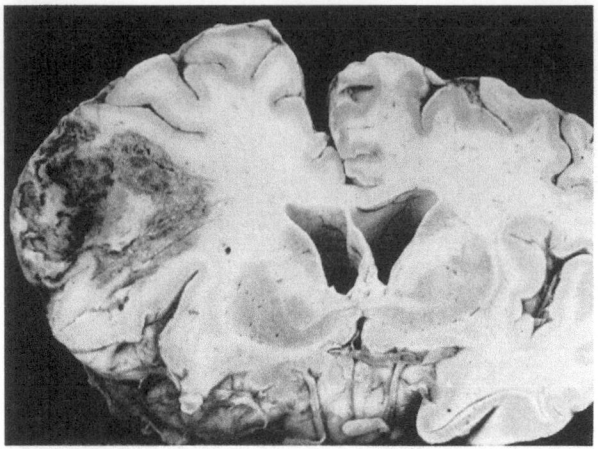

Fig. 113. Frontolateral glioblastoma with moderate brain swelling and minimal shift of the midline structures. Variegated patterns of necrosis may be seen within the tumor mass

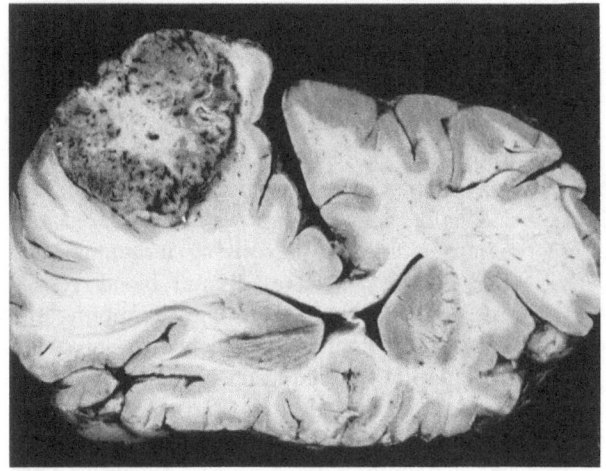

Fig. 114. Frontodorsal glioblastoma with associated cerebral edema and mass displacement to the opposite side

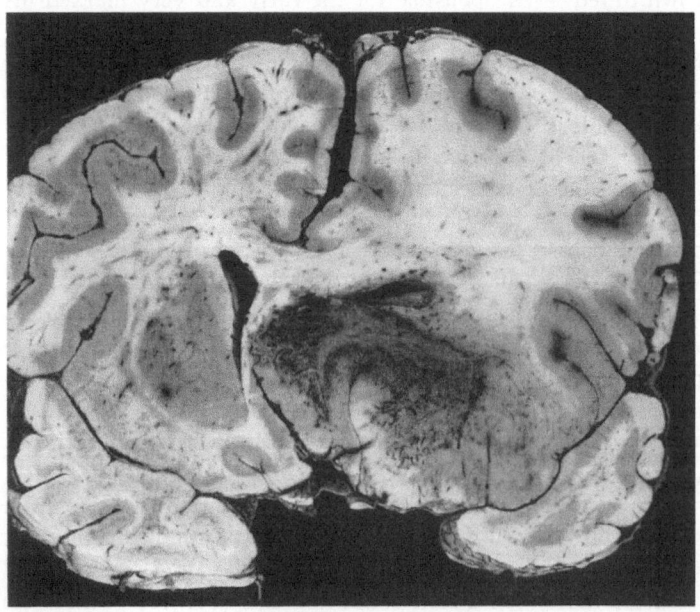

Fig. 115. Frontobasal glioblastoma with associated brain swelling and gross distortion of the ventricular system

gyrus rectus and the adjacent basolateral convolutions, from where they occasionally spread through the corpus callosum to the opposite side. More caudally, we find them in a parietolateral location (Fig. 116), extending subcortically from the foot of the third frontal convolution through the middle and inferior portions of the pre- and postcentral gyri to the inferior part of the parietal lobe; and in the parietodorsal region (Figs. 117–119), originating subcortically at the foot of the first and second frontal convolutions but this time extending through the superior third of the pre- and postcentral gyri into the superior parietal lobe. In the temporal lobe we recognize temporolateral (Figs. 121, 122) and temporomedial (Fig. 123) glioblastomas. The temporolateral glioblastoma extends from the temporal tip through the first and second convolutions and throughout all the white matter of the lobe. In this instance, the medial convolutions remain tumor-free, while they are particularly affected with the temporomedial glioblastoma. The main bulk of this latter tumor lies in the neighboring white matter with extension spreading to the temporal lobe and to the occipital lobe. Glioblastomas of the occipital lobe lie either occipitolateral (Fig. 124a, b) or occipitobasal and can grow across to the opposite side through the posterior portion of the corpus callosum. These types, however, have not been too clearly characterized. Certain glioblastomas loop from the frontal into the temporal lobe. Spread may also occur in a "butterfly" distribution from the corpus callosum (Figs. 125, 126), bilaterally extending into the depths of the adjacent white matter as in the anterior (Fig. 125) or posterior (Fig. 126) callosal glioblastomas. Infiltration may also be limited to the white matter of one side only, as in the glioblastoma of the anterior (Fig. 127) or posterior (Fig. 128) callosal radiation. Glioblastomas may grow along the fornix (Fig. 129) (particularly in its frontal, parietal, or temporal portions) and are also found in the thalamus (Fig. 130), but rarely in the region of the quadrigeminal plate (Fig. 131),

and only exceptionally in the pons and the spinal cord; they have almost never been verified in the cerebellum. Generally speaking, glioblastomas spread subcortically. On frontal section they appear wedge-shaped, like an infarct (Fig. 127), but they can also—especially in the temporal and occipital regions—assume a cylindrical form and extend along the long axis of the lobe (Fig. 116).

The glioblastomas are a tumor group occurring in the middle ages and senescence. They represent the "cancer" of the brain. They occur only rarely in the young, become more frequent after the age of 30, and have a definite peak around the ages of 45–65 (see p. 46). It is difficult to determine the actual incidence of the glioblastomas. In CUSHING's series (1932, 1935) they represented 10.3%, in our material of 9000 cases 12.2%. There were 674 males and 419 females, with a ratio of 2:1. Thus they share with the medulloblastoma not only the highest malignancy grading of any of the neuroepithelial tumors but also a definite predilection for the male sex.

The prognosis of the glioblastomas is very poor and is reflected in the survival statistics even after combined surgery cytotoxic and radiation therapy. Three main histologic subtypes are recognized, but these do not seem to vary either in growth potential or in biological behavior. Metastases within the CSF pathway may occur (Fig. 132), particularly if the parent tumor lies near the ventricular surface (Fig. 129). These appear as granular, nodular metastases (Figs. 132, 133) and sometimes resemble ependymitis. Rarely they are multilocular (Fig. 134). Metastases into body organs are not likely. Usually, such cases actually represent examples of sarcomas—as, for example, the monstrocellular sarcoma (see p. 140).

Recurrences are the rule even after so-called "complete" removals. Hemispherectomy has not changed this outcome. Glioblastoma multiforme almost seems to be a "disease" of the brain and reoperations are, therefore, practically useless.

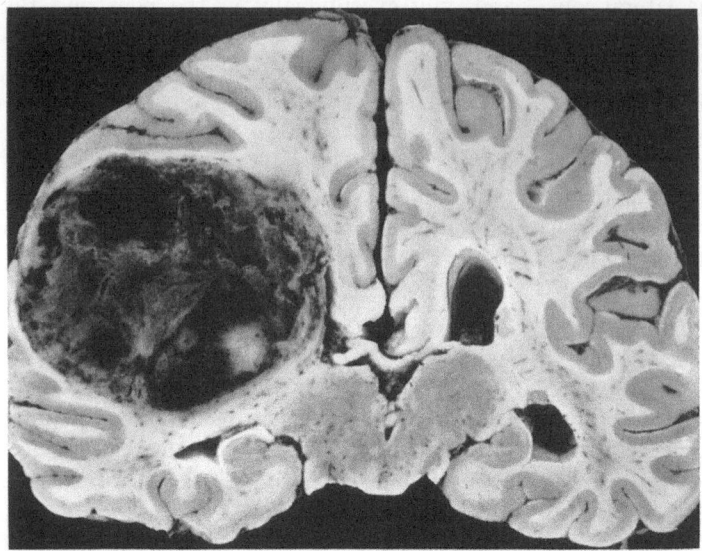

Fig. 116. Parietolateral glioblastoma with only slight midline shift. The falx has cut through the splenium of the corpus callosum

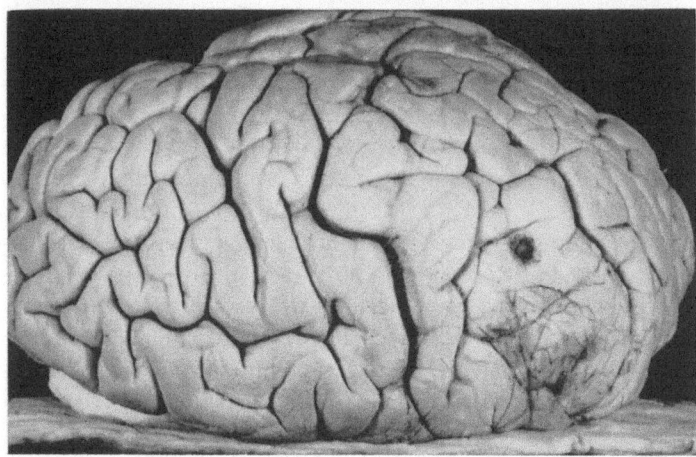

Fig. 117. Parietodorsal glioblastoma presenting on the cortical surface (see Fig. 118)

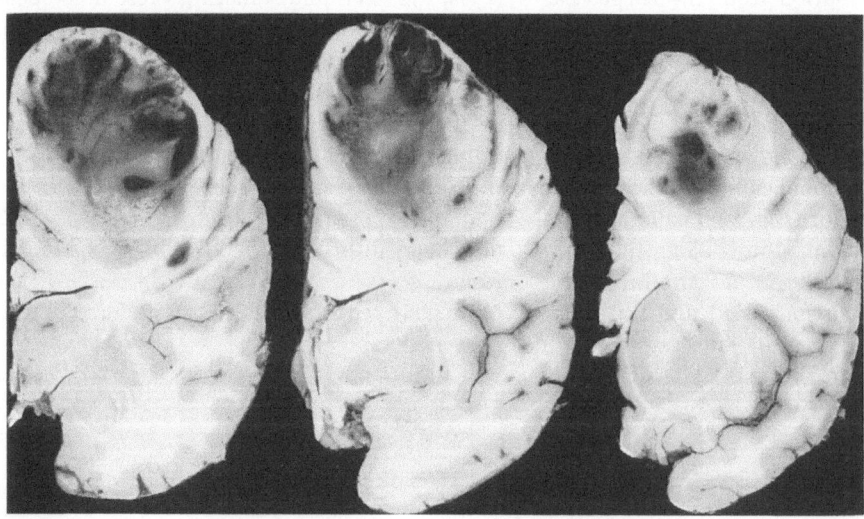

Fig. 118. Horizontal sections of previous case. Minimal shift of midline structures

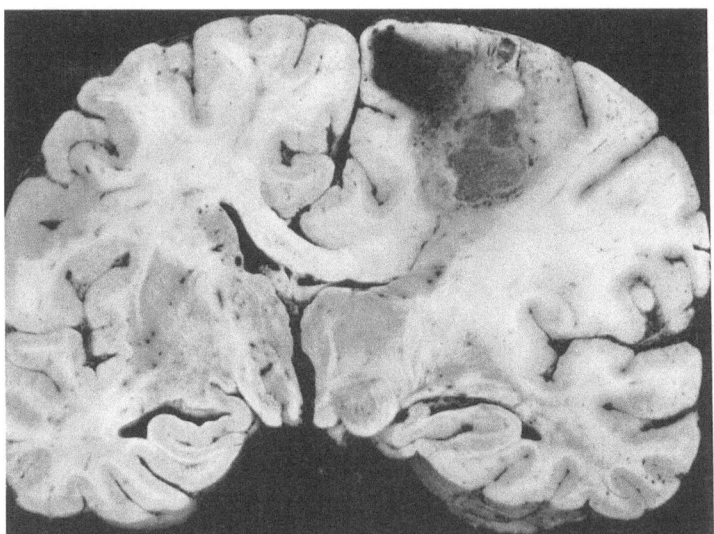

Fig. 119. Parietodorsal glioblastoma with collateral brain
edema

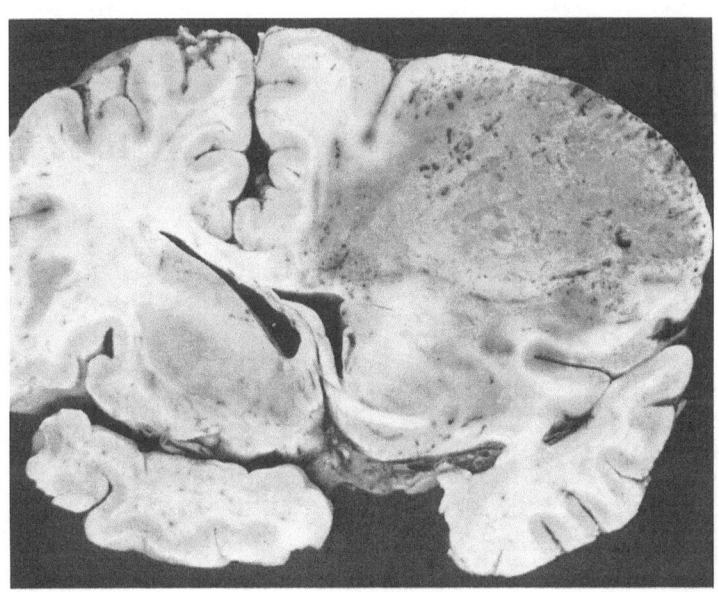

Fig. 120. Large parietolateral
glioblastoma with extensive
shift across the midline anteriorly

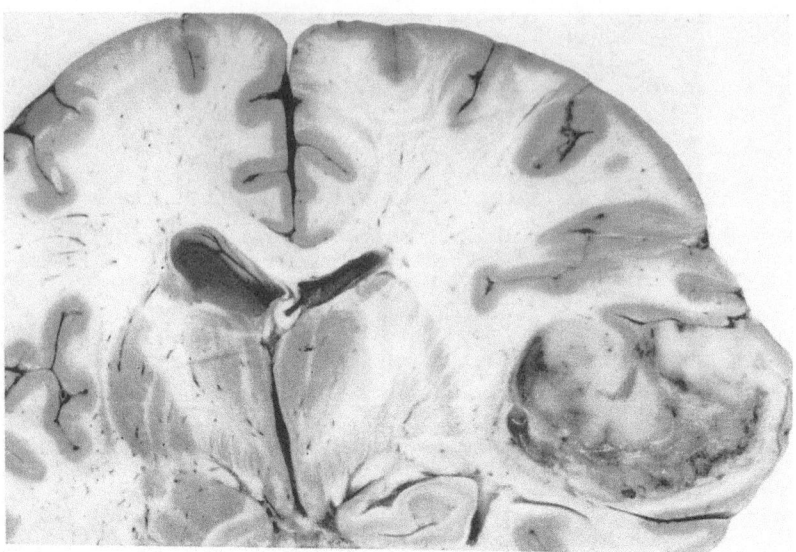

Fig. 121. Temporolateral glioblastoma with moderate cyst formation in parts

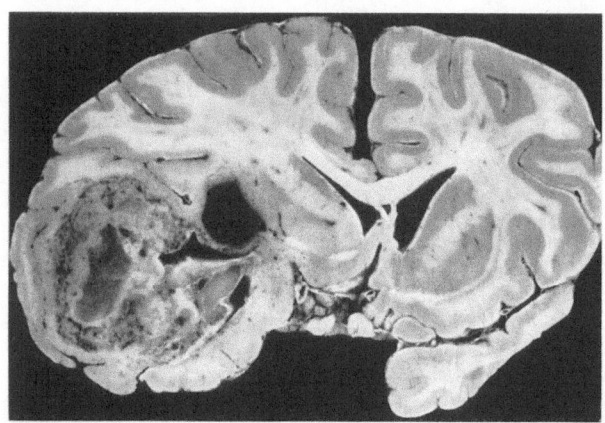

Fig. 122. Temporolateral glioblastoma with cyst formation and adjacent hemorrhage. Note herniation of gyrus cinguli

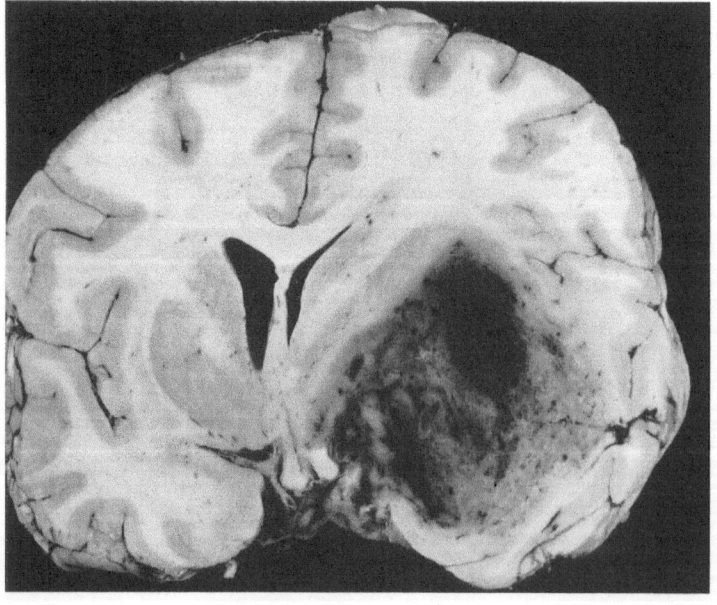

Fig. 123. Temporomedial glioblastoma which did not reach the cortex of the convexity. Note the distortion and upward displacement of the adjacent Sylvian fissure and the corpus callosum

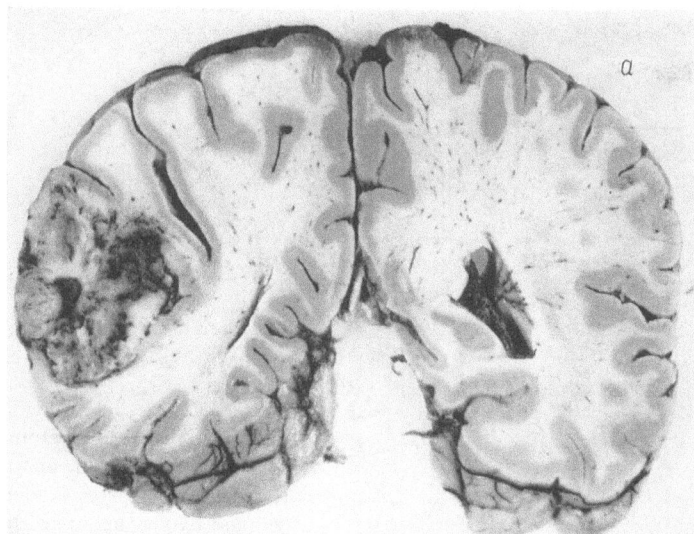

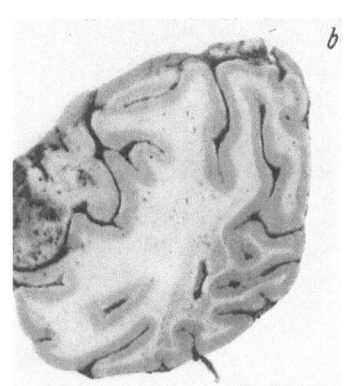

Fig. 124. Occipitolateral glioblastoma

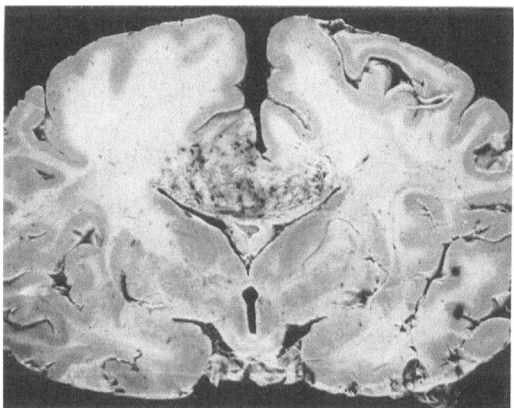

Fig. 125. Typical bilateral glioblastoma of corpus callosum ("butterfly"-distribution) with considerable adjacent brain swelling

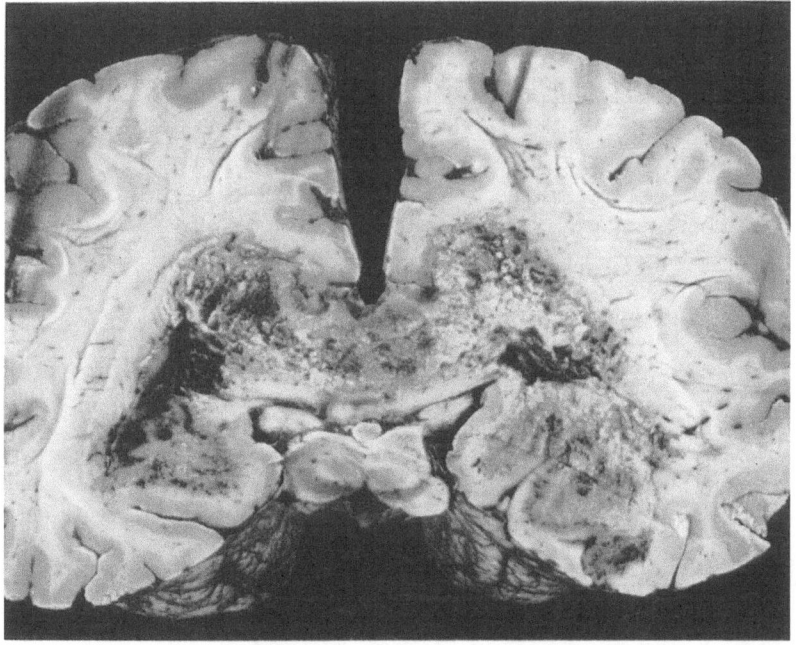

Fig. 126. Extensive bilateral "butterfly"-shaped glioblastoma of the caudal corpus callosum. Note infiltration of the medial temporal lobes

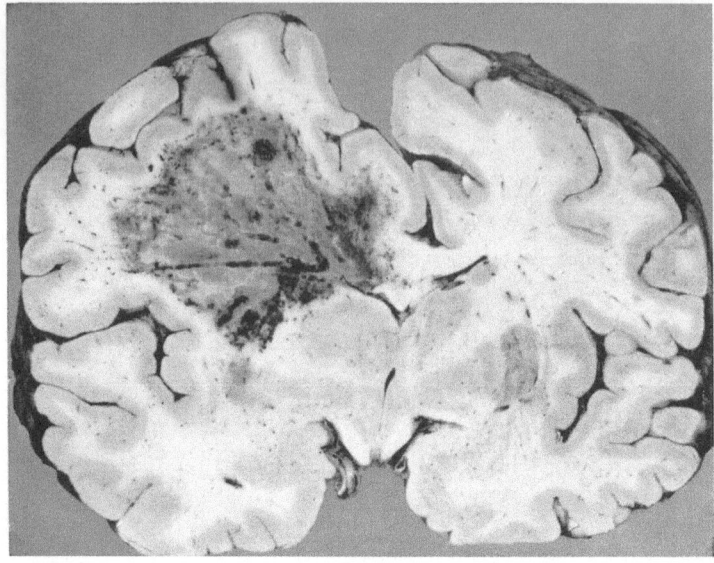

Fig. 127. Typical glioblastoma of the rostral radiation of the corpus callosum with considerable mass displacement to the opposite side

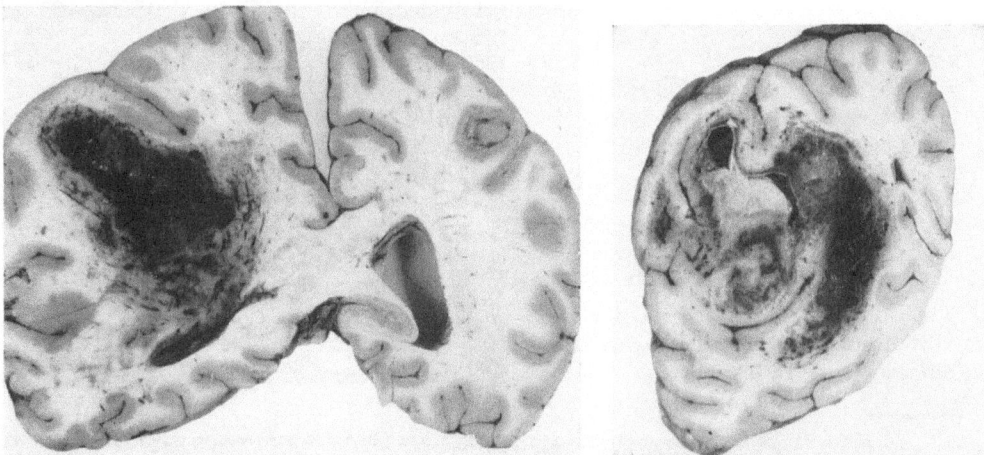

Fig. 128. Typical glioblastoma of the caudal radiation of the corpus callosum with infiltration of the occipital lobe posteriorly

a

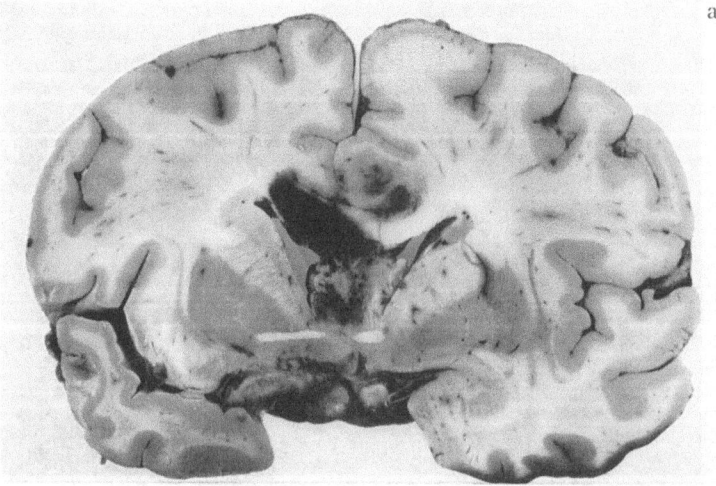

Fig. 129a, b. Glioblastoma of the fornix. In these two sections note how the tumor (with hemorrhages) follows the anterior-posterior anatomical distribution of the fornix, from the midline laterally. Note also the involvement of the temporal lobe in the posterior section

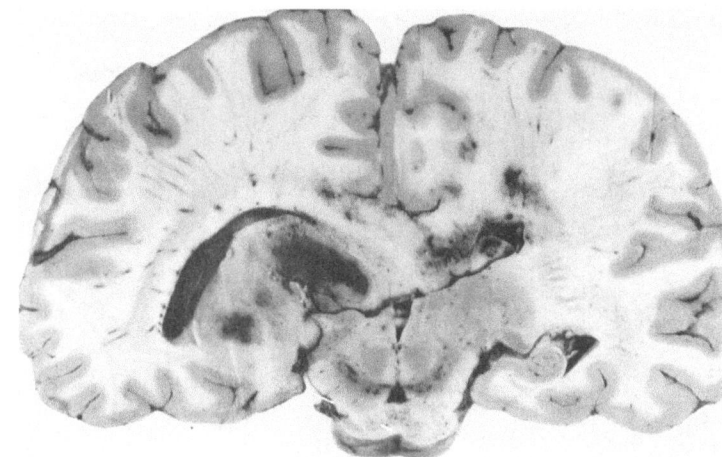

Fig. 129b. (Legend see opposite page)

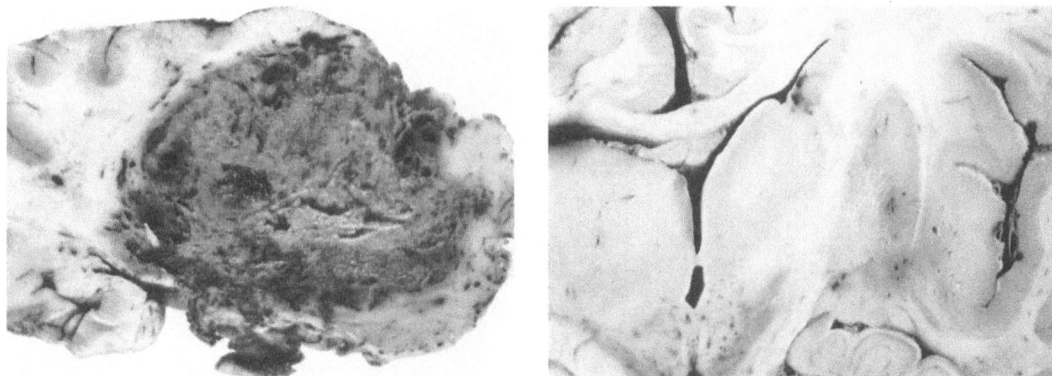

Fig. 130. Widely divergent macroscopic appearance in different glioblastomas. To the left, one sees the more common variegated pattern with necroses, hemorrhages, and fatty degeneration. Rarely, a homogenous infiltration is found, as in the thalamic glioblastoma to the right

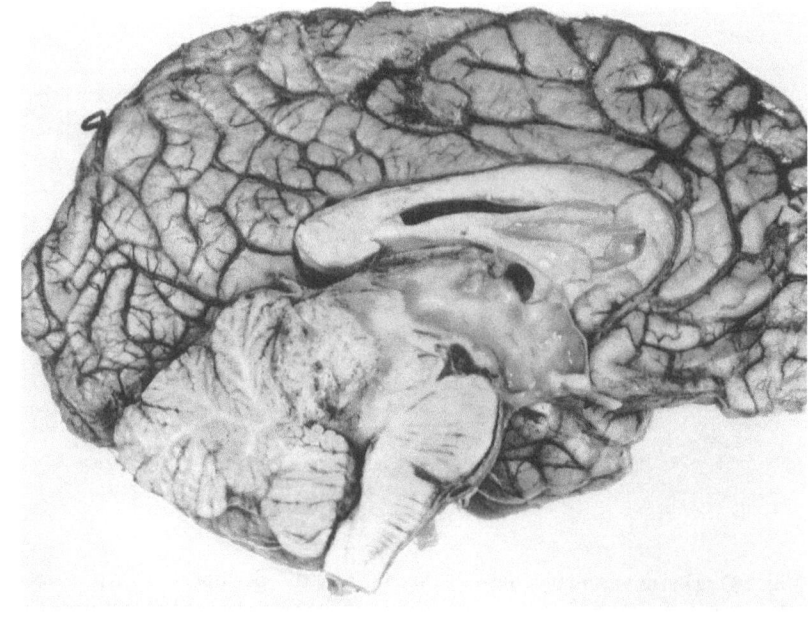

Fig. 131. Walnut-sized glioblastoma of the quadrigeminal plate with secondary obstructive hydrocephalus

91

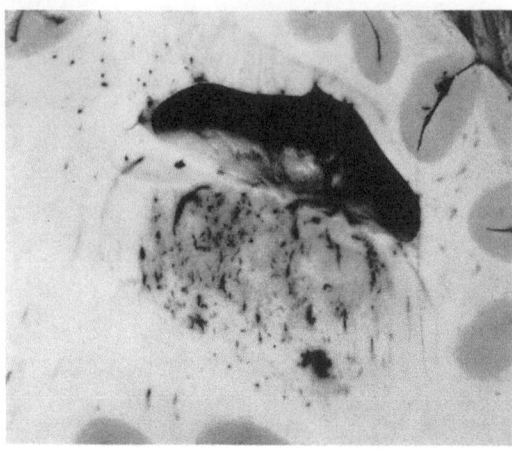

Fig. 132. Small ventricular metastasis of a glioblastoma. One sees in this early stage numerous enlarged vascular channels

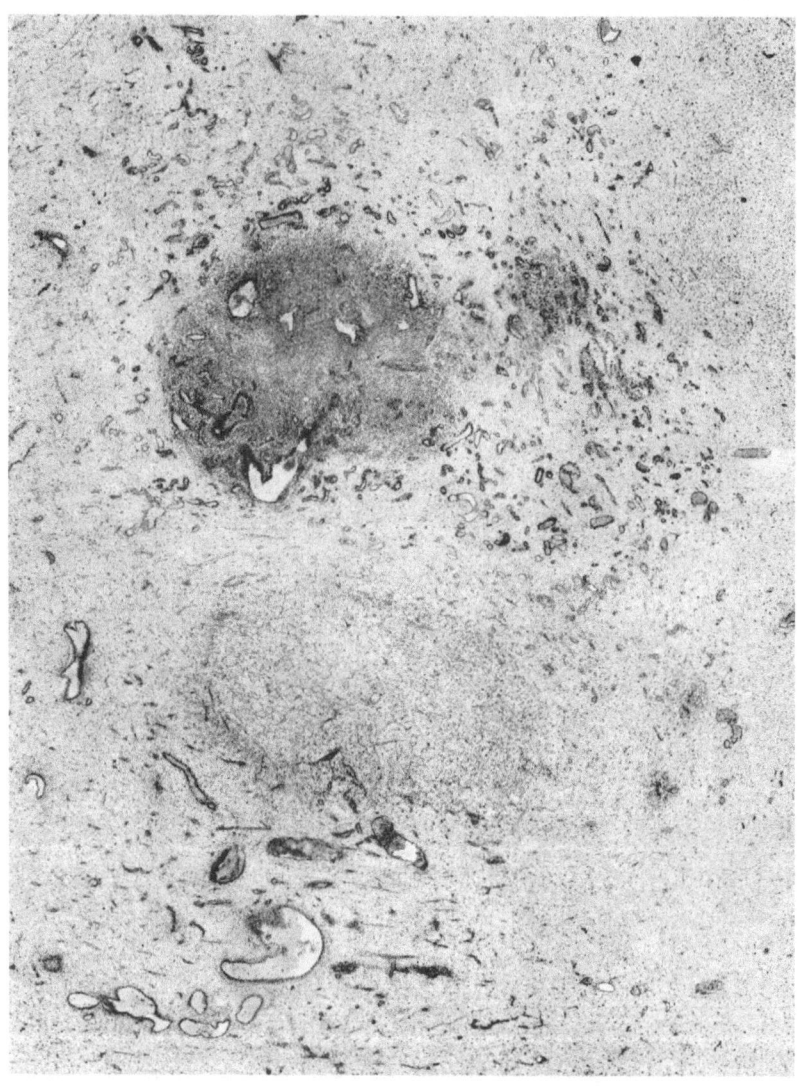

Fig. 133. Dense vascular sinusoidal pattern in the periphery of a pea-sized glioblastoma metastasis, where one sees an earlier form of the later characteristic glioblastoma vasculature

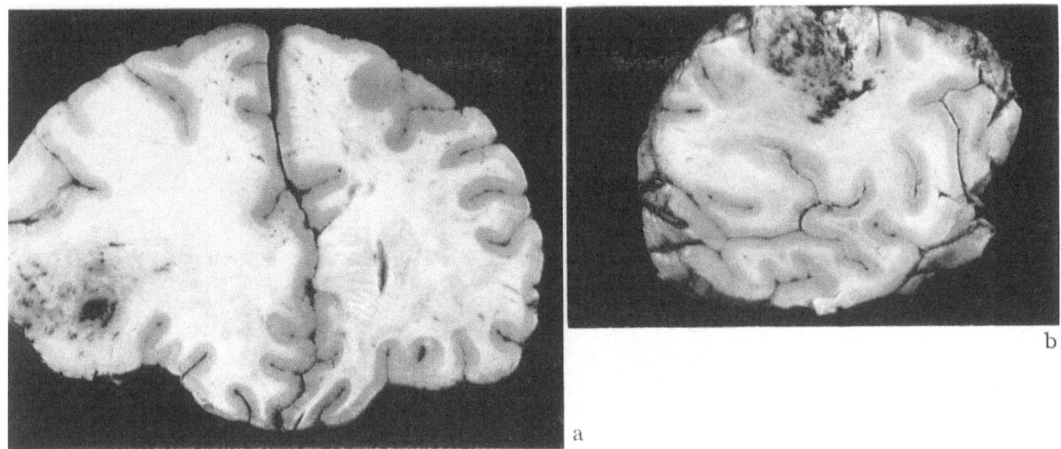

Fig. 134a and b. Two independently arising glioblastomas a) in the left frontolateral region and b) in the occipitodorsal part of the same hemisphere; no histological interconnection

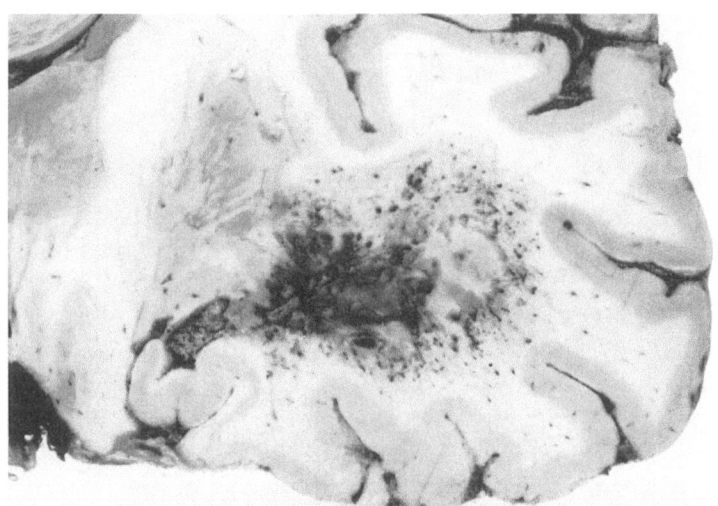

Fig. 135. Typical pattern of a glioblastoma which had a "malignant" vascular pattern on arteriography corresponding to the large area of central necrosis surrounded by a mantle of fistulous vessels

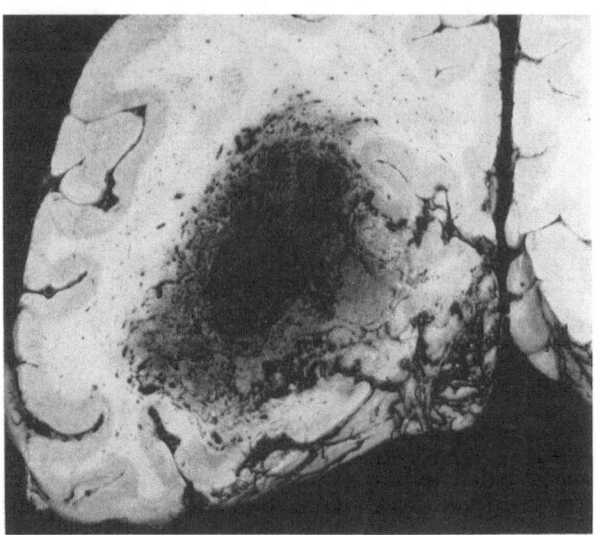

Fig. 136. Glioblastoma with mass hemorrhage into the center of the tumor. A typical mantle zone of fistulous and lacunar vessels is apparent

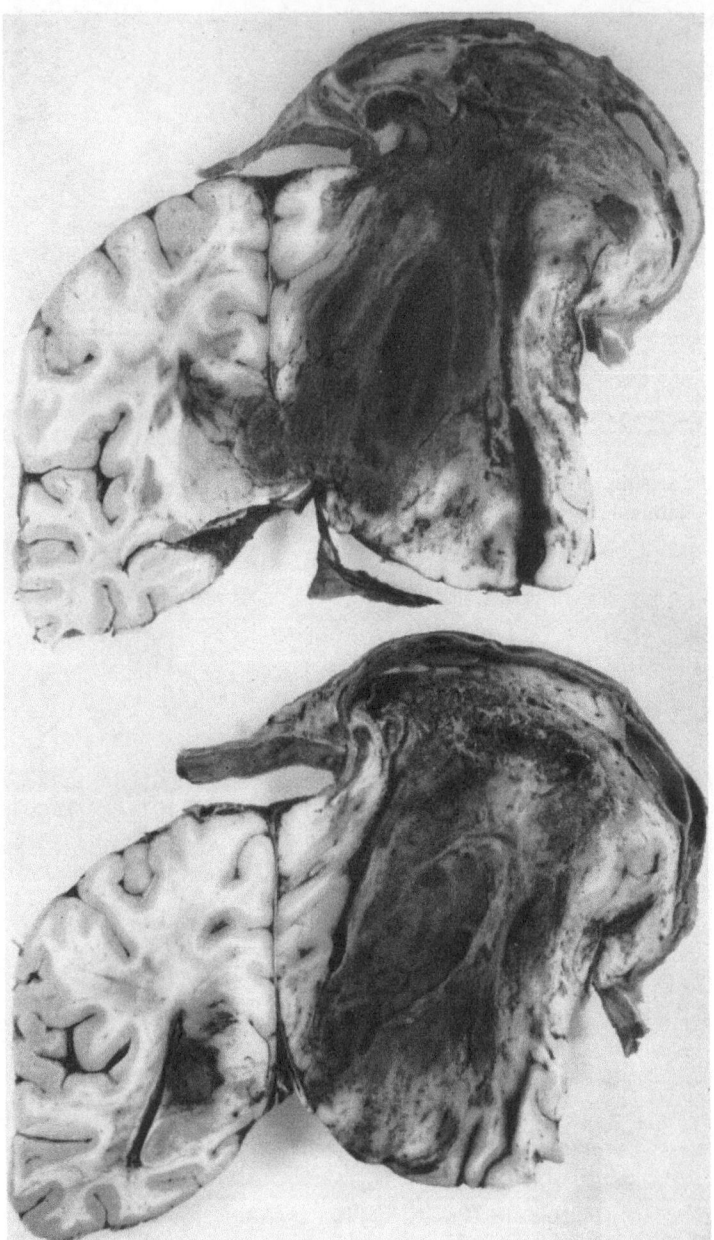

Fig. 137. Grotesque prolapse after craniotomy for a glioblastoma through the operative site. The tumor had invaded practically the entire hemisphere on one side and had extended to the opposite side via the corpus callosum

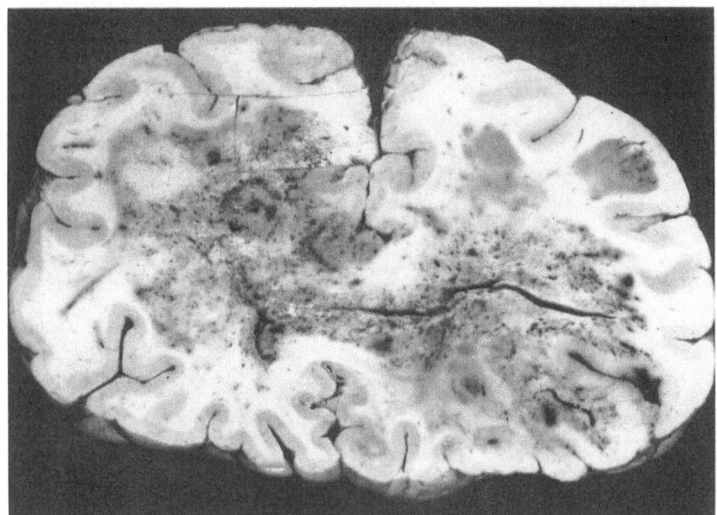

Fig. 138. Enormous expansion of a butterfly glioblastoma predominantly within the white matter simulating hemorrhagic encephalitis

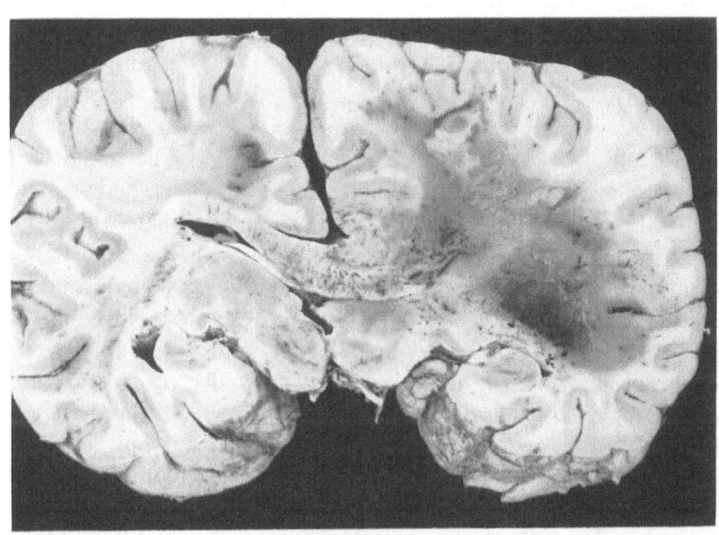

Fig. 139. Little hemorrhages and engorged vessels in a glioblastoma of the white substance

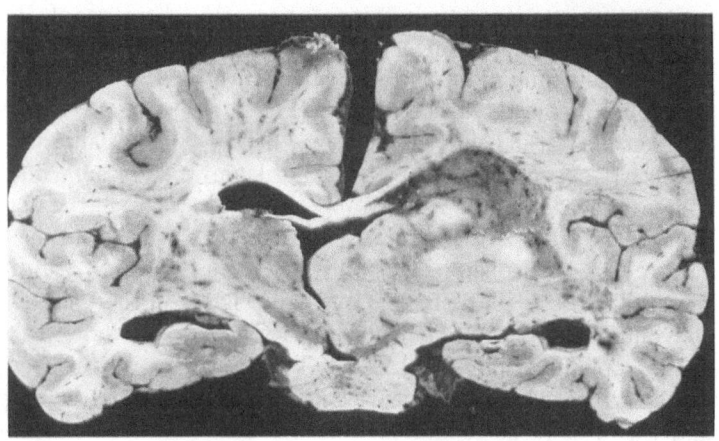

Fig. 140. Glioblastoma of the thalamus. Extensive necrosis of the adjacent corpus callosum

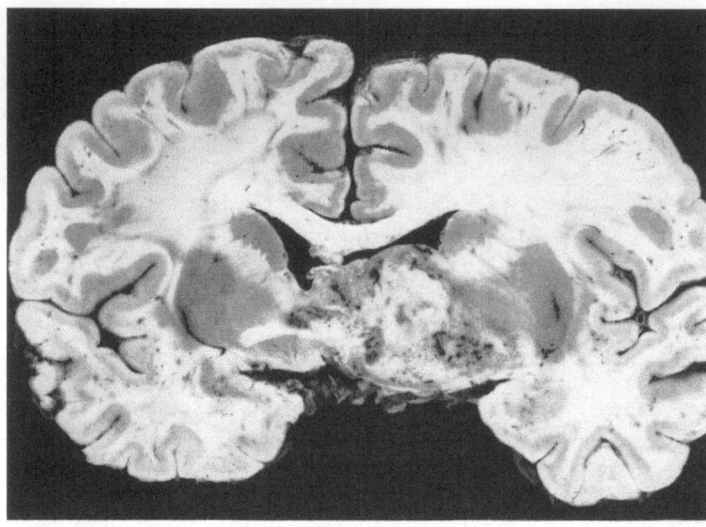

Fig. 141. Glioblastoma of the right basal ganglion

The Polar Spongioblastomas (Piloid/Pilocytic Astrocytomas, Astrocytoma of Juvenile Type, Cerebellar Astrocytomas, Optic Nerve Gliomas)

The spongioblastomas are well-circumscribed, infiltrating tumors of variable size. The line of cleavage (Fig. 142) from adjacent tissues (apart from the cases growing in the optic nerve, chiasm and pons) is usually very sharp. They are greyish-pink, sometimes translucent, and have a tough, elastic or occasionally mucoid consistency. Degenerative cysts of all sizes (Figs. 143–145, 150) are often present, as well as an occasional small hemorrhage within the tumor tissue or a brownish discoloration of the cyst wall (Fig. 143). Spongioblastomas mainly grow by expansion although they infiltrate at the margins (see, however, the spongioblastomas of the anterior optic system, "the optic nerve gliomas", and the pons) (Figs. 155–158).

The most important type of spongioblastoma lies in the cerebellar midline (Fig. 143) (the so-called "cerebellar astrocytoma"). They frequently expand into one or the other hemisphere and at operation often appear in the "cerebellar lobes"; they may even reach the surface of a hemisphere (Fig. 142) where their presence causes a flattening of the cerebellar convolutions (Fig. 145). Tumor size varies from that of a plum to that of a hen's egg (Figs. 142, 145). They tend to be well-demarcated tumors and can usually be separated from the cerebellar folia by peeling, as one peels an onion (Fig. 142), the correct plane of dissection being readily apparent. In addition, they may appear encapsulated (Fig. 146) as a result of the manner in which they grow into the leptomeninges. The majority are cystic (Figs. 143–147, 150). These cysts can exceed the size of the tumor many times (Fig. 144) and may extend far into the cerebellar hemispheres (Fig. 145); sometimes a small mural nodule is all that remains of the solid tumor (Fig. 143) and in this respect they resemble the hemangioblastomas. However, in contrast to the Lindau tumor, the mural nodule of the spongioblastoma is not blue in color and is only slightly vascularized. Usually the cyst contains an amber, protein-rich fluid which coagulates after aspiration. Although most spongioblastomas are only sparsely vascularized, some parts may be very vascular. They can be distinguished from the medulloblastoma grossly because of the latter's granular, soft consistency.

Of importance is the relationship of the tumor to the floor of the fourth ventricle. There is usually no adherence. However, in long-standing "midline" cases, the tumor may adhere to the floor, and in rare cases can actually arise from the floor and fill the fourth ventricle (Fig. 147). Adherence to the floor is never seen in the "lateral" cases, the average ratio of the "midline" to "lateral" cases being about 3:2.

In the spongioblastoma of the optic system ("optic nerve glioma") the bulk of the tumor lies over the chiasmal region (Fig. 148), in the

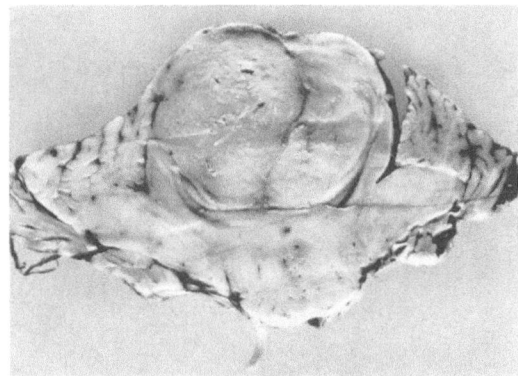

Fig. 142. Circumscribed spongioblastoma in the anterior-superior vermis with distortion of adjacent midbrain

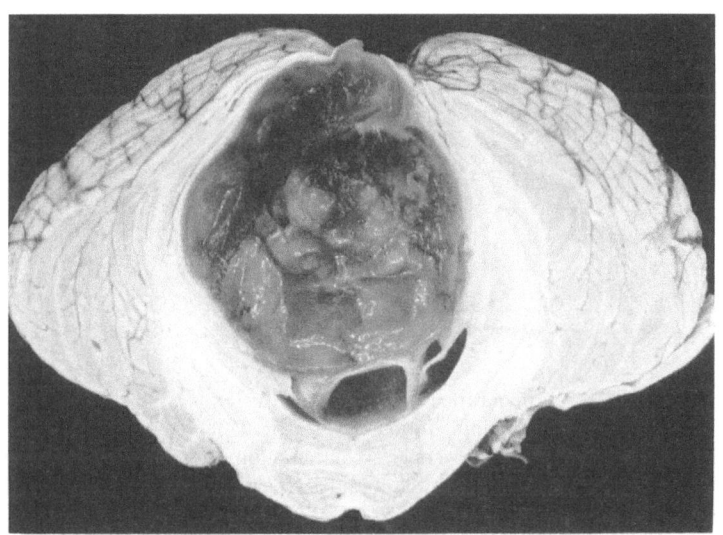

Fig. 143. Large spongioblastoma of the midline cerebellum with prominent cyst formation

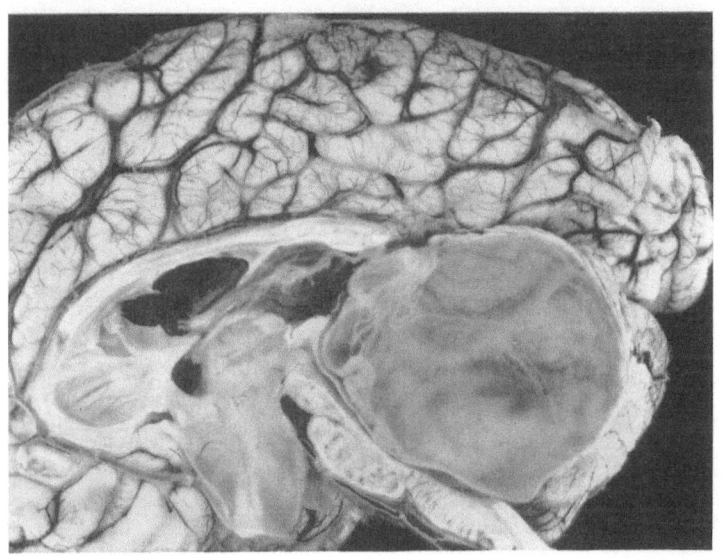

Fig. 144. Enormous cystic spongioblastoma of the midline cerebellum. Note the small mural nodule on the anterior-superior cyst wall and the secondary hydrocephalus of the third ventricle (patient $1^1/_2$ years old)

97

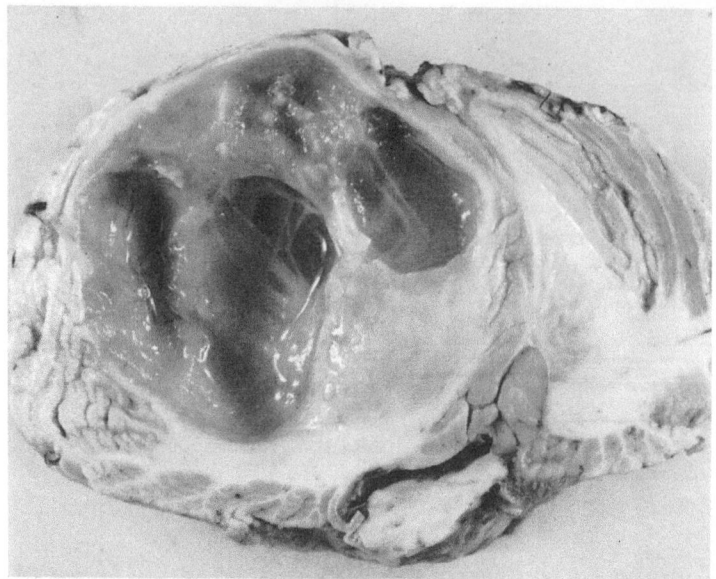

Fig. 145. Huge cystic spongioblastoma of the right cerebellar hemisphere. Mural nodule visible at right lower corner of cyst

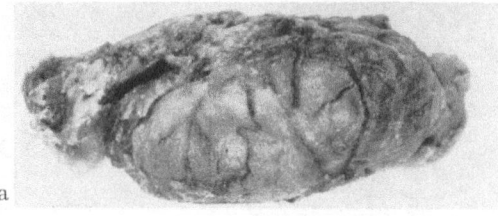

a

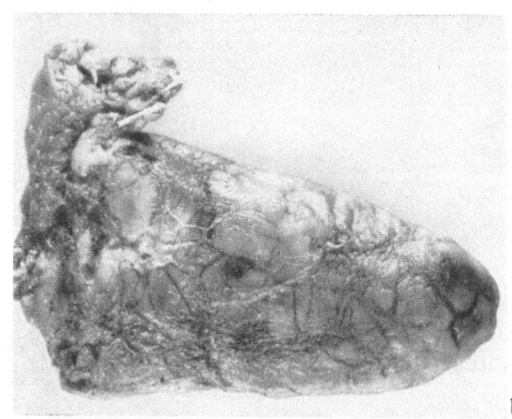

b

Fig. 146. Gross appearance of two surgically excised cerebellar spongioblastomas. Note the well-formed capsules which consist of enveloping leptomeninges in which arachnoidal vessels are seen

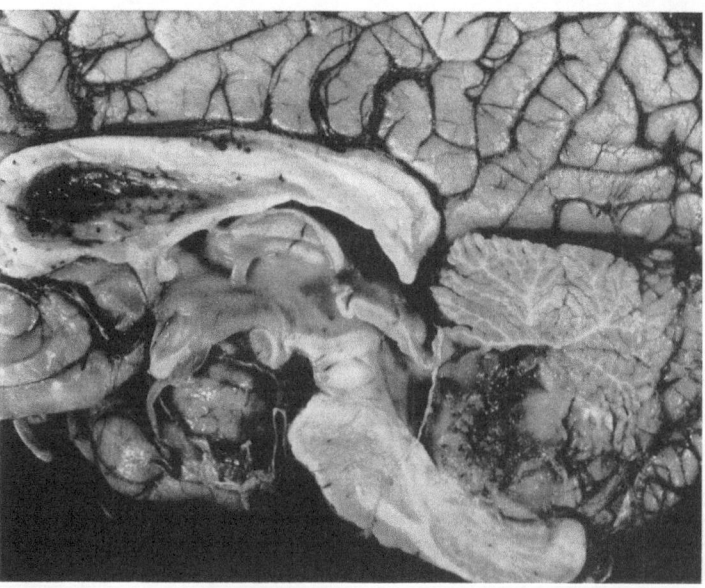

Fig. 147. Spongioblastoma in the lumen of the fourth ventricle

hypothalamus (Fig. 149), in the chiasm itself (Fig. 148), or in the optic nerves (Fig. 159). Tumor may fill the third ventricle (Fig. 149) and can extend through the foramina of Monroe into the lateral ventricles (Fig. 150). In the optic nerve, they can occur either in its orbital portion alone, on both sides of the optic foramen taking the shape of an hour-glass (here the nerve may appear abnormally enlarged) (Fig. 159), or predominantly in the chiasm (Fig. 149) which they can blow up to enormous dimensions (Fig. 148). Or, the chiasm may be relatively uninvolved and may appear as a flat band at the base of the tumor (Fig. 149). Spongioblastomas expand the arachnoid sheath of the optic nerve by infiltration (Fig. 159).

In rare cases, they may grow on the outer wall of the lateral ventricle (Fig. 151) in the same position as the more common "extra-ventricular" cerebral ependymoma (see p. 57 ff.) and may so resemble this latter tumor that distinction is frequently possible only on histologic grounds. Large cysts commonly accompany spongioblastomas in this location and may reach the size of a fist. The tumors are well-demarcated and are easy to remove after aspiration of the contents of the cyst. Spongioblasto-

mas may be found in the aqueduct, reaching the size of a pea (Fig. 152), and are the most common tumor in this location. They can also infiltrate the quadrigeminal plate (Figs. 153, 154) and here may attain the size of a walnut.

Spongioblastomas of the pons are not uncommon. Two types prevail; one grows more diffusely through the whole organ (Fig. 155), the other shows a more nodular growth (Figs. 156, 158). More caudally they cover the medulla oblongata (Fig. 158).

Finally, they may be found growing as large or larger than a pencil in the central portion of the spinal cord (Fig. 159), rarely also as small intraventricular growths (Fig. 160). The spongioblastomas are a tumor group of infancy and adolescence having a definite peak around the ages of 10 to 25 years (see p. 46). It is difficult to determine the actual incidence of polar spongioblastomas, because of the differences in nomenclature (see p. 96). In CUSHING's series (1932, 1935) they represented around 6.1%, in our material of 9000 cases 6%. There were 270 males and 268 females for a ratio of 1:1. This figure is somewhat in contrast to our earlier figures, which showed a prevalence of the female sex in a ratio 11:9.

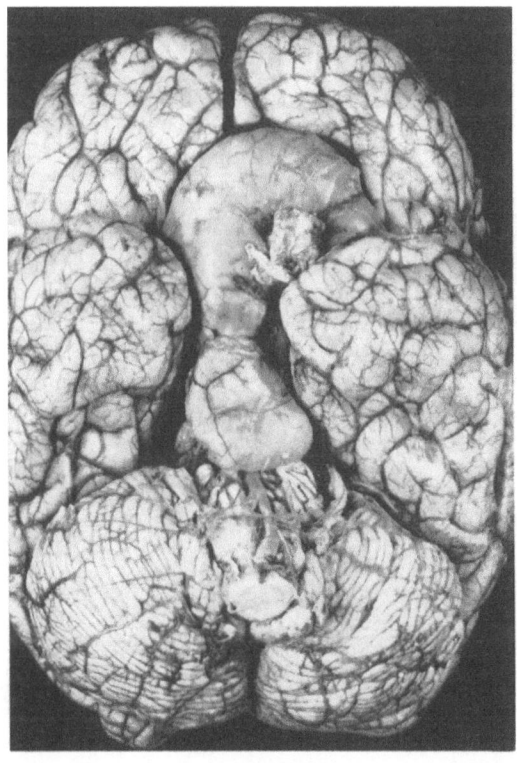

Fig. 148. Huge amorphous spongioblastoma of the base of the brain enveloping chiasm, optic nerves, and mammillary bodies

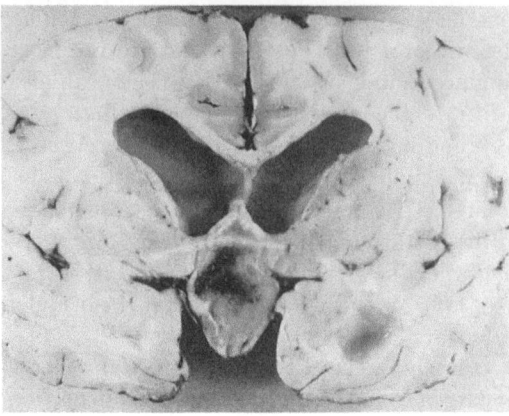

Fig. 149. Frontal section through a spongioblastoma of the chiasm and hypothalamus. Note elevation of the anterior commissure and secondary occlusive hydrocephalus. Mucous degeneration within the tumor has occurred

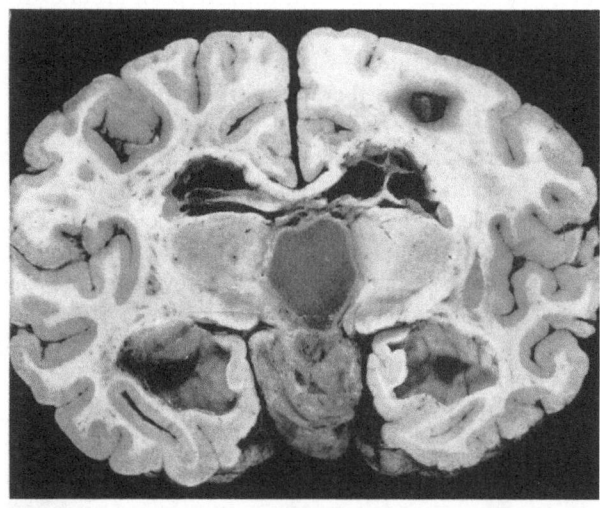

Fig. 150. Spongioblastoma of chiasmal region which has broken into the 3rd ventricle and filled it with a glassy fluid. Mucoid tumor masses have also extended through the foramina of Monro and can be seen coating the walls of the adjacent lateral ventricles

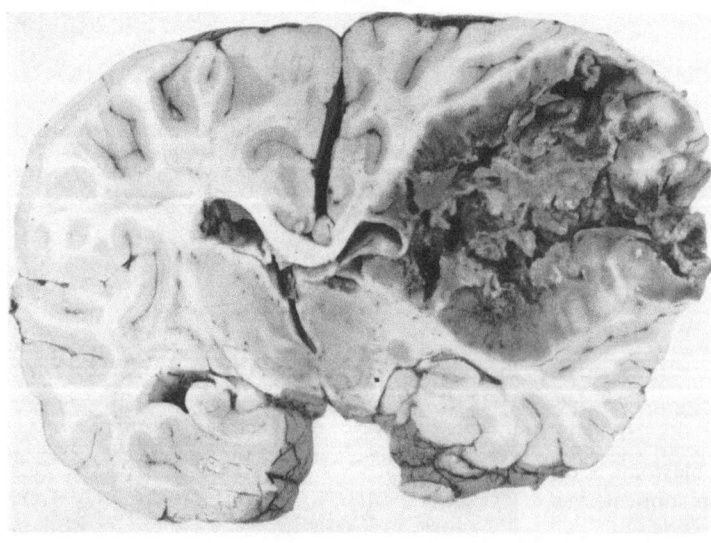

Fig. 151. Large cystic extraventricular spongioblastoma of the parietal lobe, macroscopically mimicing an extraventricular ependymoma

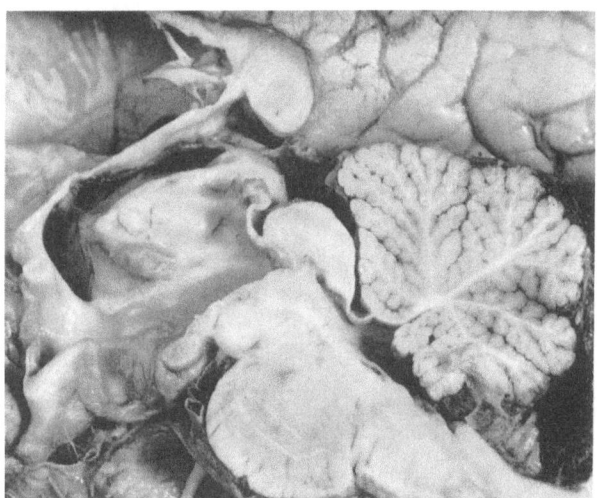

Fig. 152. Small spongioblastoma arising
in the region of the aqueduct and diffusely
infiltrating the midbrain

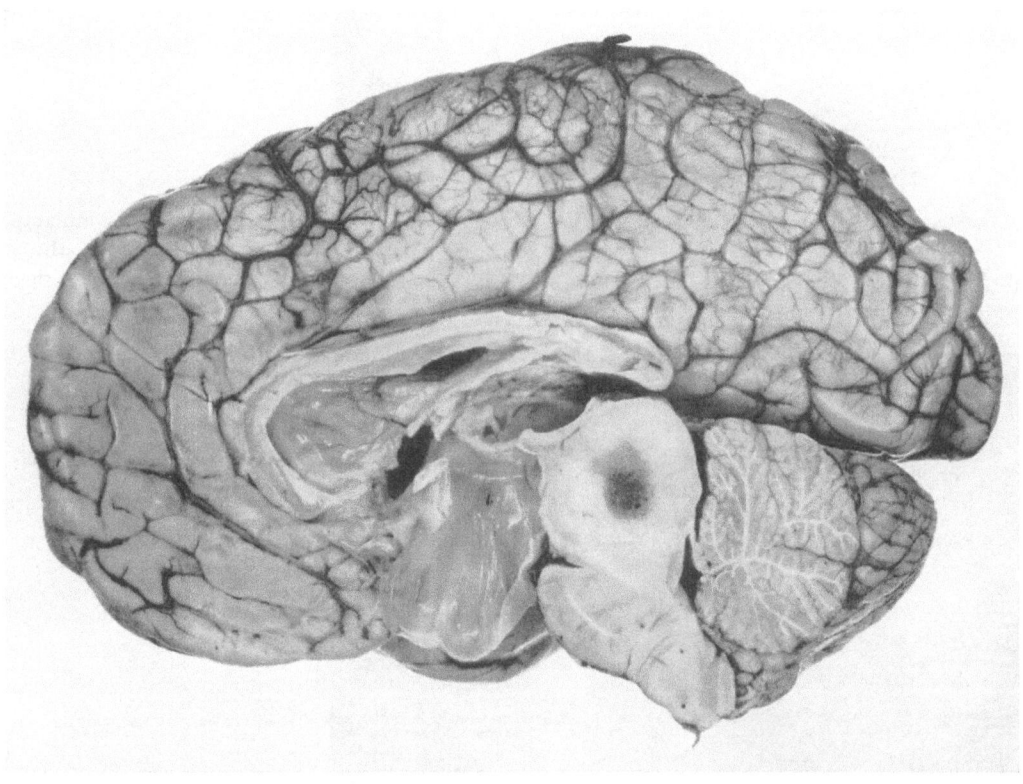

Fig. 153. Walnut-sized spongioblastoma of the midbrain with small central hemorrhage. Note thinning
of the wall of the 3rd ventricle secondary to obstructive hydrocephalus

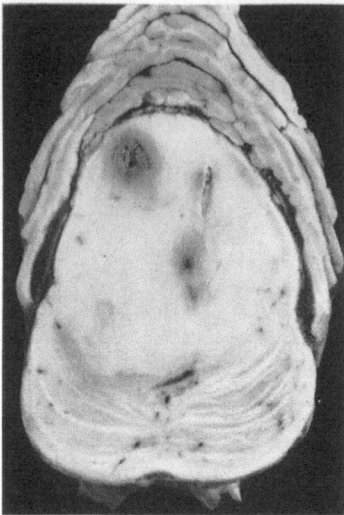

Fig. 154. Large spongioblastoma of the midbrain with lateral displacement of the aqueduct to the left

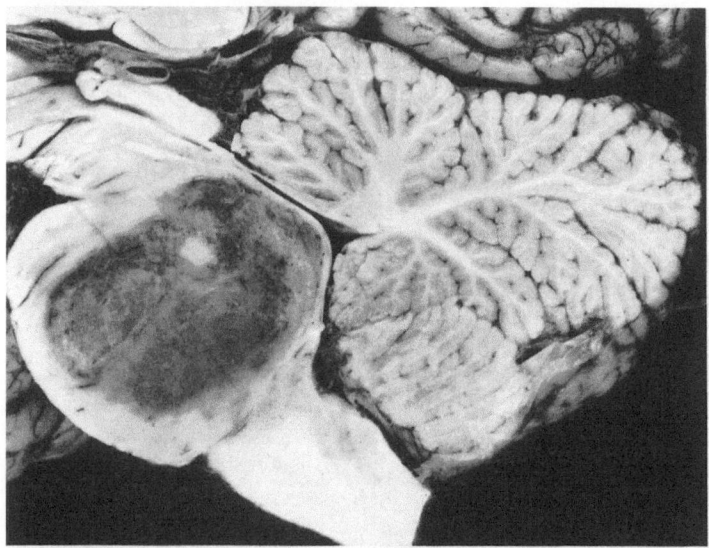

Fig. 155. Large nodular polar spongioblastoma of the pons with foci of malignant degeneration

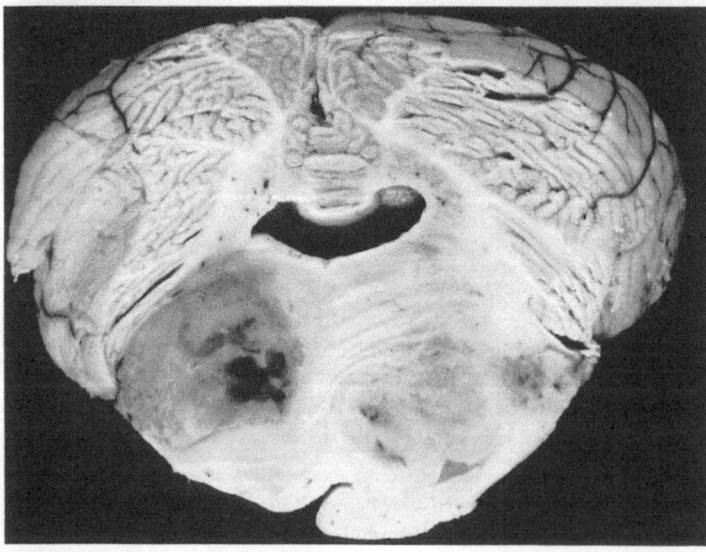

Fig. 156. Large spongioblastoma with malignant degeneration and hemorrhage into cystic areas

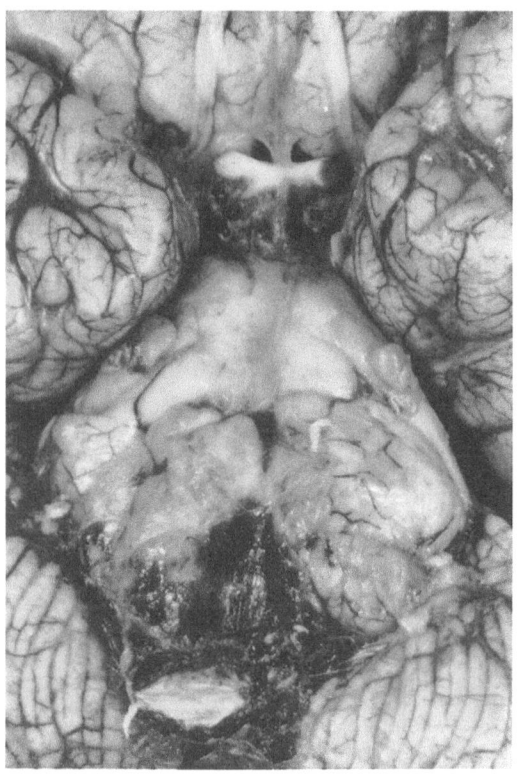

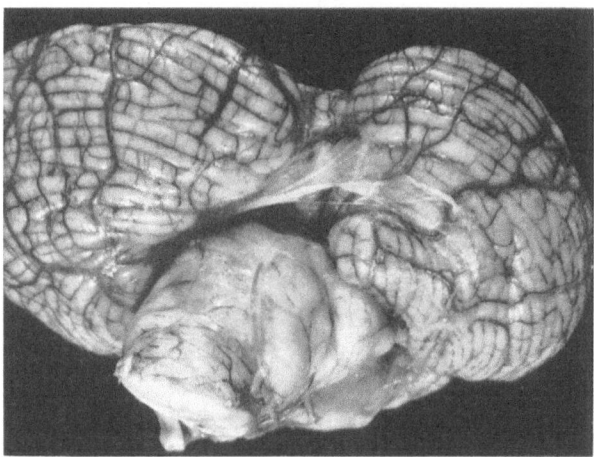

Fig. 158. Nodular spongioblastoma of the pons and medulla oblongata with extension caudad to the upper cervical cord

Fig. 157. Spongioblastoma diffusely infiltrating the pons

Fig. 159. *Left upper:* Spongioblastoma of the optic nerve which has infiltrated the optic sheath with resultant swelling and distortion of the nerve. *Right upper:* Spongioblastoma of the aqueduct presenting through an enlarged orifice. *Left lower:* Spongioblastoma of the dorsal columns of the spinal cord. This portion of tumor was not connected to the main tumor mass in the pons and medulla (c.f. Fig. 158). *Right lower:* Spongioblastoma of the spinal cord, the so-called "pencil" glioma

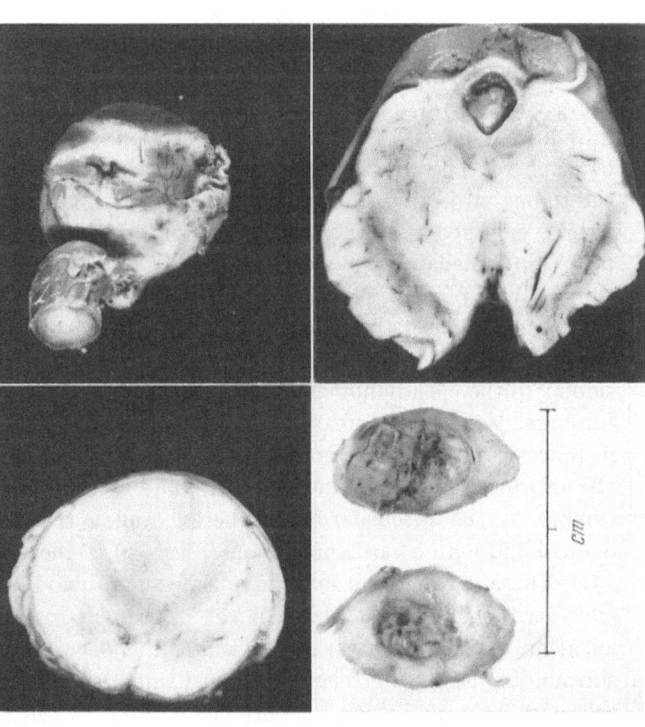

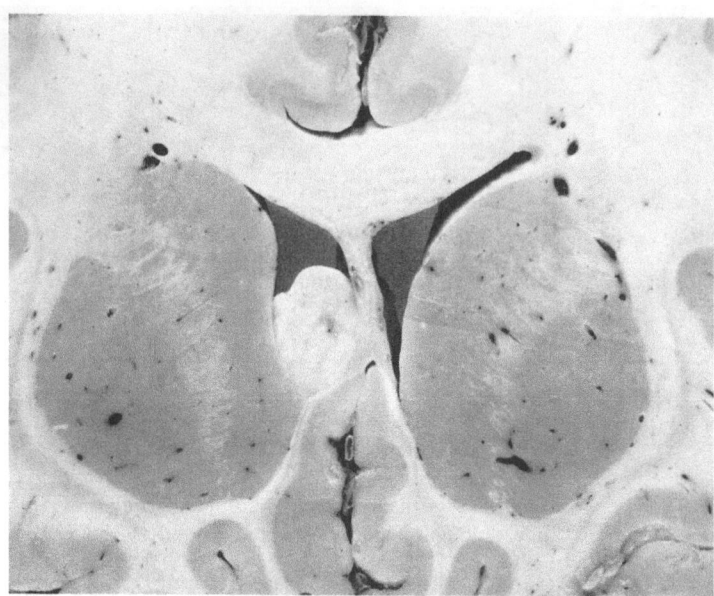

Fig. 160. Acorn-sized spongio-blastoma in the region of the foramen of Monro (incidental finding)

The Medulloblastomas

This group, described as an entity in 1924 by BAILEY and CUSHING, is well defined in its occurrence as the malignant cerebellar tumor of childhood and adolescence.

Medulloblastomas of the cerebellum lie mainly in the inferior cerebellar vermis, into which they spread from the roof of the posterior part of the fourth ventricle (Figs. 161, 162); they may reach the size of a tangerine. From here they can expand in all directions, but only infrequently lie with their main portion in one hemisphere. The fourth ventricle, filled with the tumor projecting from above (Fig. 162), is usually enlarged and the vermis is compressed to a thin lamella on the upper surface of the tumor. With further growth, tongues of tumor may push between the cerebellar tonsils into the cisterna magna (Fig. 163) in a fashion similar to the ependymomas of the foramen of Luschka. Medulloblastomas may, in very rare instances, originate in the pons (Fig. 164). There are also more superficial medulloblastoma-like tumors of the cerebellar hemispheres, well-defined and with a hard consistency (Figs. 240, 241). These, however, usually have a peculiar and very characteristic histological appearance: an extensive network of reticulin fibers surrounding islands of "clear" enlarged tumor cells within the meshwork, but with no reticulin fibers between individual clear cells. These were interpreted as "cerebellar arachnoidal sarcomas" (see p. 140) by FOERSTER and GAGEL (1939) and as a "desmoplastic" variant of the medulloblastoma by RUSSELL and RUBINSTEIN (1971). Their real nature is not yet well defined. Grossly, even medulloblastomas in the vermis often appear well-circumscribed (Figs. 165, 166), however, at their margin they grow diffusely into the surrounding tissue and arachnoidal space. The cerebellar folia with their leptomeninges are thus engulfed in tumor mass. The tumors are not very vascular; their consistency is usually soft, and firmer only when a lot of connective tissue has been included and multiplied by a stromal reaction to the presence of neoplastic cells in its midst. The medulloblastoma may freely spread within the spinal fluid compartments even metastasizing upstream to the aqueduct, infundibulum (Fig. 168), and floor of the lateral ventricles (Fig. 169) or downstream to the dorsal surface of the cerebellum (Fig. 170), to the cerebral hemispheres, to the dorsal surface of the spinal cord, and to the cauda equina. In these areas they assume the form of buttons, plaques, nodules (Figs. 169, 171), or spread diffusely like frosting (Fig. 170).

The peak of incidence falls between the ages of 7–12 years (see p. 46). However, occasional cases occur into in the fourth decade as well.

In our series of 9000 tumors they comprised 4.2%, in CUSHING's series (1932, 1935) 4.5% and in RINGERTZ' (1950) 6.5% of the total cases. However, in a series consisting only of *gliomas* (1792 cases of various authors) 10% were medulloblastomas. They make up 20% of all brain tumors of childhood and adolescence [also in McCRAIG *et al.* (1949) 20.1%], but only 0.8% of those occurring after 20 years of age. The average age was in INGRAHAM's series (1948) 7.5 years, in RINGERTZ' (1950) 13.8 years, and in our series 14.2 years.

Of our 373 cases of medulloblastoma, 251 were males and 122 females giving a sex ratio of 2:1. Males also predominated in CUSHING's series, three to one.

Metastases to other organs—cervical lymph nodes, lumbosacral vertebrae, or into the pelvic bones (probably along peripheral nerve roots)—are quite rare, but do occur. Some other tumors of early infancy and childhood—i.e., of the retina (retinoblastoma with or without true rosettes), the pineal region (pinealoblastoma) or the sympathetic trunk and adrenals (sympathoblastomas)—are histologically very similar to the cerebellar medulloblastomas. They are biologically also very malignant and their tendency to metastasize is even more pronounced. The tumors of the eyes and adrenals directly invade tissue of a different embryonic origin (mesoderm) or metastasize to it—retinoblastoma, particularly to the bones and lymph nodes, and sympathoblastoma to the bones, lymph nodes and liver. The pineoblastoma does not metastasize except via the CSF.

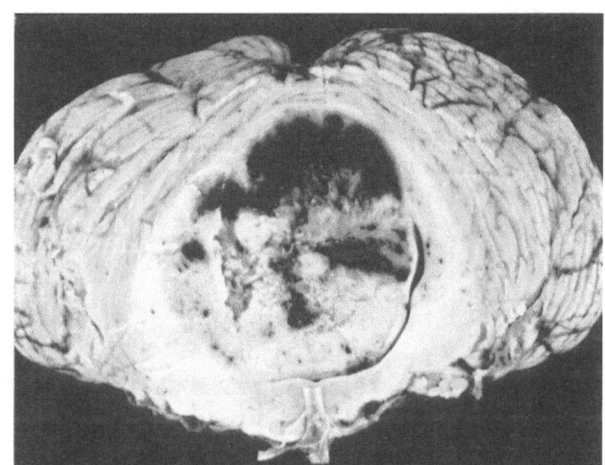

Fig. 161. Medulloblastoma arising from the roof of the fourth ventricle on the right. Hemorrhage into the tumor mass followed attempts at surgical excision. Note sharp demarcation of tumor from surrounding cerebellar tissue

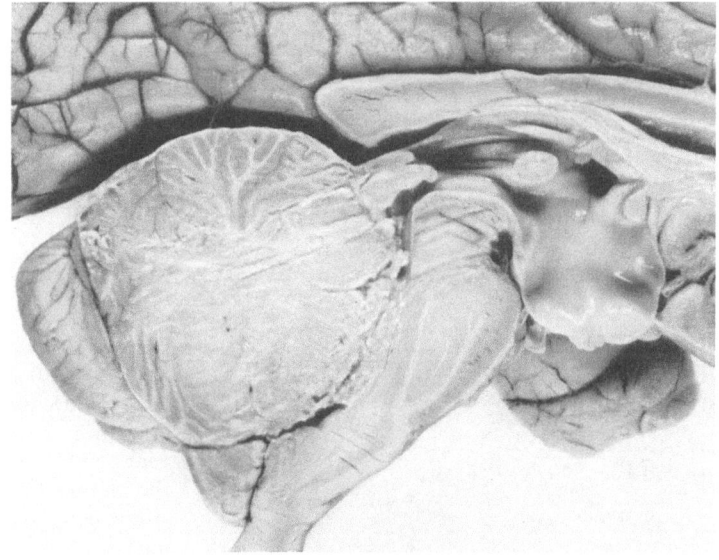

Fig. 162. Typical medulloblastoma situated in the lower vermis with extension into the 4th ventricle and infiltration of its floor. Secondary occlusive hydrocephalus with dilatation of the 3rd ventricle, the floor of which is paper-thin

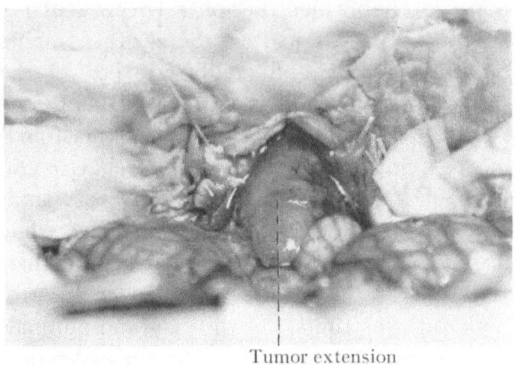

Tumor extension

Fig. 163. Operative photograph of a medullo-blastoma from above. Note extension of tumor process separating tonsils and reaching to the C_2 level

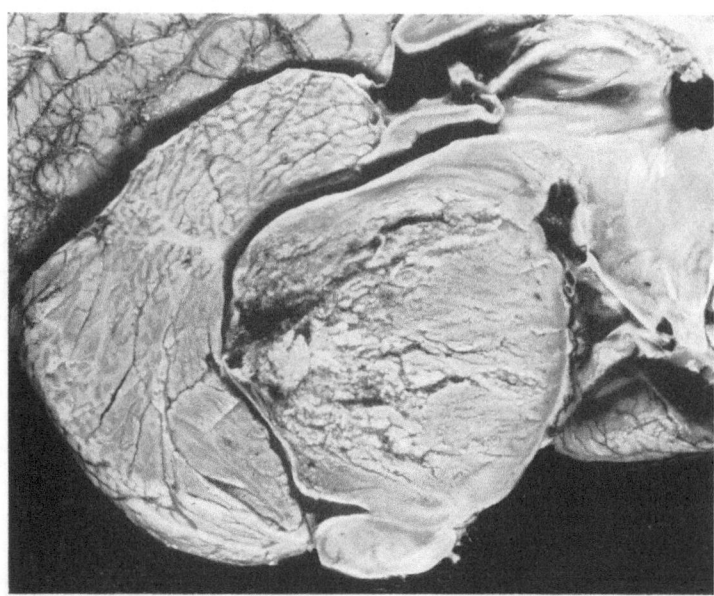

Fig. 164. Giant medulloblas-toma of the pons. The fourth ventricle is seen as a narrow cavity outlining the tumor

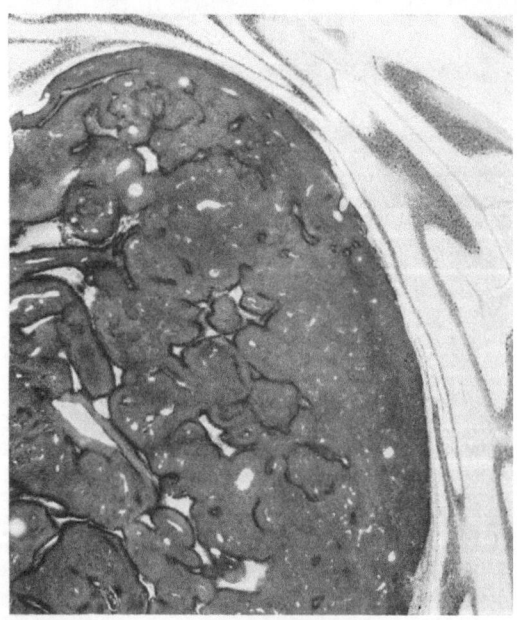

Fig. 165. Densely cellular medulloblastoma which appears to be sharply demarcated from the adja-cent cerebellum, yet is extensively infiltrating in the marginal zone. Note necrotic areas of varying size which are outlined by dark rings of pyknotic nuclei

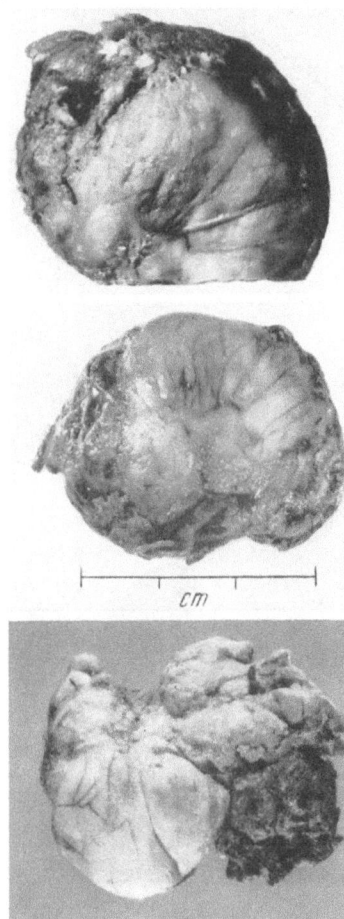

Fig. 166. Operative specimen following macroscopic "total" excision of a medulloblastoma. Note the apparent capsule in this specimen

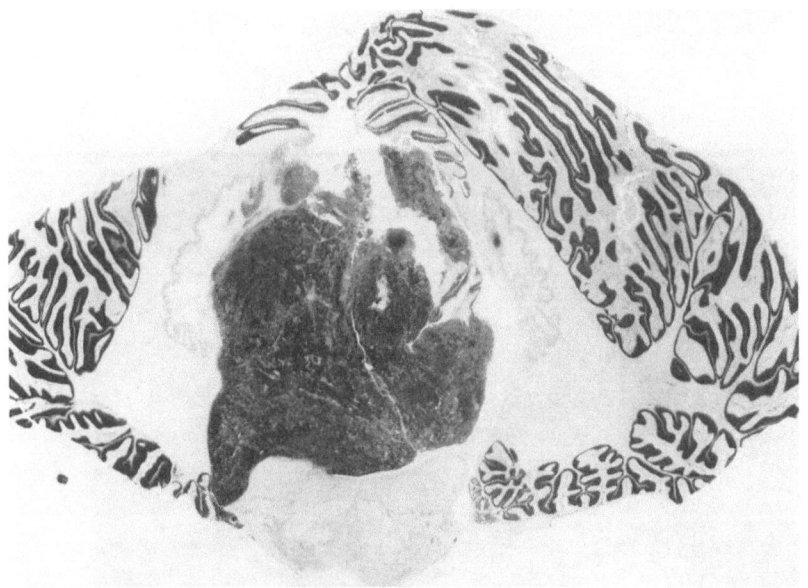

Fig. 167. Section through a medulloblastoma which occupies the area of the 4th ventricle and has even extended through the lateral recess externally. Note the absence of macroscopical necrosis which was confirmed microscopically

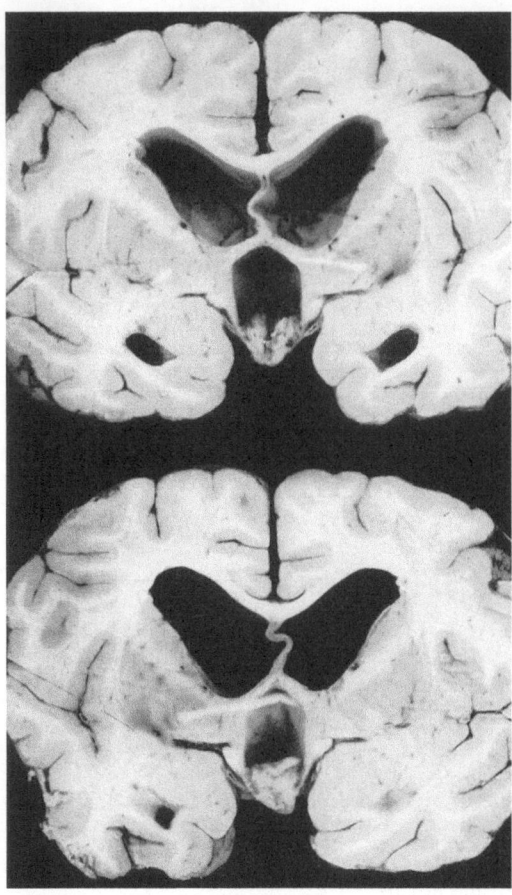

Fig. 168. Metastasis of a medulloblastoma to the floor of a dilated third ventricle (infundibular recess)

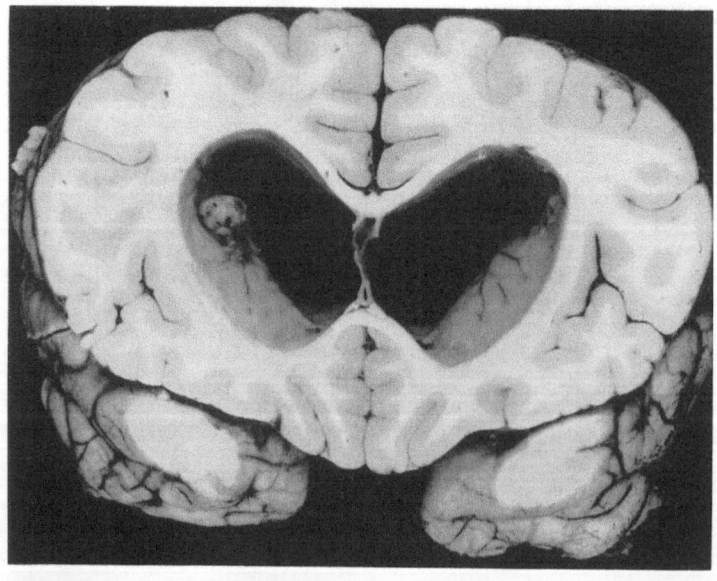

Fig. 169. Nodular metastasis of a medulloblastoma into a dilated right lateral ventricle

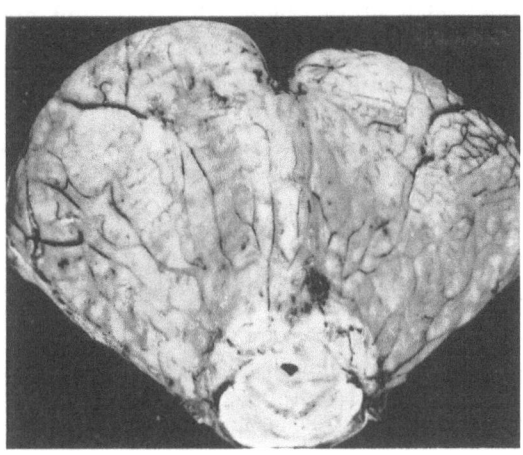

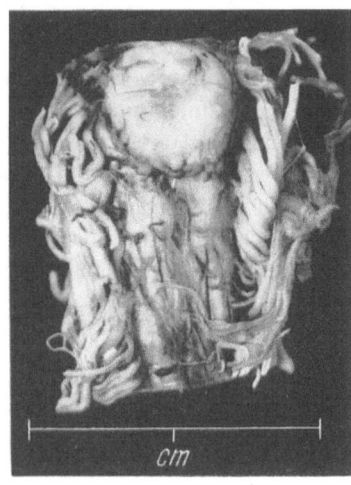

Fig. 170. Diffuse metastases of a medulloblastoma in the leptomeninges of the dorsal surface of the cerebellum

Fig. 171. Nodular metastasis of a medulloblastoma to the dorsal surface of the cervical cord. This particular tumor was most unusual in that it was calcified

1.2.5 Peripheral Nerves and Nerve Sheaths

The Neurinomas (Schwannomas, Neurilemmomas, Neurofibromas)

The neurinomas are smooth, well-encapsulated tumors often with a fine nodular appearance (Fig. 172). In the arachnoid capsule course the feeding branches of the vascular supply. The color of the tumor varies from a reddish-gray-yellow to a deep yellow to a translucent gray. Consistency will also vary and depends on the extent of the regressive changes—particularly fatty degeneration—that have taken place. It may be harder and fibrous or rubbery in the marginal zone close to the capsule, but friable and softer in its center, so that intracapsular curettage may be easily accomplished. Cystic degeneration is common in the large spinal tumors, but rare in the cerebellopontine types. They usually start growth within the internal auditory meatus and later enlarge it (Fig. 177). The neurinomas occur most frequently in the vestibular part of the acoustic nerve. They may form tumors of hazel and chestnut size (Figs. 172–174) in the cerebello-pontine angle, but with modern otological and neuroradiological

diagnostic techniques are often found when they are much smaller (Fig. 173). Neurinomas never infiltrate adjacent tissues, but may deform the brainstem (Fig. 175), indenting the pons and medulla and displacing them in such a manner as to form a large groove (Fig. 172). They may also displace the cerebellar hemisphere superiorly and inferiorly and may thus create cerebellar pressure cones (Fig. 174) of the incisura of the tentorium ("upwards") and in the foramen magnum ("downwards"). The seventh and later the fifth cranial nerves may be thinned out and may be found running over the tumor capsule. Primary neurinomas of the trigeminal nerve are rare.

As a result of these pressure changes and the accompanying circulatory disturbances, small areas of softening may occur in the pons. A small or large arachnoidal cyst may cover the tumor (Fig. 174). Bilateral acoustic neurinomas occasionally occur (Fig. 172) and are looked upon as a "forme fruste" of von Recklinghausen's neurofibromatosis.

Neurinomas in the spinal canal are one of the most common tumors in that location. They may be distributed over one or more segments, are attached to the posterior roots or cauda equina (Fig. 176), and may be finger-shaped if large or may resemble a lima bean. Dumbbell forms are not uncommon and arise when the tumor grows through an intervertebral foramen. These tumors may be accompanied by a large segmental artery, which may be inadvertently divided and lead to subsequent neurological deficit. Spinal neurinomas more often show mucoid degeneration and cyst formation, occasionally with various sized hemorrhages into these cysts. In the course of von Recklinghausen's disease neurinomas may be present on every cranial, spinal, or peripheral nerve. Solitary neurinomas of the peripheral nerves can provoke the formation of an abundant collagenous fibrous stroma in which case the name "neurofibroma" is preferred. Solitary neurinomas occur particularly in the middle and later decades of life with a peak around 35–40 years (see p. 146) and are only rarely seen in childhood. They may also occur in the latter decades of life as incidental findings in the region of the cauda (Fig. 176) and are asymptomatic. The neurinomas comprised 8.7% in CUSHING's series and 6.8% of all our intracranial tumors (9000 cases). Of our patients 213 were males and 401 were females, neurinomas in females predominating by a margin of roughly 2:1.

The neurinomas are one of the most frequent benign groups of intracranial and intraspinal tumors. Malignant cases do occur; however, these are very rare. Malignant degeneration is also seen in unilocular neurinomas of the peripheral nerves. In fact, in von Recklinghausen's disease "sarcomatous" transformation of a neurofibroma is not at all uncommon in the course of the disease. In such cases, the capsules are lost and invasive growth occurs. Metastases of neurinomas are unknown.

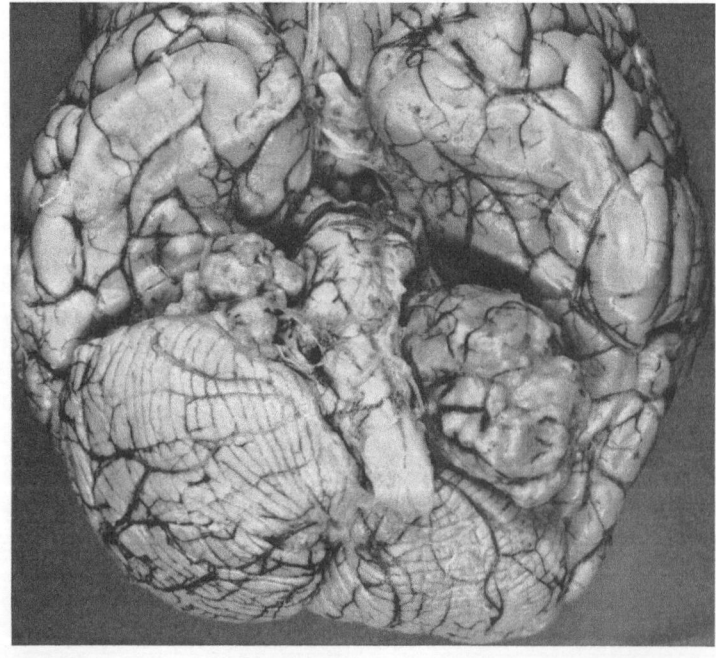

Fig. 172. Bilateral acoustic neurinomata with massive displacement of the pons in a non-surgical specimen

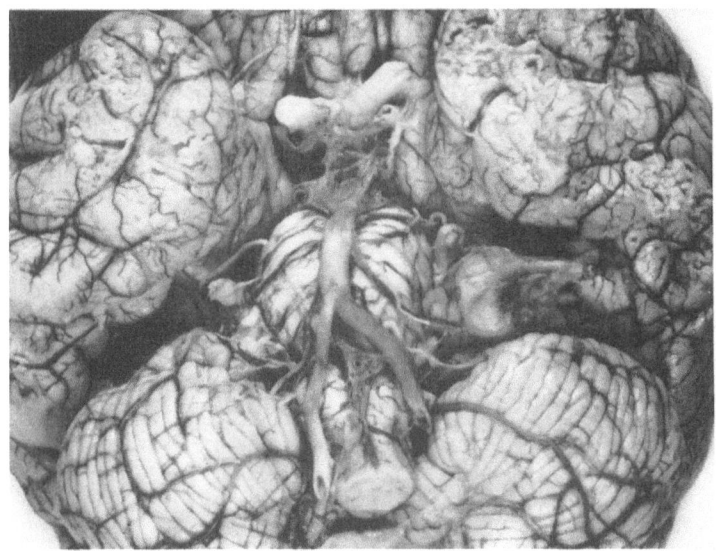

Fig. 173. Cherry-sized cere-bellopontine angle neurinoma

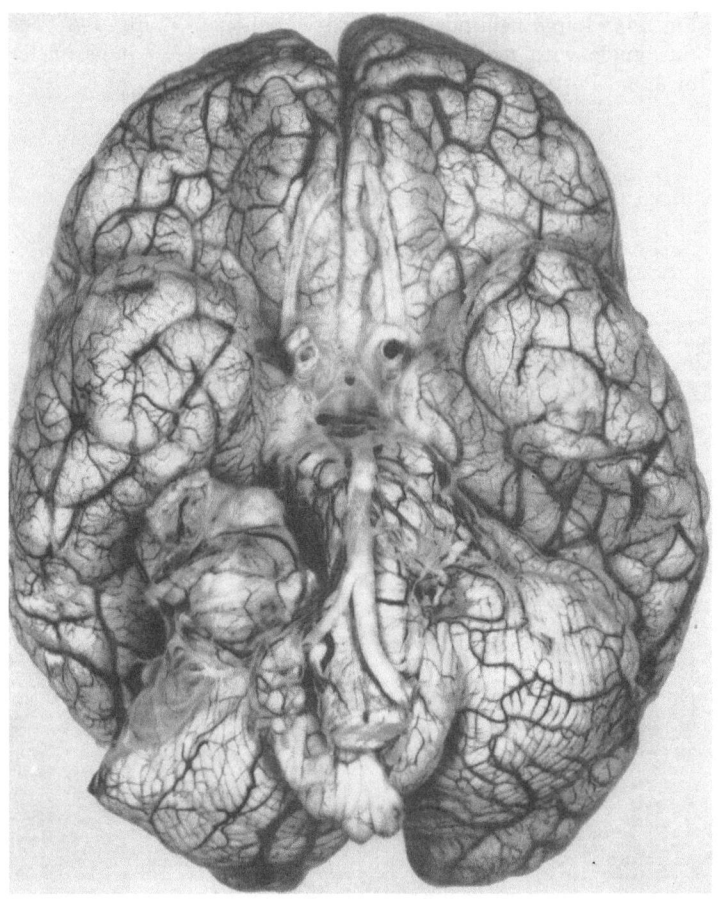

Fig. 174. Large acoustic neuri-noma with a small arachnoid cyst located in its posterior portion in a non-surgical speci-men. A marked cerebellar pressure cone had occurred with mass shifting from right to left. Arteriosclerosis of the vertebro-basilar system is seen

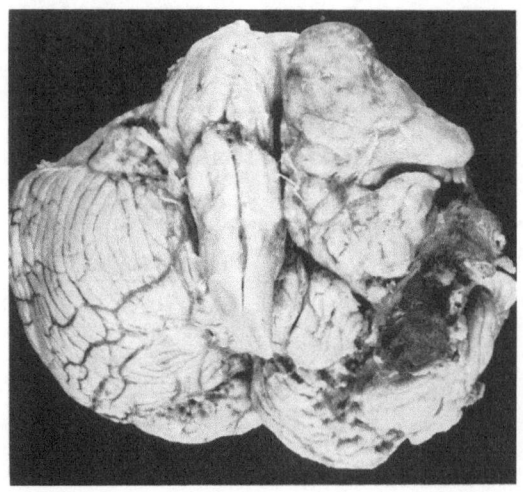

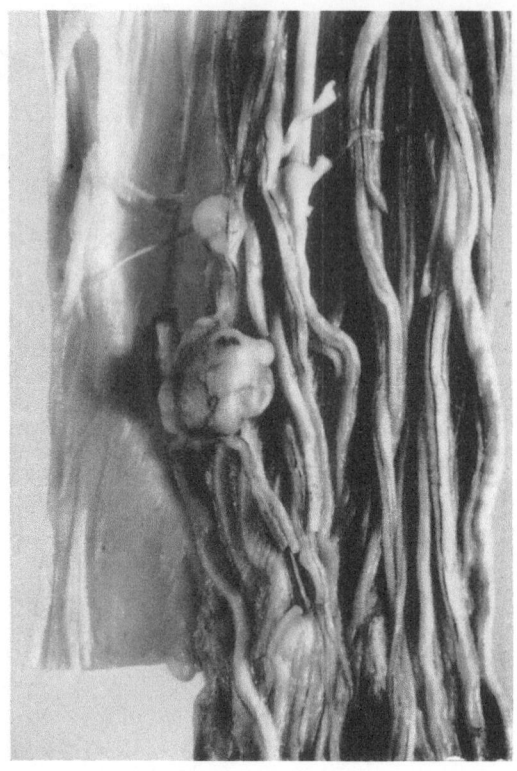

Fig. 175. Large neurinoma of the cerebellopontine angle with marked shift of the pons and medulla. Post-operative state

Fig. 176. Two small neurinomas of the cauda equina (incidental finding)

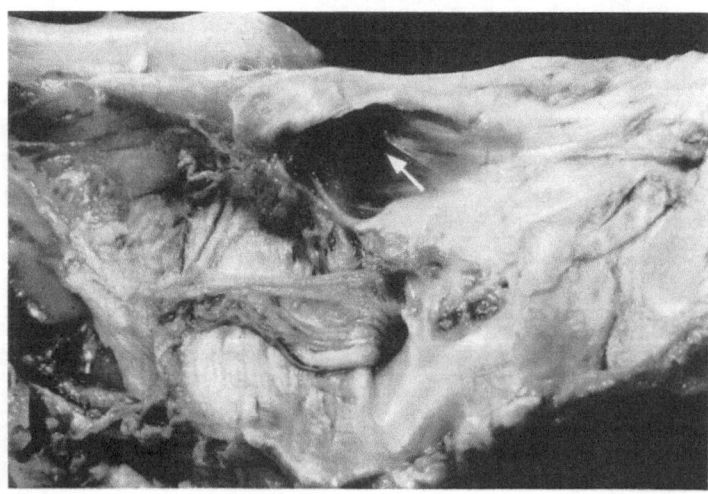

Fig. 177. Enlargement of the left internal acoustic meatus (arrow!). The tip of the petrous bone is seen in the upper right corner. Portions of the IXth, Xth and XIth nerves are clearly visible below the foramen

1.2.6 Meninges, Vascular Structures of the Central Nervous System and Connective Tissue

The Meningiomas (meningotheliomatous, fibrous, transitional, psammomatous, angiomatous, hemangiopericytic, anaplastic), Exothelioma, Meningeal Fibroblastoma

The meningiomas are encapsulated benign tumors, which do not invade the brain and do not recur when they are completely removed.

The fresh operative specimen is dark red with lighter translucent parts; the cut section is coarsely fibrous (Fig. 178), and cysts are only rarely found. The angioblastic type may be recognized by the coarse vascular meshwork on the cut surface. Meningiomas range in size from a pinhead to a man's fist (Fig. 189), depending on the location and the type of growth (Fig. 180). Their form may be spherical, hemispherical or conical, or they may grow out "en plaque" or in carpet-like manner (Figs. 179, 211, 213). Rarely are both types of growth combined, a conical tumor growing out of a flat one. The hyperostosis (Fig. 178) which they not infrequently induce leaves a corresponding impression, an umbilication (Fig. 178c), in the tumor. When meningiomas sit astride a bony ridge such as the sphenoid wing or petrous ridge, or even the falx, a corresponding saddle-shaped impression results. If the growth takes place in two directions, as it does in tumors of the tentorium, a dumbbell form develops (Fig. 196). The weight of the meningiomas in our series ranged from a few grams to 835 g

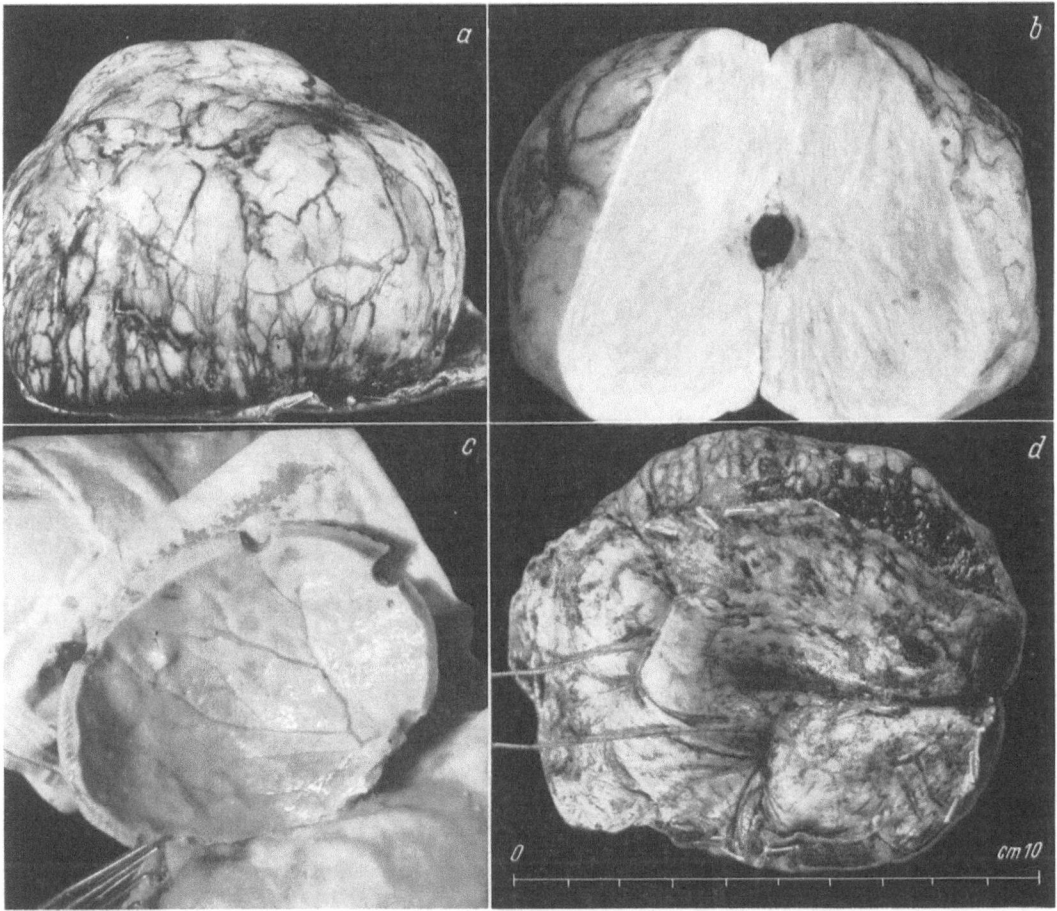

Fig. 178. a) Typical spherical meningioma with a richly vascular capsule. b) The cut surface shows a finely fibrillated appearance. c) Typical hyperostosis ("spicula") usually adherent to the tumor nidus (see d). Note the peripheral widening of the grooves of the middle meningeal artery. d) The nidus of the meningioma in the center is seen as a shallow central groove

(Fig. 218), and in one case even reached 1 300 g including the infiltrated bone; the average weight was 50–300 g. Meningiomas are smoothly encapsulated (Fig. 178), or coarsely (Figs. 211, 219), or finely nodular. The consistency varies depending on size, the amount of degeneration (hyalinization, cyst formation), the formation of fibers and calcification, and is described as rubbery or hard. At the site of dural attachment, where the connective tissue of the meninges radiates into the tumor, meningiomas are often harder than in other regions. The brain substance adjacent to the meningioma can either be pushed aside and compressed or it can be both softened (Fig. 212) and edematous, particularly by infarction after involvement of the carotid

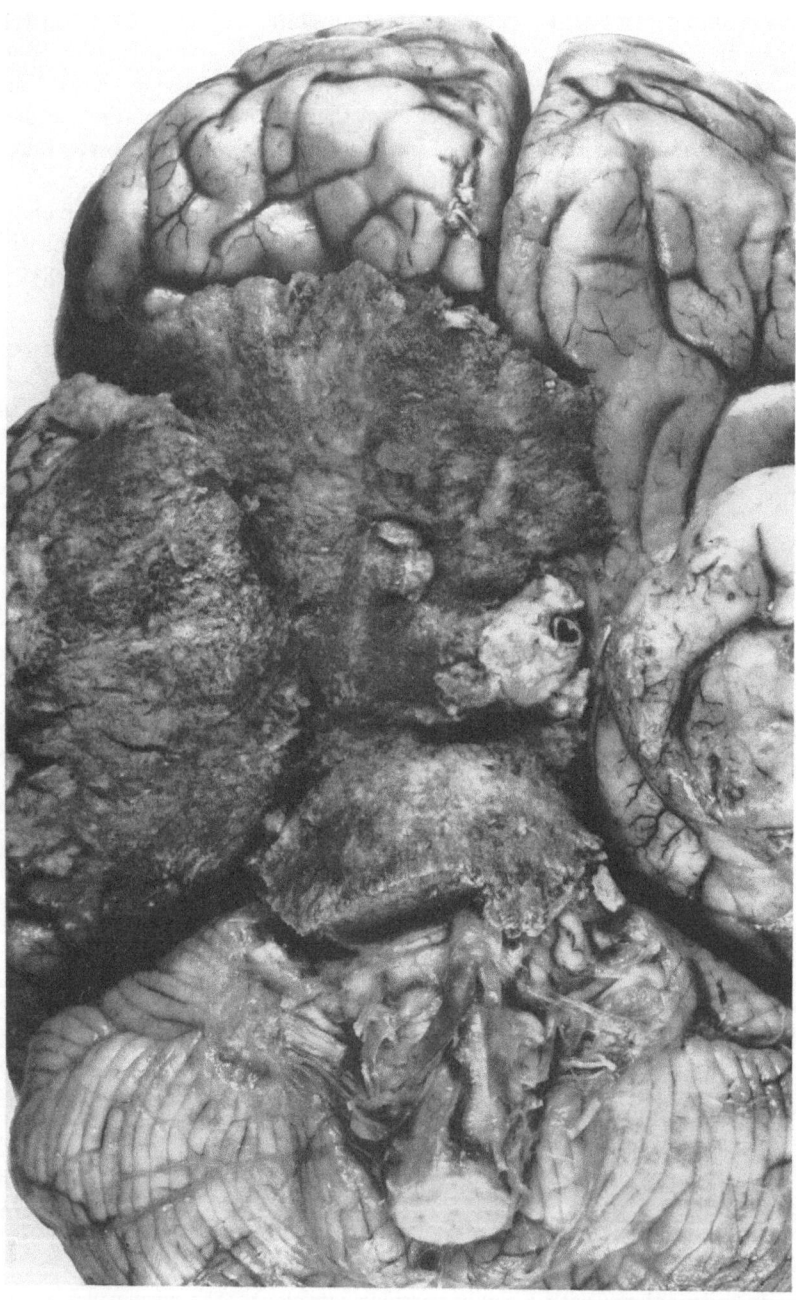

Fig. 179. Giant "en plaque" meningioma arising in the middle fossa which has enveloped both carotids and the chiasm. A posterior extension along the clivus has compromised the pons. Note the small defects on the base of the left temporal lobe

or middle cerebral arteries in sphenoid ridge meningiomas; it may even have undergone cystic degeneration (Fig. 212). The vascular supply comes most often only from the dural vessels (Fig. 214), but may in rarer (and more malignant) cases arise as well from internal carotid branches.

The increased frequency of meningiomas in certain regions is well known and corresponds to the distribution of the arachnoidal granulations (see SCHMIDT, 1902; CUSHING, 1922). Arranged in order of frequency, we have the following groups (here we have followed CUSHING's groupings with only slight changes) (see p. 36ff.):

1. Meningiomas of the Sagittal Sinus or Parasagittal Region (of the Anterior, Middle, and Posterior Thirds of the Sagittal Sinus). These tumors may reach the size of a tangerine or an apple and usually lie in the angle formed by the falx, the sinus and the dura of the convexity (Fig. 184). They are commonly spherical and often somewhat lobulated. They are most common in the middle third of the sinus (Figs. 8, 9, 184, 185), less common in the anterior third (Figs. 180–183) and rare in the posterior third (Fig. 186). The overlying bone is often invaded by the tumor or hyperplastically thickened (hyperostosis) (Figs. 216, 218, 219). They may occur bilaterally (Fig. 187) (this may be a

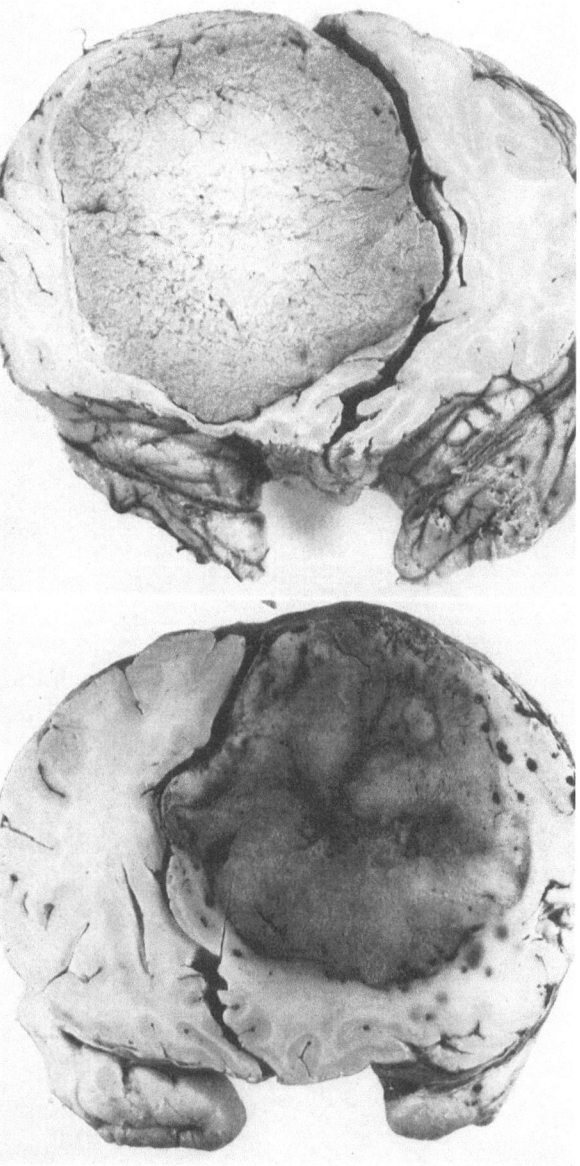

Fig. 180. Fist-sized meningioma of the anterior third of the sagittal sinus with massive brain distortion

primary or a secondary extension) and in these cases, the sinus is commonly invaded and occluded. However, unilateral parasagittal meningiomas can also lead to an occlusion of the sinus (Fig. 213).

The meningiomas of the anterior third ("frontodorsal" meningiomas) (Fig. 183) grow fairly large (up to the size of an apple) and if they are situated near the frontal pole, they tend to displace it posteriorly; if growing more posteriorly, the frontal lobe is displaced later-ally. When situated near the middle third of the sinus ("parietodorsal" meningiomas) (Figs. 8, 9, 185), they are usually symptomatic earlier and therefore sometimes smaller. The adjacent parietal lobe is displaced laterally and inferiorly, the lumen of the ventricle being at times almost obliterated (Fig. 9).

The meningiomas of the posterior third ("occipitodorsal" meningiomas) tend to displace the brain anteriorly (see p. 9) and inferiorly.

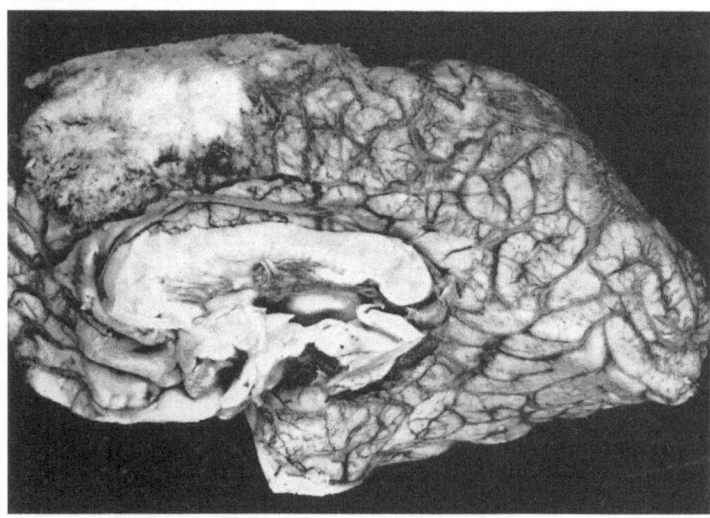

Fig. 181. Large right parasagittal meningioma of the anterior third of the sinus. Medial view

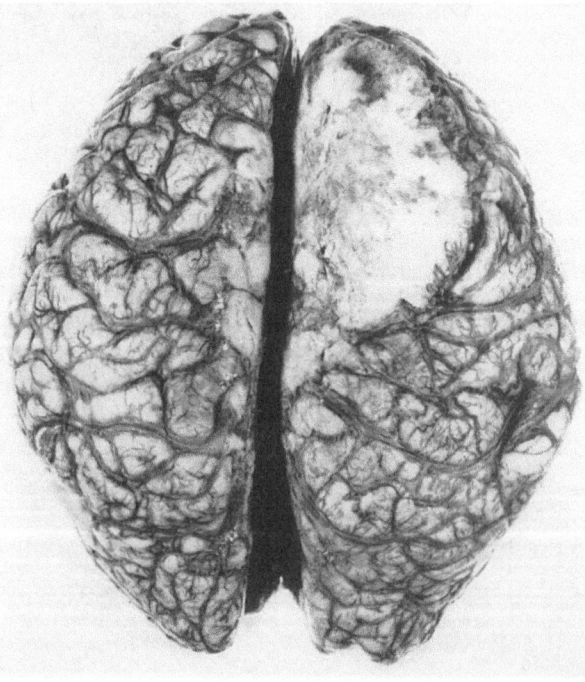

Fig. 182. View from above of parasagittal meningioma (see Fig. 181)

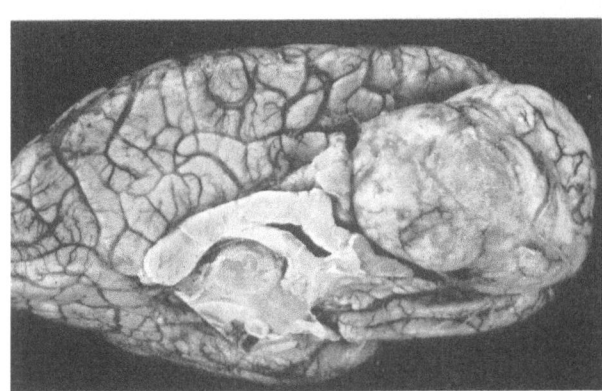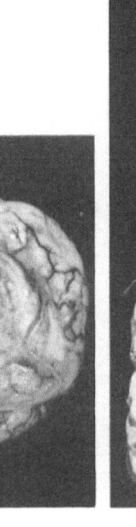

Fig. 183. Fist-sized left parasagittal meningioma. The corpus callosum is displaced posteriorly and inferiorly

Fig. 184. Two cross sections through an apple-sized meningioma of the middle third of the sagittal sinus. Note marked distortion of the adjacent brain and ventricular system

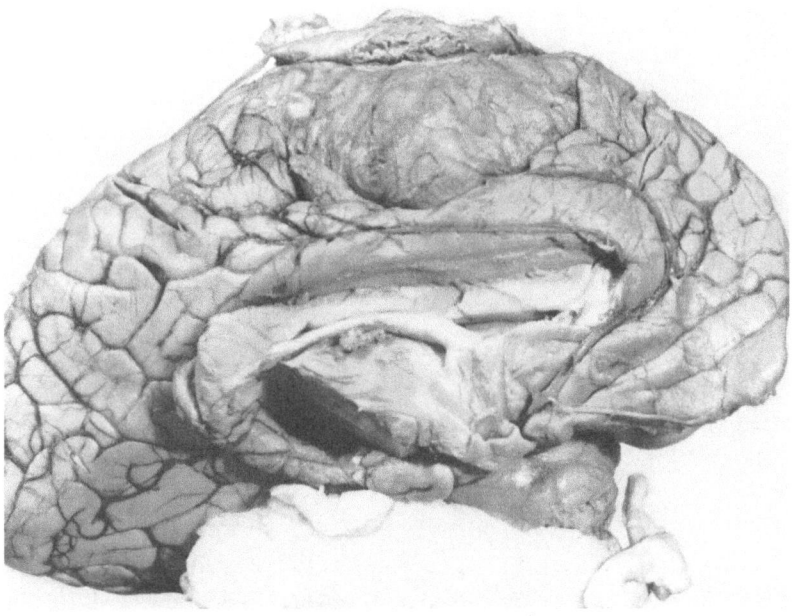

Fig. 185. Parasagittal meningioma of the middle third of the sagittal sinus, with extensive subfalceal and transtentorial herniations

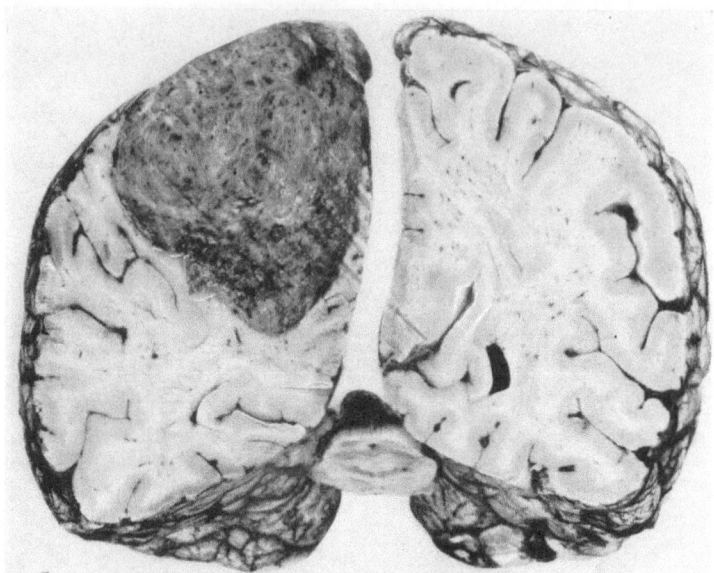

Fig. 186. Anterior view of a meningioma of the posterior third of the sagittal sinus

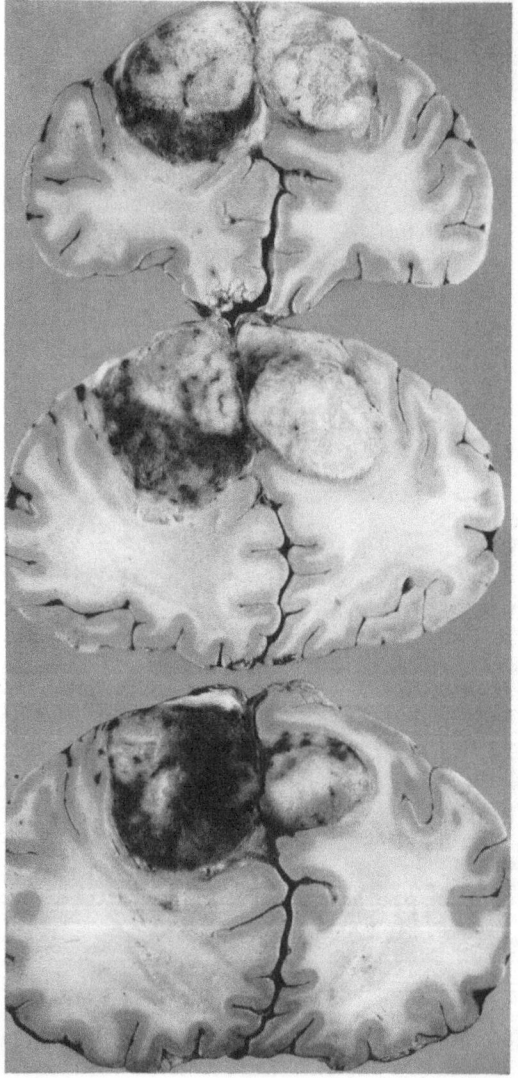

Fig. 187. Bilateral parasagittal meningiomas of the anterior third of the sagittal sinus. The left tumor is larger than the right and has considerably more associated edema causing a marked left to right shift

2. The Meningiomas of the Falx. These may be distinguished from the parasagittal meningiomas by the fact that they are extensively attached to the falx (Figs. 188–190). They commonly extend bilaterally (Fig. 190) and are covered superiorly by a mantle of brain tissue (Fig. 189). The attachment to the falx is therefore at some distance from the sinus. Most of them occur anterior to the central fissure. They are usually spherical and produce an inferior displacement of the adjacent brain, with characteristic distortion of the anterior horns of the ventricles in the ventriculogram.

3. Meningiomas of the Convexity. These meningiomas differ from the foregoing types by their lack of any type of relationship to the falx. They are distributed over the whole convexity, with the majority lying anterior to the Rolandic fissure. Here too, we find local or diffuse hyperostoses, with or without actual infiltration of the bone (Fig. 178). A particularly typical and common example of the convexity meningioma is the tumor situated around the third frontal convolution ("F₃" or "frontolateral" meningioma; Figs. 191, 192). The inferolateral mass displacement produced by this tumor often leads to the "tentorial notch" (where the peduncle of the opposite side is pressed against the tentorial edge (Fig. 32) and, therefore, results in ipsilateral symptoms (see p. 14).

4. Meningiomas of the Olfactory Groove (or of the Cribriform Plate). These lie on the lateral or medial floor of the anterior fossa ("frontobasal" meningiomas; Figs. 193, 194) and their attachment to the floor of the anterior fossa is over the cribriform plate. They usually reach the size of a tangerine (Fig. 193), are hemispherical in shape, displace the brain superiorly, and may extend posteriorly to the optic nerve and the chiasm, depressing them and pushing them backward.

The base of the frontal lobe is lifted upward (typical convex deformity of the anterior cerebral artery on arteriography) and there is an associated upward movement of the tips of the anterior frontal horns. The tumors may even straddle the falx. A small hyperostosis at the base may be found indicating the point of tumor attachment.

5. The Meningiomas of the Tuberculum Sellae (Suprasellar or Prechiasmal Meningiomas). These meningiomas lie in the midline, posterior to those of the olfactory groove. They are usually the size of a cherry or a tangerine (Fig. 195), definitely smaller than the olfactory meningioma (early optic or chiasmal symptomatology!), and often have a fine nodular surface. They displace the chiasm posteriorly, the carotids and optic nerves laterally and upwards, and the adjacent brain structures superiorly; in the olfactory groove meningioma, on the other hand, the displacement of these structures is downward. In later stages the sphenoid sinus may be invaded or the pituitary gland compressed.

There are some rare meningiomas situated in the vicinity of—but not attached to—the tuberculum sellae and olfactory groove, as well as meningiomas of the sheath of the optic nerve. The latter grow from the optic sheath, which they may then envelop and reach the size of a plum. Furthermore, in the orbital roof itself, a meningioma may grow "ectopically".

6. The Meningiomas of the Sphenoid Ridge and the Sylvian Fissure. These meningiomas lie along the sphenoid ridge either "medially" or "laterally" (Figs. 27, 196). They may be round and spherical (Fig. 197) or flat (Fig. 198) like a carpet ("meningioma en plaque"). They may extend either more into the anterior or middle fossa and some of them grow equally into both fossae (Fig. 197). The large, carpet-like tumors may reach the chiasm, orbital roof, or even the posterior fossa (Fig. 198). Vessels and cranial nerves can be surrounded. More than any other type, these meningiomas tend to produce hyperostosis of the sphenoid wing (Fig. 198) and of the base of the skull which can often be demonstrated in the AP x-rays, or produce visible deformities of the forehead, face and orbit (exophthalmus). The medially situated tumors may encase the carotid artery and the optic nerve, and displace them medially and superiorly (stretching the siphon of the carotid artery, the middle cerebral artery, and the medial and lateral striatal vessels). Only rarely are the vascular structures not involved.

Meningiomas lying more laterally around the Sylvian fissure (Fig. 199) merge with the group over the convexity (they are a posterior extension of the F_3 group of meningiomas). If flat and more "en plaque", there may be portions of the tumor which interdigitate with the brain. The lateral sphenoid wing (pterion) tumor may invade the ridge (hyperostosis, see above) or in rare cases the bones of the convexity and the temporal muscle, but involvement of vessels and nerves fails to occur.

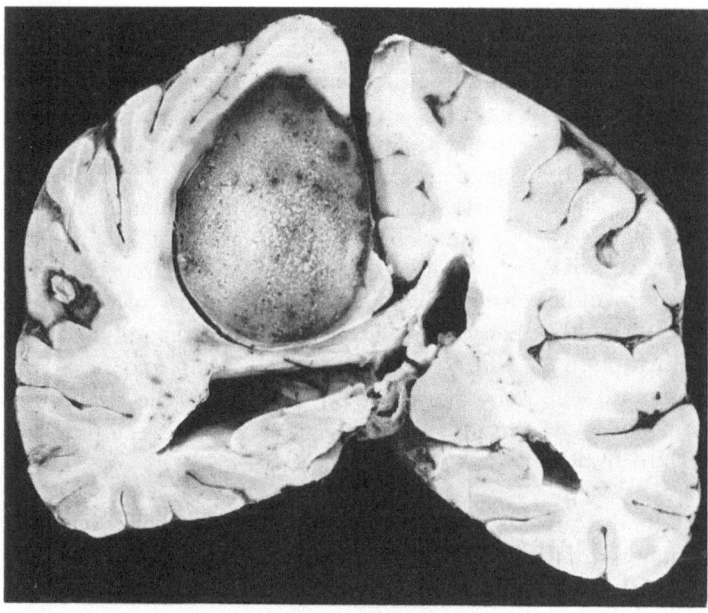

Fig. 188. Falx meningioma of the posterior third of the sagittal sinus

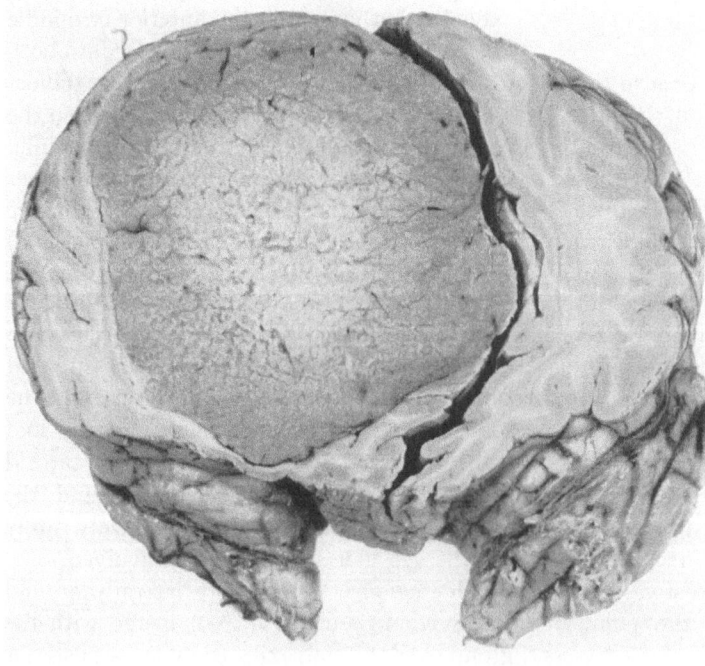

Fig. 189. Colossal meningioma of the right falx with massive distortion of the opposite frontal lobe

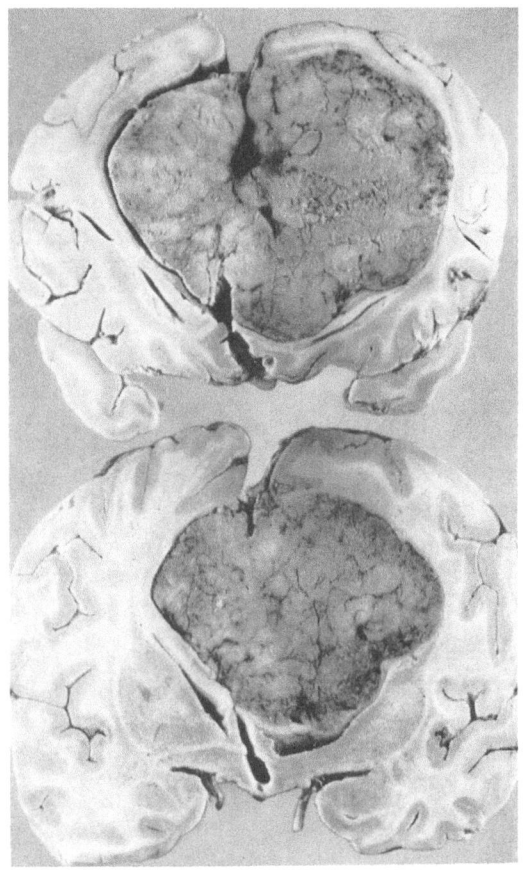

Fig. 190. Huge meningioma of the falx with bilateral growth, more on the right side than on the left

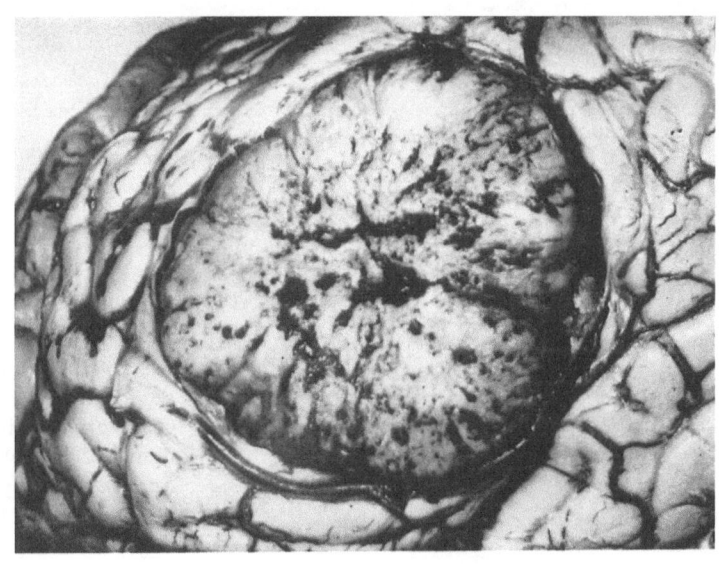

Fig. 191. Large frontolateral meningioma, in its typical location in the third frontal convolution (see Fig. 192). Such a meningioma commonly results in mass shifting with a resultant involvement of the contralateral cerebral peduncle ("tentorial notch", see Fig. 32)

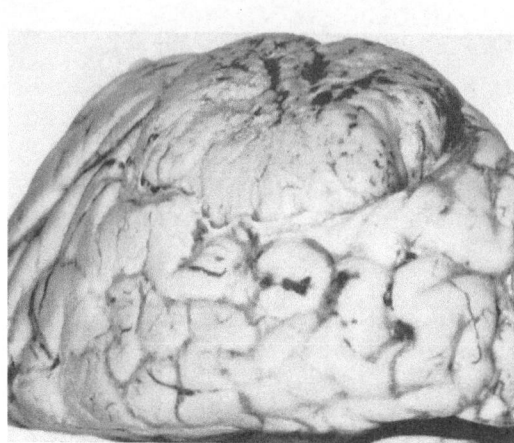 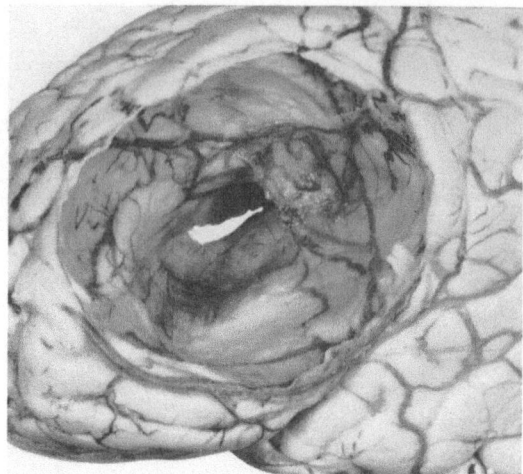

Fig. 192. Same case as Fig. 191. The left figure is the view from above. After extraction (right) one can see the anterior horn of the lateral ventricle through the tumor bed (see Fig. 191)

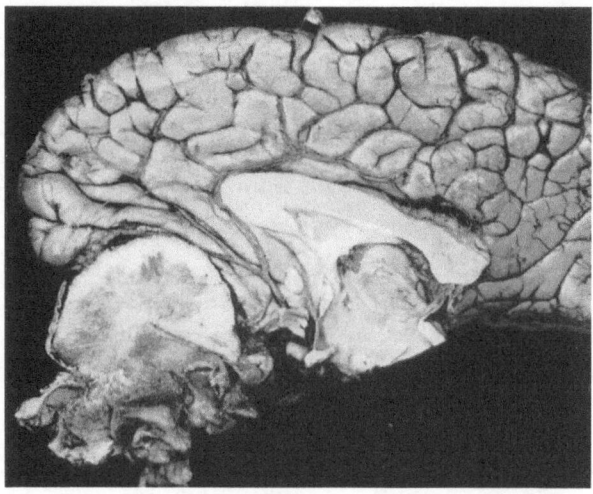

Fig. 193. Olfactory groove meningioma the size of an apple with typical distortion of the base of the frontal lobe

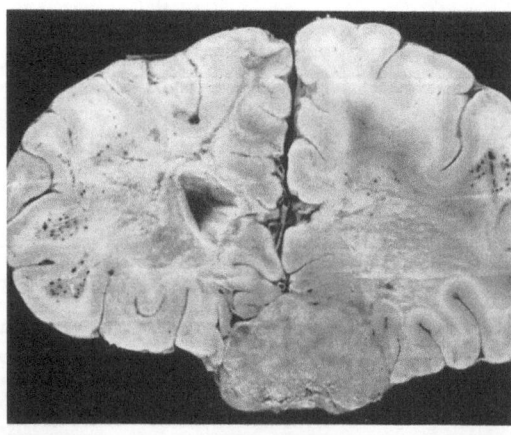

Fig. 194. Walnut-sized olfactory groove meningioma in a case of intensive radiation therapy. The entire white matter has been extensively damaged and softened to a gelatinous consistency. Scarring and cystic degeneration are apparent, as well as some flea-bite hemorrhages in the subcortical white matter

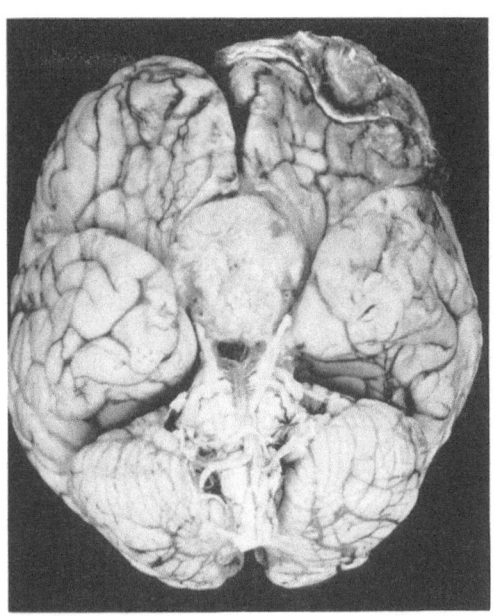

Fig. 195. Tangerine-sized meningioma of the tuberculum sellae. Post-operative state

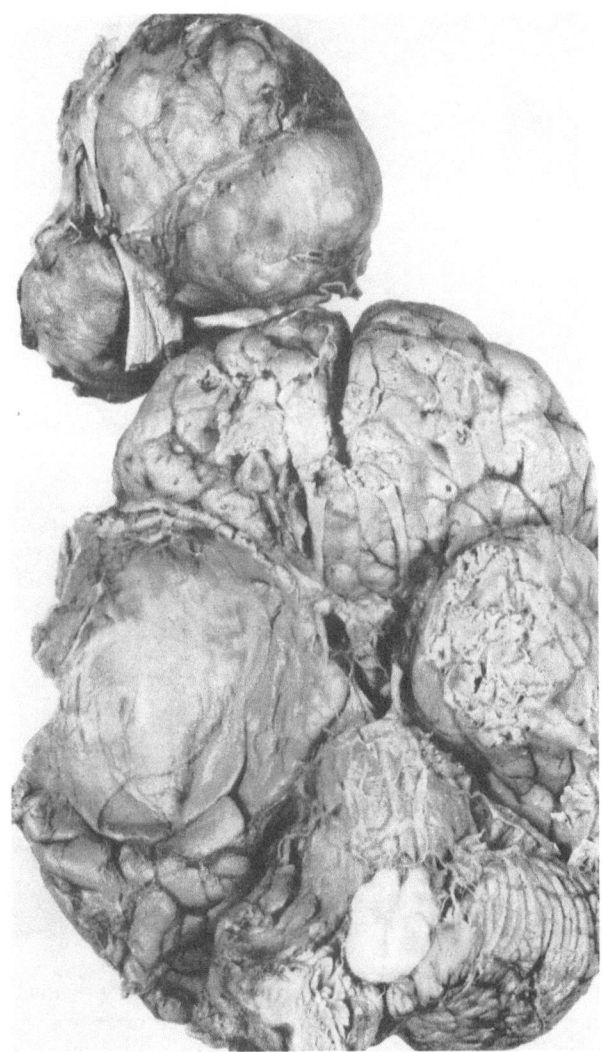

Fig. 196. Dumb-bell shaped meningioma of the right tentorium. The larger portion extended into the middle fossa, the smaller into the posterior fossa. Massive shifting of the adjacent brain has occurred. Note the numerous little holes perforating the base of the brain (c.f. Fig. 218 for an explanation)

123

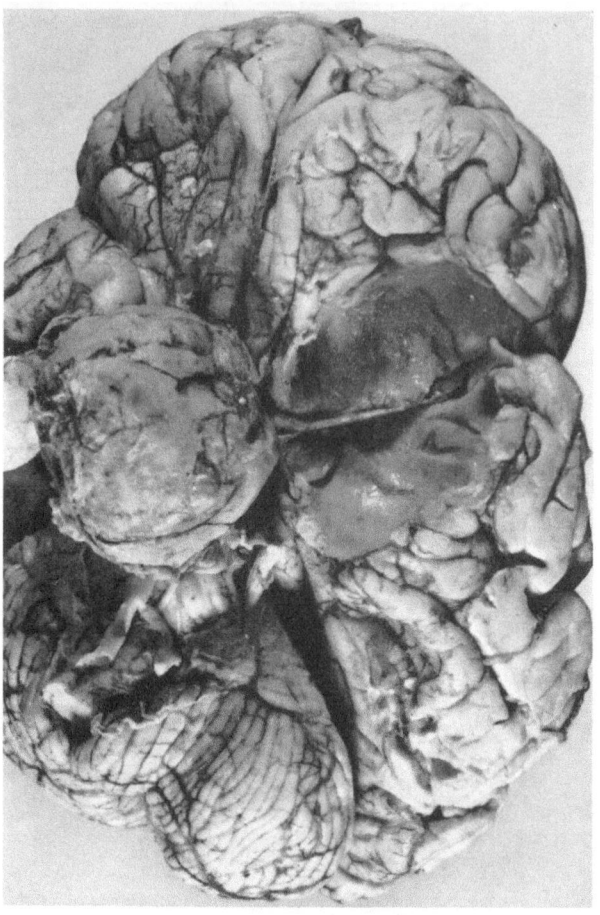

Fig. 197. Apple-sized meningioma of the middle third of the sphenoid ridge, which had compromised the left middle cerebral artery

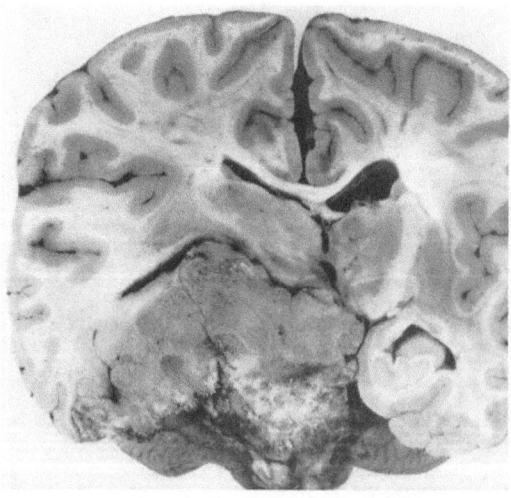

Fig. 198. Flat meningioma near the sphenoid ridge (note indentation in tumor) with associated mass effect

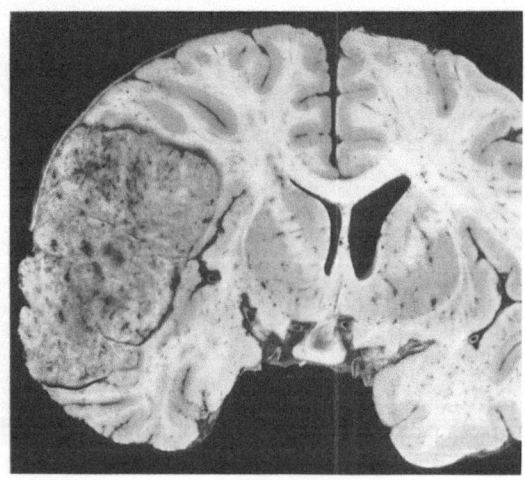

Fig. 199. Temporolateral meningioma (meningioma of the Sylvian fissure)

7. Meningiomas of the Temporal Fossa and Meckel's Cave. These tumors lie beneath the temporal lobe at the base. They are round, spherical and are positioned between the meningiomas of the sphenoid anteriorly, the cerebellopontine angle meningiomas posteriorly, and Meckel's cave meningioma medially. Here the meningioma may occur "en plaque" at the petrous tip and may send processes into the surrounding regions (Fig. 198).

8. Meningiomas of the Cerebellopontine Angle. These meningiomas lie along the medial portion of the petrous pyramid (Figs. 200–203)—i.e., in the posterior fossa. They may resemble the acoustic neurinoma in size and in extension. However, they do not enlarge the internal acoustic meatus, more often growing toward the tentorial hiatus (Fig. 200).

9. Meningiomas of the Tentorium (Peritorcular Meningioma) — Meningiomas of the Cerebellar Convexity. These meningiomas either grow supratentorially (expanding beneath the temporal or occipital lobes) or infratentorially (over the superior surface of the cerebellum; Fig. 206). They may also grow in both directions and assume the shape of a dumbbell (Fig. 196). In general they are most frequent around the torcular herophili.

Not common are meningiomas of the cerebellar convexity, which have no relation to the various venous sinuses.

10. Meningiomas of the Ventricles. The meningiomas of the lateral ventricle occur as egg-shaped tumors that reach the size of a fist and lie mainly in the trigonal region, where they are firmly attached to the choroid plexus and often calcified. Meningiomas of the velum interpositum project into the third ventricle.

11. Meningiomas of the Clivus, or Craniospinal Meningiomas (Including Meningiomas of the Foramen Magnum). These proceed from the lateral or medial clivus (Figs. 204, 207) toward the temporal lobe, anterior surface of the cerebellum, or the pontine region, and may send a tongue of tumor down into the foramen magnum or the spinal canal (Fig. 207).

12. Meningiomas in the Hiatus Tentorii. Rarely meningiomas occur near the V. magna Galeni extending over the quadrigeminal region (Fig. 208).

13. Spinal Meningiomas (or Meningiomas of the Cord). These are bean or acorn-sized (Fig. 209) occasionally finger-shaped (Fig. 210), and extend over several segments. They are most common in the thoracic region, but most extensive in the cervical or caudal regions. They are firmly attached to the dura, usually dorsolaterally, but occasionally elsewhere. At times they cannot be distinguished macroscopically from neurinomas (here the site of attachment may be of some help) (Fig. 209). Curiously, they tend to have a high frequency in women in the 5th or 6th decade where they lie in the thoracic segments. These tumors are heavily calcified.

On rare occasions meningiomas are multiple (Fig. 215), their size ranging from that of a cherry-pit to an apple, and are encountered in any of the above-mentioned sites; there may be as many as 100 of them (Fig. 215). They are often associated with acoustic nerve tumors, or other neurinomas and neurofibromas in von Recklinghausen's neurofibromatosis (see p. 109, 110). Some authors apply the term *diffuse meningiomatosis* to the primary tumors involving the dura (Fig. 215).

The histological subdivisions are of little concern to the neurosurgeon apart from the angioblastic variant, which has a slightly more unfavorable prognosis. Otherwise, they behave biologically in a similar way and will not recur if completely removed. However, the "polymitotic" variety may recur at frequent intervals if any tumor tissue at all is left behind, and may show a slightly different histological picture each time (Figs. 216, 217). Some exceptionally rare cases may completely alter their biological behavior, recur after 5–10 years, and at this time even metastasize outside of the central nervous system. In the latter types there is a gradual transition to the fibroblastic sarcoma of the dura which lacks a capsule, invades the brain freely, and varies in histology.

The meningiomas comprise around 16% of the bigger tumor series (see p. 48) and are the largest group of operable intracranial tumors. They show a clear predilection for the middle and later decades of life (see p. 46). They begin to become more frequent only in the third decade—a fact that may be useful in differentiating them from other tumors, particularly in the region of the chiasm. However, there may be great variance as to age of preference depending on whether the cases come from a neurosurgical series, from general autopsy material, or from autopsies in a mental institution. In our collection the peak of incidence lies around the age of 45 years. The average age of CUSHING's patients was 46.6 years for both sexes, for male alone 52, and for females 42.9 years. The sex ratio of our patients was 532 males and 960 females—roughly 5:9. However, in some localizations it is quite different (suprasellar 1:4 = males:females), and even up to 1:8 or 1:20 in some papers on spinal meningiomas. In CUSHING's series (1932, 1935) the meningiomas accounted for 13.4%, in OLIVECRONA's 18.4% (see CASTELLANO *et al.*, 1952), in KERNOHAN's and SAYRE's 17.2% (1952), and in our series of 9000 for 16.6% of all tumors. However, in spinal tumor series the figure is far higher—for instance, in 979 spinal tumors in the Mayo Clinic series 25.9% were meningiomas.

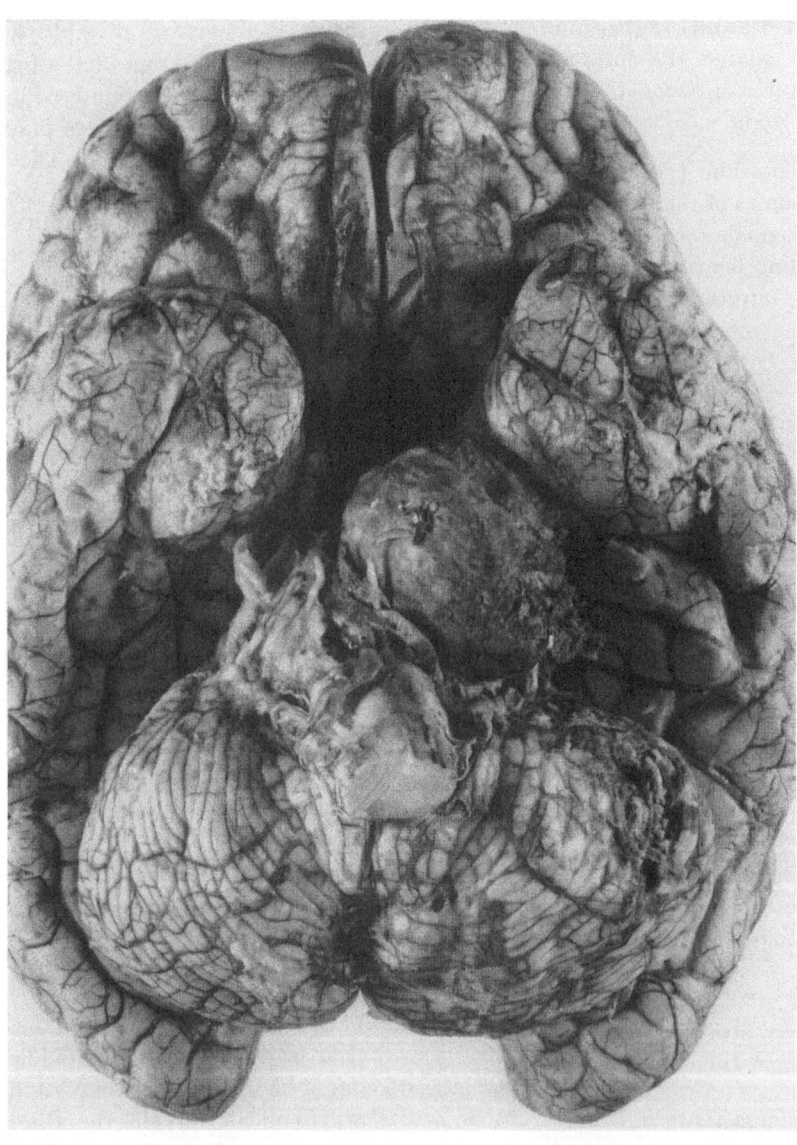

Fig. 200. Meningioma of the tip of the petrous bone which has compromised the midbrain and pons. A previous attempt at surgical excision had been made

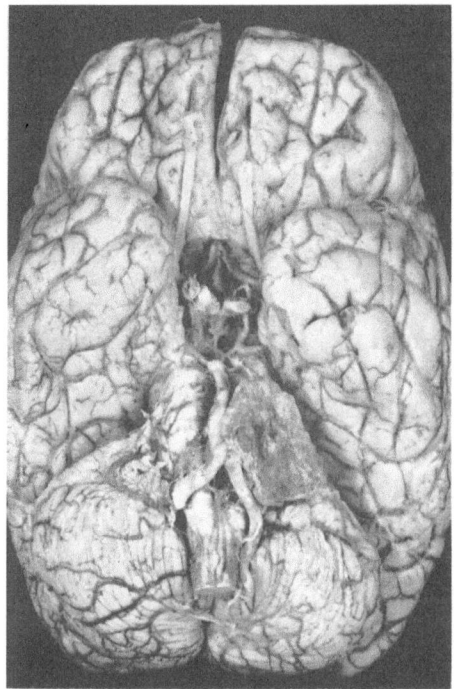

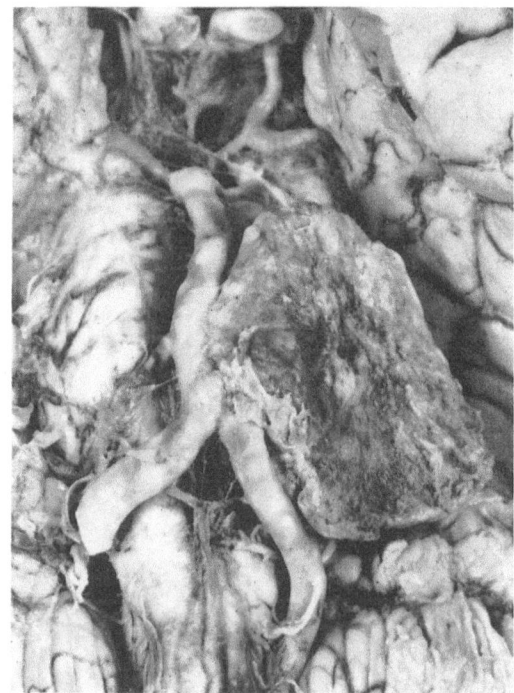

Fig. 201. Meningioma in the cerebellopontine angle. Basal view of lesion in situ. High degree of basal arteriosclerosis

Fig. 202. Close-up view of Fig. 201

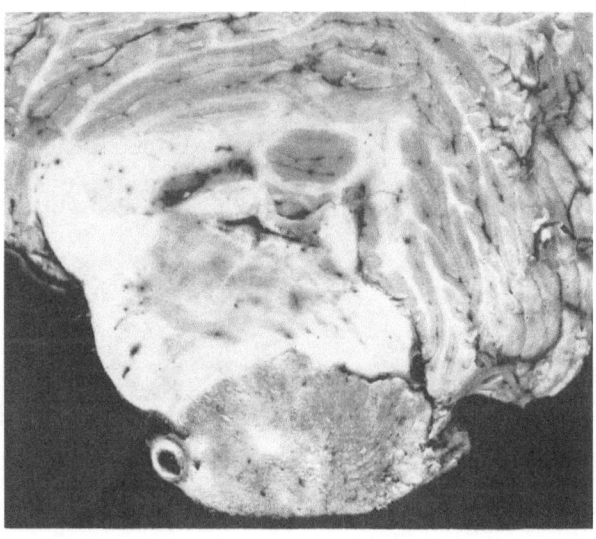

Fig. 203. Section showing displacement of the pons by a meningioma in the cerebello-pontine angle (see Figs. 201, 202)

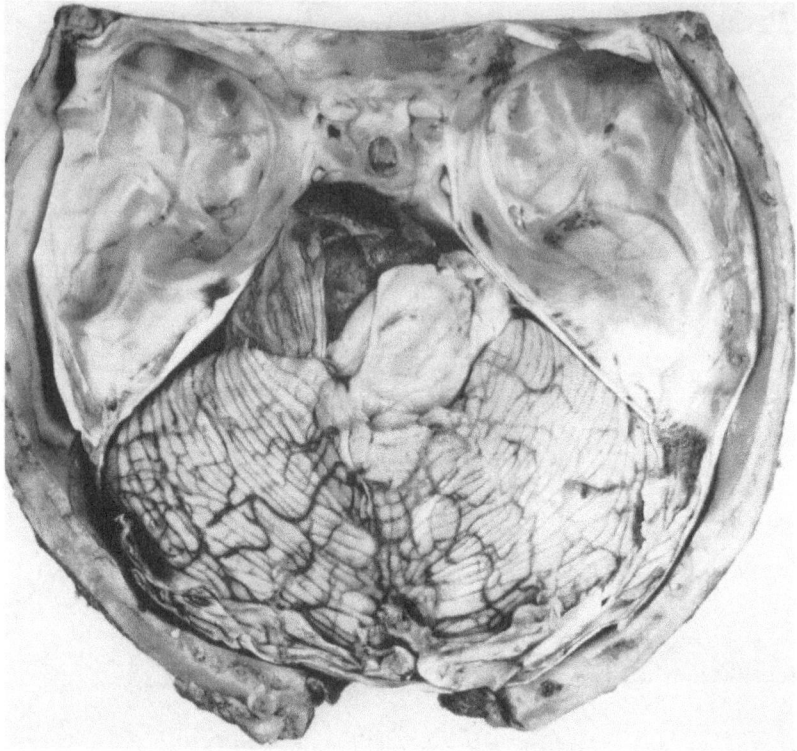

Fig. 204. A meningioma of the left upper clivus markedly displacing the pons and midbrain, viewed from above. Note the stretched cranial nerves over the lateral aspect of the tumor

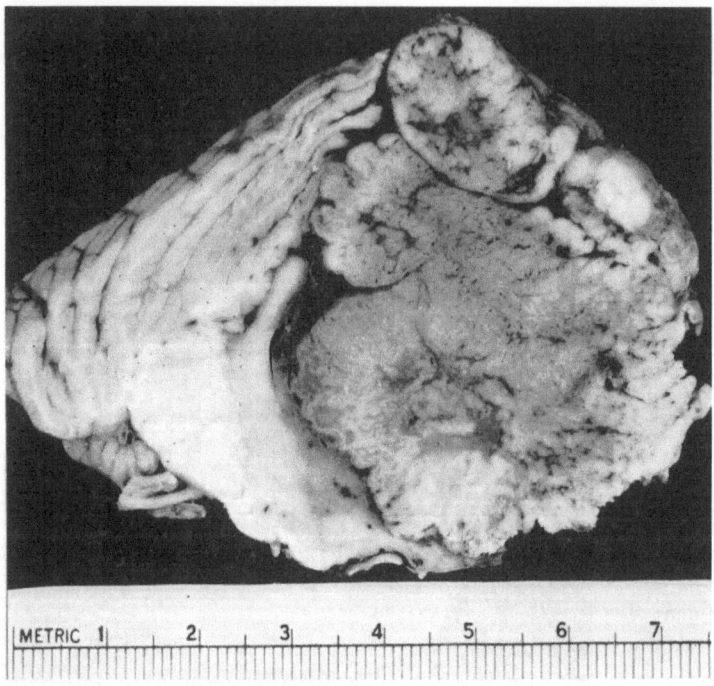

Fig. 205. Angioblastic meningioma of the cerebellopontine angle. View depicting extensive destruction and pressure atrophy of adjacent pons

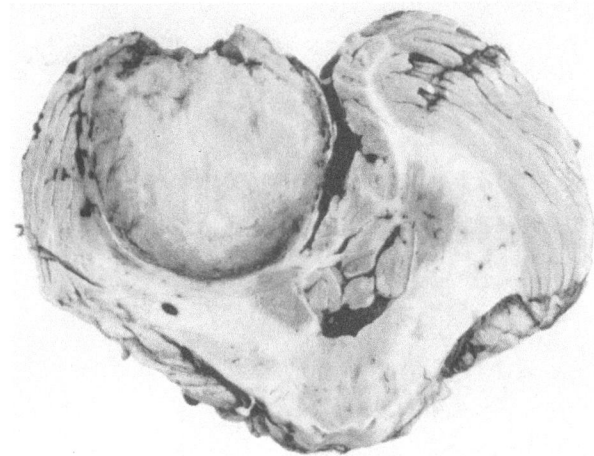

Fig. 206. Tentorial meningioma extending into the posterior fossa (so-called peritorcular meningioma)

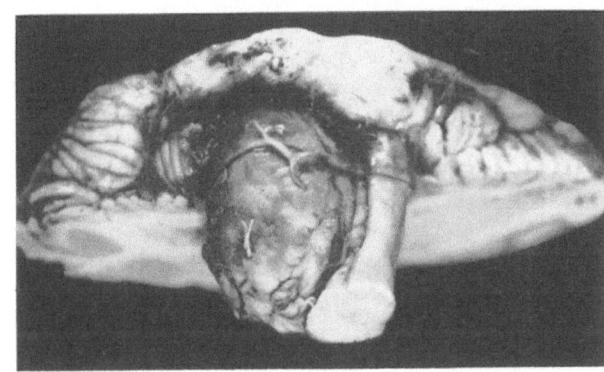

Fig. 207. Typical right-sided "craniospinal" meningioma (meningioma of the foramen magnum) with associated distortion of the pons and medulla oblongata

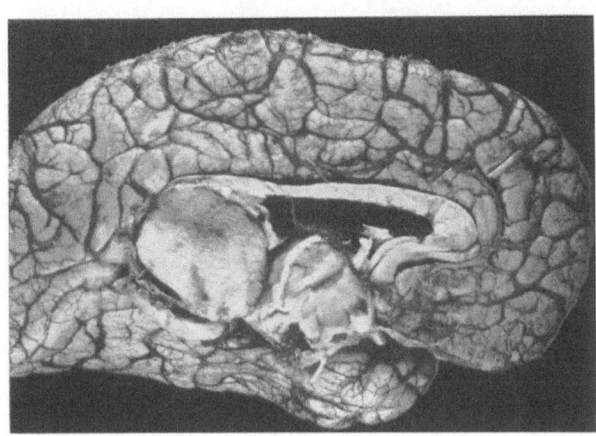

Fig. 208. Walnut-shaped meningioma arising from the tentorium in the region of the midbrain

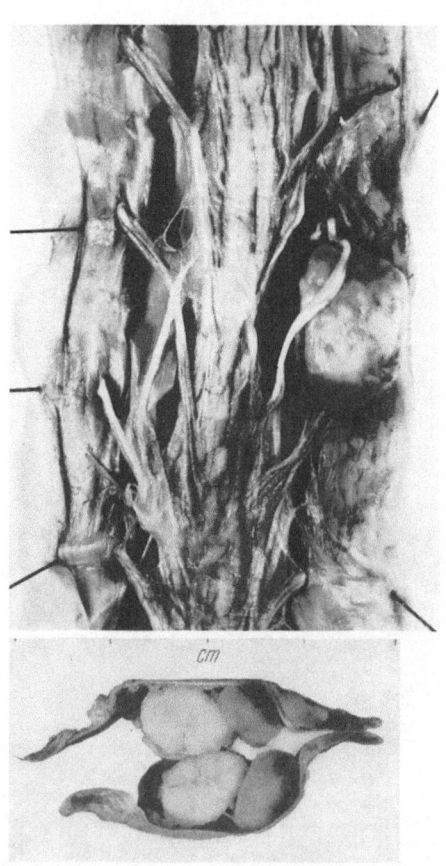

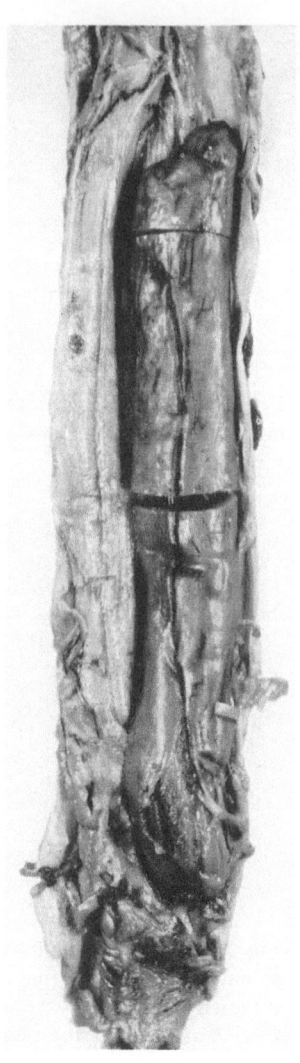

Fig. 209. Two meningiomas of the spinal canal without clinical symptoms (incidental findings)

Fig. 210. Unusually long finger-like meningioma extending over approximately 10 spinal segments

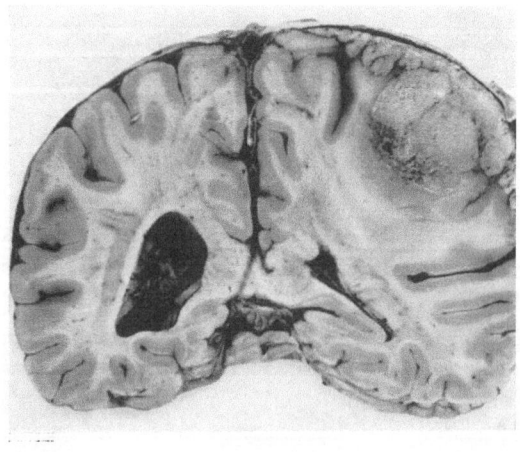

Fig. 211. Rare type of meningioma, which demonstrates both a plaque-like outer shell and a central nodule in the right convexity

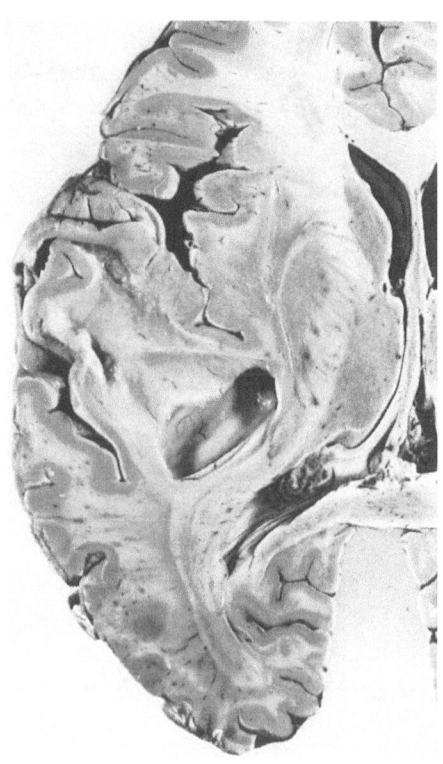

Fig. 212. A large cystic infarct in the area of distribution of the middle cerebral artery which had been compromised by a meningioma

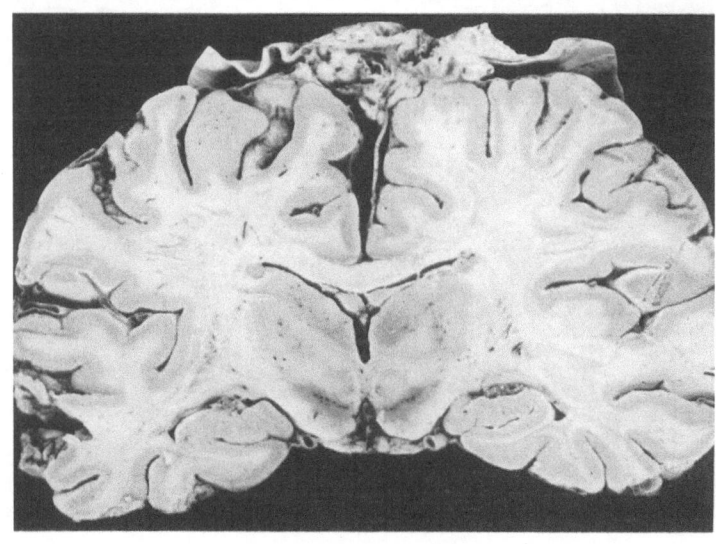

Fig. 213. Intra- and extradural extension of a small plaque-like meningioma originating from the middle third of the sagittal sinus

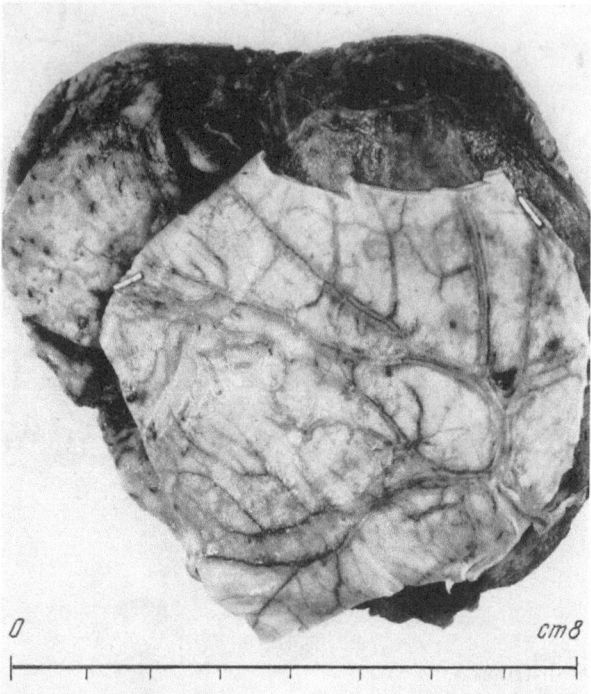

Fig. 214. Surgical specimen of a meningioma demonstrating the vascular pattern in the dura, which corresponds to the radiologically-described "star" formation of meningeal arteries

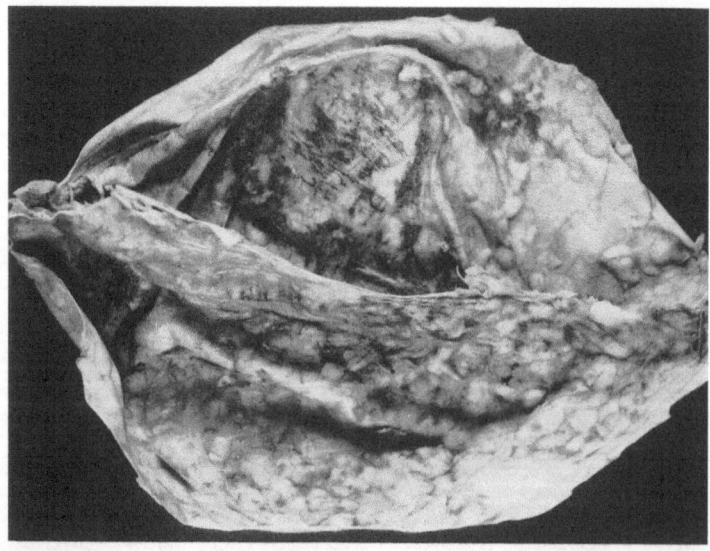

Fig. 215. Numerous small meningiomas, some of which are plaque-like, others more nodular in appearance, involving the dura and falx (so-called meningiomatosis)

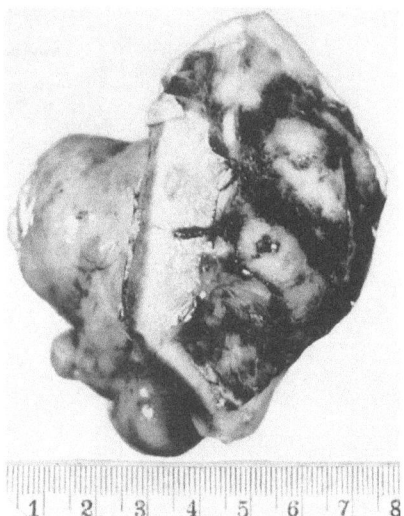

Fig. 216. Malignant meningioma with late metastases to the lung (after 22 years of growth!). The tumor and adjacent bone flap have been removed together

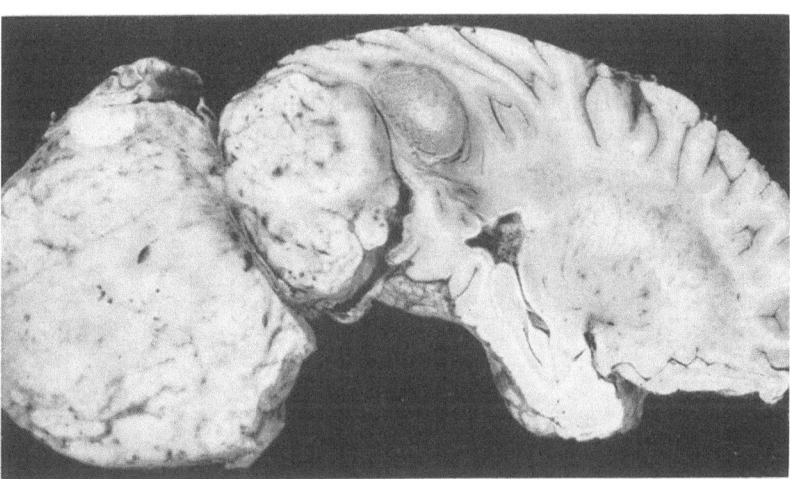

Fig. 217. Recurrent peritorcular meningioma years after an attempted total excision. The bulk of the tumor mass is now extracranial, having escaped through a surgical defect in the skull (note constriction in tumor)

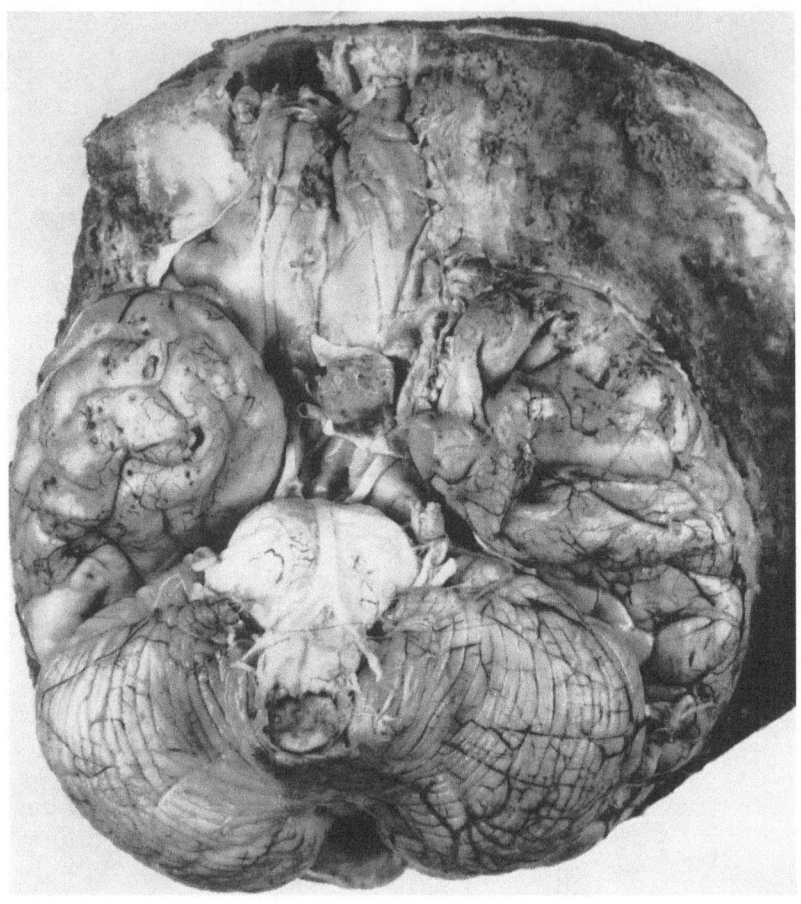

Fig. 218. Giant meningioma diffusely covering the entire left hemisphere (c.f. Fig. 219). At the base of the contralateral temporal lobe one may note small defects, which were consequent to a shearing off of small pedicles of brain substance which had herniated through perforations in the dura. This may be seen in cases where there has been long-standing increased intracranial pressure (c.f. Fig. 196)

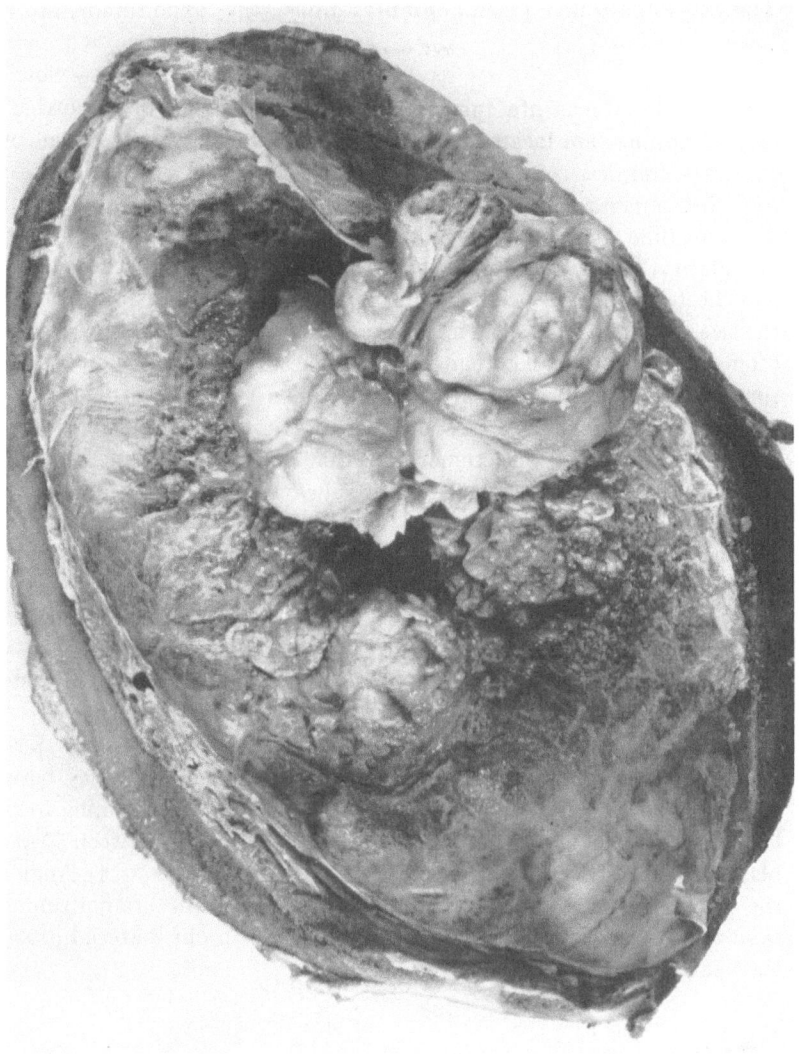

Fig. 219. Part of the giant meningioma of the convexity and falx seen in Fig. 218. In this picture one sees many large tumor nodules and the prominent hyperostosis of the overlying cranium is particularly well demonstrated

The Angioblastomas (Hemangioblastomas, Lindau Tumors)

The angioblastomas are tumors which, with rare exceptions, are located only in the posterior fossa and (less commonly) in the spinal canal. The tumor is recognized by its bright bluish-red color (like a cherry) which is due to its rich vascularity. The solid tumors can be as large as a chestnut, while associated cysts may attain the size of a child's fist. The mural nodules are often as small or smaller than cherries. These tumors are frequently covered by many tortuous cortical vessels (Fig. 223). In some cases there may be more than one tumor, so that in case of a "recurrence" one must always consider this possibility.

The angioblastomas lie either (1) in the cerebellar hemisphere (Fig. 220) and vermis or tonsils (Figs. 225, 226), or (2) in the roof of the fourth ventricle (Fig. 224). In the cerebellar hemispheres we usually find them near the cortex, and more often cystic (Figs. 221, 222) than solid. The cysts, in fact, may be many times larger than the solid portions and are usually unilocular (Fig. 221), rarely multilocular (Fig. 223). The second group of hemangioblastomas lie between the tonsils (Fig. 224) and the exit of the fourth ventricle, the underlying cysts sometimes firmly interdigitating with the ventricular floor.

The tumors are well-circumscribed and largely cystic, with a cyst fluid which may vary in color from yellow to black, depending on the degree of hemorrhage present. This fluid may coagulate spontaneously.

In the spinal cord, the tumor often assumes the shape of a pencil and the large cystic part may mimic a syringomyelia (as do the spinal spongioblastomas and ependymomas on occasion).

There are only a few rare examples of true hemangioblastomas occurring in the cerebral hemispheres.

In the full-blown Lindau's syndrome cysts of the pancreas and kidney are also found. There may be an association with retinal angiomas, the so-called retinal angiomatosis of von Hippel (he named this syndrome "angiomatosis of the nervous system"). This may, in rare instances, be hereditary (v. Hippel-Lindau's disease), as also the occurrence of isolated cerebellar angioblastomas may be hereditary in rare instances.

There is a peak in age incidence of angioblastomas between 35 and 45, with the curve beginning to rise steeply at 20 and trailing off between 50–60. There is a preponderance of males (2:1). Angioblastomas comprised 1.2% of intracranial tumors in CUSHING's series and in our material (9000 cases) 1.3%.

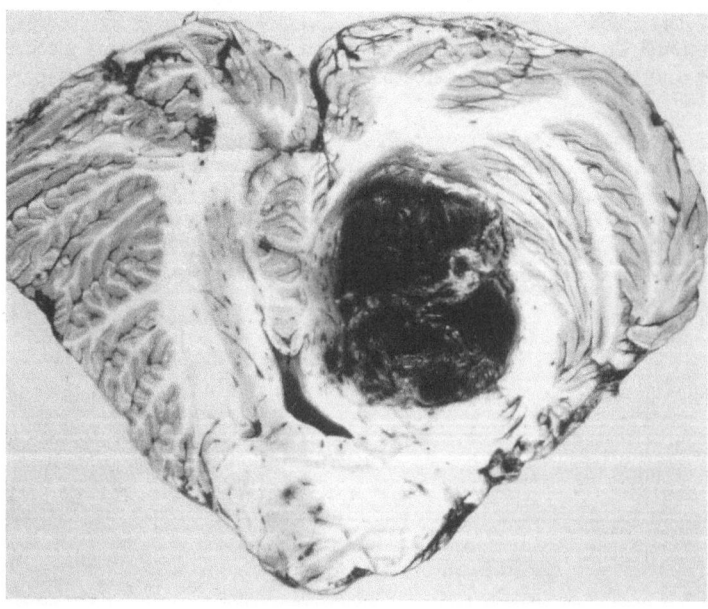

Fig. 220. Circumscribed, partly-cystic angioblastoma with intrinsic hemorrhage. A marked shift of the fourth ventricle has occurred

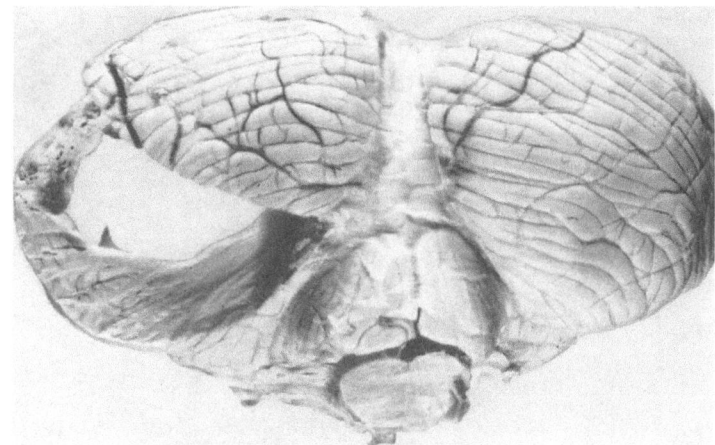

Fig. 221. Large cystic angioblastoma with the typical
small mural nodule. Very
marked tonsillar herniation is
noted

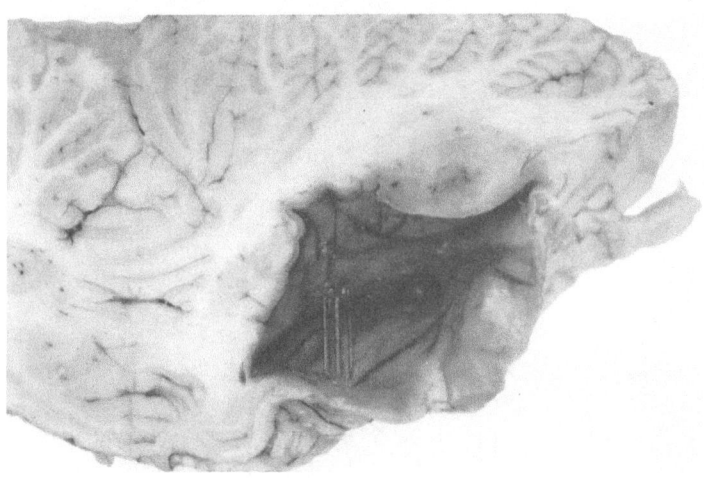

Fig. 222. Cystic angioblastoma
with a bean-sized mural nodule on its superior wall

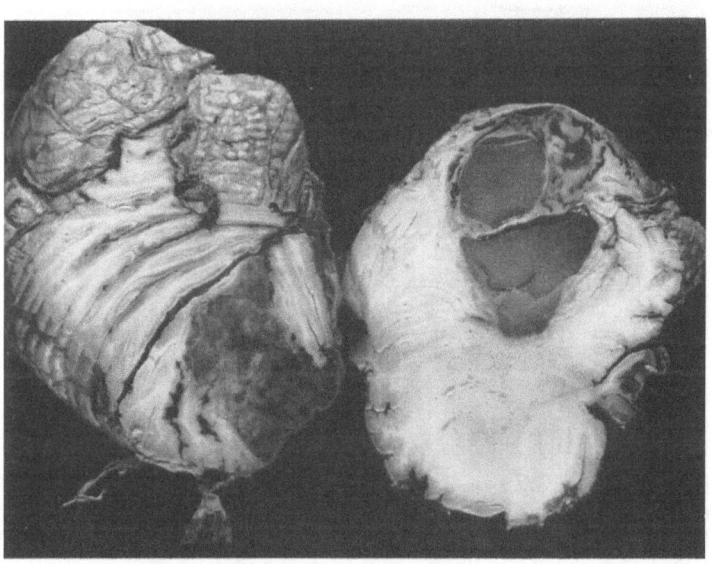

Fig. 223. Multiple cerebellar
angioblastomas. Note the en-
gorgement of the vessels of
supply

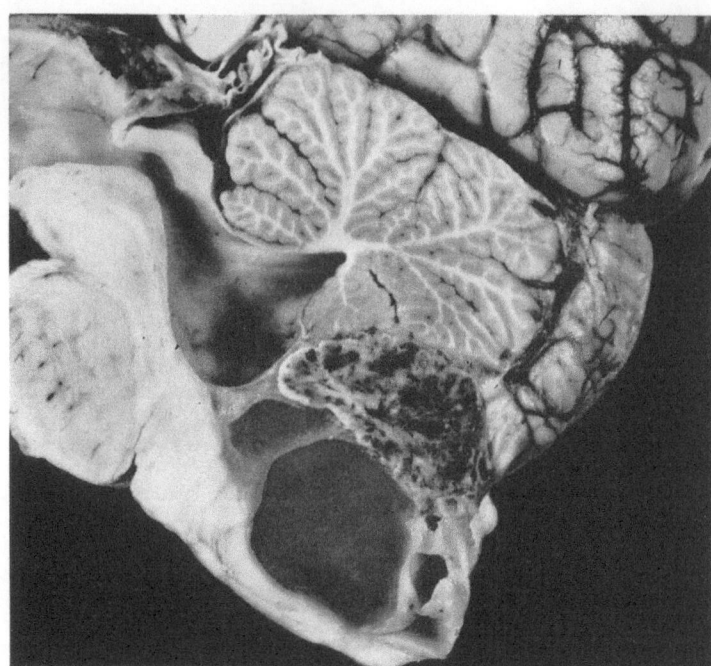

Fig. 224. Plum-sized angio-blastoma at the caudal end of the fourth ventricle (area postrema). Two cysts have developed within the tumor and have greatly flattened the medulla oblongata

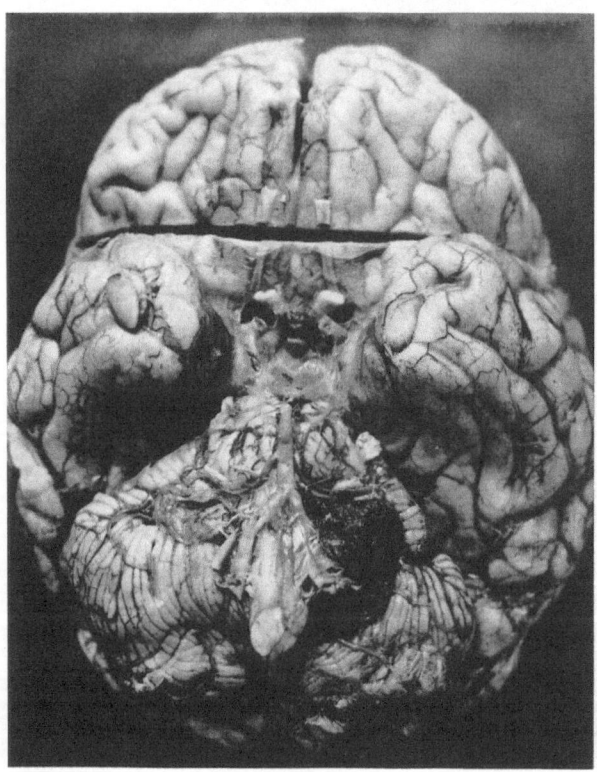

Fig. 225. Angioblastoma of the cerebellar tonsil which intermittently compromised the vertebro-basilar system (confirmed by arteriography!)

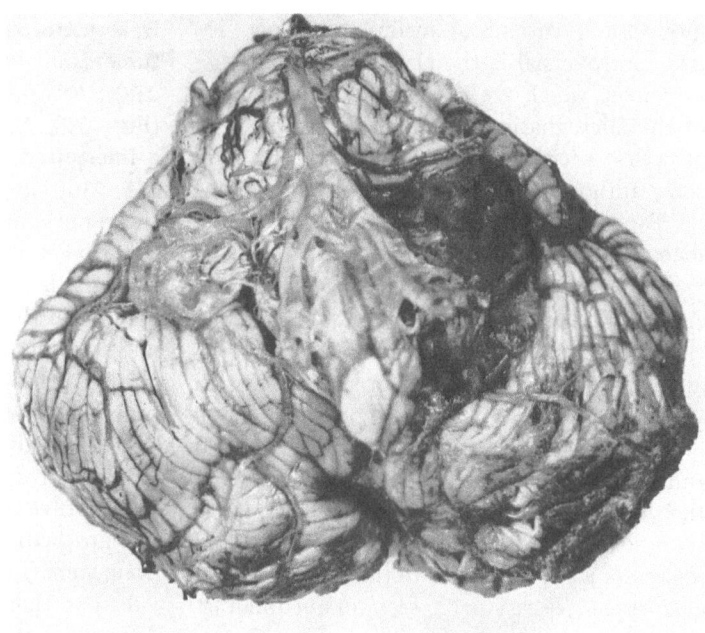

Fig. 226. Close view of Fig. 225

Sturge-Weber's Disease

Sturge-Weber's disease (angioma capillare et venosum calcificans), when full-blown, presents a true syndrome in the same manner as Lindau's disease and consists of glaucoma, nevus flammeus of the face, and calcified angioma of the brain. Other vascular malformations can also occur. Attention has been called to the parallel nerve supply to both leptomeninges and skin by branches of the trigeminal nerve ("encephalo-trigeminal angiomatosis"). However, "full-blown" cases are rare; the facial nevus alone is most common, followed by the combination of facial and cerebral nevi. There is increased vascularity in the leptomeninges, and a sinuous network of venous and large capillary vessels, no thicker than matches, overlies the cerebral cortex. The brain parenchyma is atrophic, scarred, and grossly calcified. Heterotopias are also encountered. The outcome of the controversy regarding the primary or secondary nature of the parenchymal changes seems to favor their regressive (secondary) origin. The characteristic double-contour shadows on x-rays are explained by the particular projection of the calcified gyri.

The Sarcomas

The primary sarcomas of the nervous system are rare and may be divided into two broad categories and six sub-types, as follows:
A. Diffusely growing sarcomas—i.e., sarcomatosis
    1. Primary meningeal sarromatosis; diffuse sarcomatosis of the meninges or
    2. Periadventitial diffuse sarcoma.
B. Circumscribed sarcomas
    3. Fibrosarcoma (of the dura);
    4. Monstrocellular (giant-cell) sarcoma;
    5. (so-called) Circumscribed arachnoidal cerebellar sarcoma;
    6. Reticulo- (reticulum-cell) sarcoma.
    7. Carious malignant lymphomas.

All classifications suffer from over-simplification by failing to give proper emphasis to areas of dispute. One of the sarcomas, the fibrosarcoma of the dura, may be considered in many aspects as a highly malignant variant of the meningioma. In fact, sometimes there is a definite transition from one into the other. Others, such as the "cerebellar arachnoidal sarcomas" are still controversial—as, for example, whether or not they are simply a ("desmoplastic'') variant of medulloblastoma. No less controversial is the classification of other sarcomas, which are considered to be tumors of the microglia in their more diffuse form of growth (''periadventitial diffuse sarcoma'') by some authors.

The various forms of sarcoma differ in their macroscopic appearances.

A₁ Diffuse Sarcomatosis of the Meninges. Here the leptomeninges are clouded as in meningitis and the thickened cisterns are plugged with whitish tumor masses (Fig. 227). Single small nodules may occur, but large circumscribed tumors are not found. This is a tumor found in the young and in the middle aged and affects both sexes equally. This form is grossly and microscopically so similar to the diffuse meningeal spread occasionally seen in medulloblastomas that they are often confused with one another, when only seen at operation in the cerebral cortex.

A₂ Periadventitial Diffuse Sarcoma. The gross appearance may be that of a cerebral inflammatory process (Fig. 228) whereby confluence of diffusely infiltrated perivascular zones may lead to real ''granulomas''. Cases with a more condensed perivascular spread may even resemble some of the glioblastomas (see p. 95). This tumor may be grossly distinguished from the preceding one by the way it restricts itself to infiltration around intracerebral vessels, while the leptomeninges are either uninvolved or (rarely) invaded secondarily.

B₃ Fibrosarcoma (of the Dura). The fibrosarcomas grow both inside and outside the dura (Fig. 229) but tend to infiltrate the adjacent brain tissue despite their fairly circumscribed appearance. They can provoke massive edema (Fig. 230). Their main distinguishing feature from the meningioma is that they lack a definite capsule. Otherwise, they can have the same firm consistency as the meningioma so that macroscopic distinction may not be possible (Fig. 229)—particularly if a zone of infiltration in the depths is not apparent. Fibrosarcomas rarely result from malignant transformation of scar tissue after radiation therapy (''scar-sarcomas'') (Figs. 231, 232). Fibrosarcomas demonstrate no age or sex predilections.

B₄ Monstrocellular (Giant-Cell) Sarcoma. These tumors may be fairly well-delineated (Figs. 233, 238), occasionally resembling a metastasis (Figs. 238, 239). They are fleshy tumors with a fine-tufted, fibrous, and asbestos-like (Figs. 233, 239) cut surface. The variegated color of the glioblastoma is not seen (Fig. 235), the sarcoma being a uniform gray-pink. Nor are the necrosis, fatty degeneration, and hemorrhagic foci of the glioblastoma very evident. They are not infrequently cystic (Figs. 233, 235, 236). Their consistency is firmer than that of the brain itself and may often be termed tough, due to the abundance of reticulin fibers. Monstrocellular sarcomas occur in all age groups and involve all areas of the brain (Fig. 234), perhaps with a certain predilection for the brain stem (Fig. 236). Their malignancy is equivalent to that of the glioblastoma multiforme. Apart from its uniform color this form of sarcoma also differs from the glioblastomas by its massive invasion of the dura (Fig. 239). Metastases into body organs outside of the nervous system are rarely encountered, as is pre- or postoperative diffuse seeding (Fig. 237) of the CSF. In some circles the monstrocellular sarcomas are regarded as mixed tumors, being a variety of glioblastoma multiforme with a sarcomatous component.

B₅ Circumscribed Cerebellar Sarcomas. These are sharply circumscribed (Figs. 240, 241), nodular tumors often spreading over the surface of the cerebellum like a mushroom (Fig. 241) and similar in many respects to a superficial metastasis (Fig. 240). They always occur in the cerebellar hemispheres, are harder than cerebellar tissue, and macroscopic ''total'' removal is often accomplished—however, the remaining adjacent cerebellar tissue is usually infiltrated with tumor so that actual complete excision is rarely achieved. Their firm consistency may be ascribed to the content of reticular fibers. There is no age or sex predilection in contradistinction to the usual medulloblastoma and though the tumor is highly malignant, it is not usually as malignant as the medulloblastoma. There is still discussion as to whether this tumor may be a desmoplastic variant of medulloblastoma, although its location in the cerebellar hemispheres and its particular architectural pattern differs significantly from the medulloblastoma.

B₆ Reticulosarcomas (Reticulum-Cell Sarcomas, Primary Malignant Lymphomas). The true reticulosarcomas have no unique macroscopic features. However, they are well-characterized by their location and their infiltrative growth. They commonly occur in the superior pharynx and neighboring portions of the base of the skull and are commonly seen in the posterior epidural space of the spinal canal. They may also occur as a diffusely-spreading tumor which may condense to more circumscribed lesions inside the brain and cerebellum. There are no predilections as to age or sex of the patients. This latter variety is related in some ways to the "microgliomatosis" of RUSSELL and RUBINSTEIN (1971), and "periadventitial diffuse sarcoma" (see p. 140).

The number of primary sarcomas totalled 283 of 9000 cases or 3.1%, excluding the monstrocellular type which was represented by another 89 cases (∼1%); there was a slight male prevalence both in the total series (211 males, 161 females) and in the monstrocellular subtype (48 male, 41 female). There was no age preference noted.

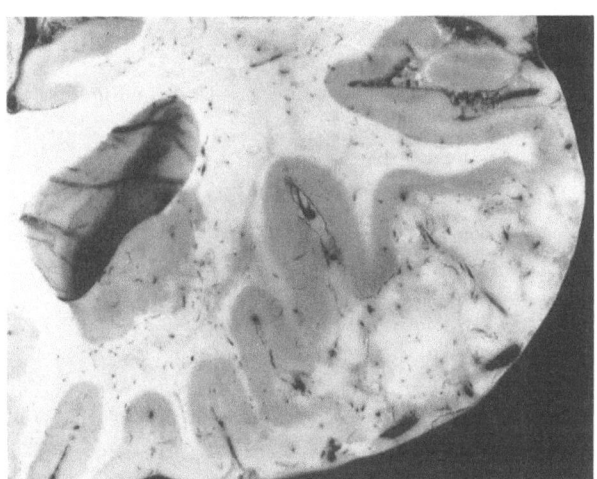

Fig. 227. Sarcomatosis of the meninges. The frontobasal convolutions and gyri are markedly infiltrated

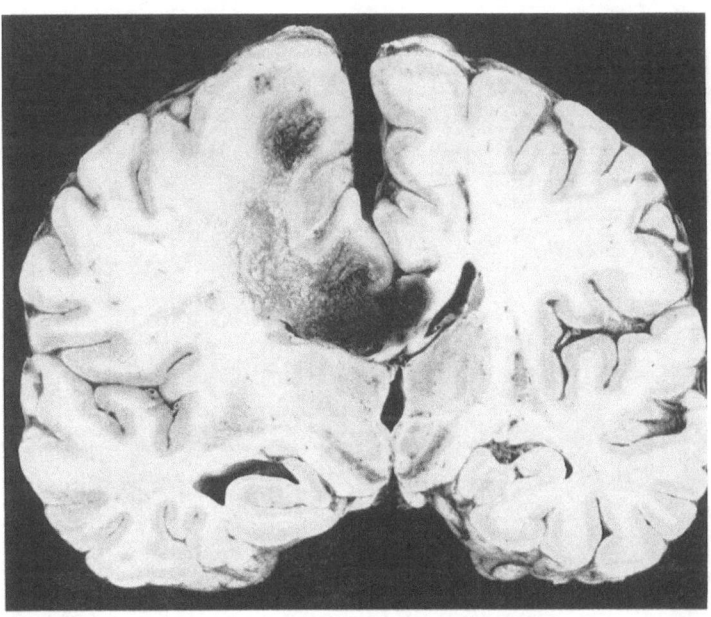

Fig. 228. Typical case of a periadventitial sarcoma predominantly involving the white matter

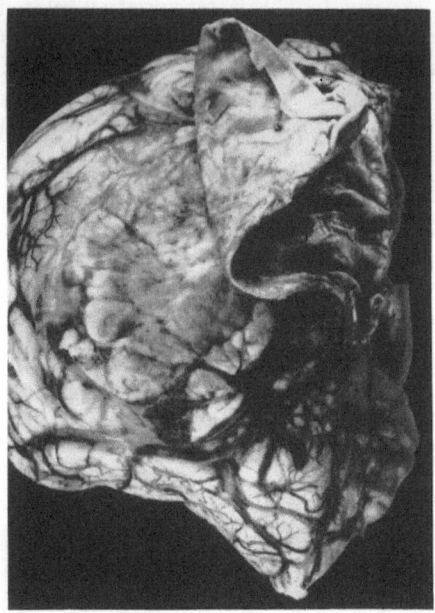

Fig. 229. Large right frontal fibrosarcoma of the dura

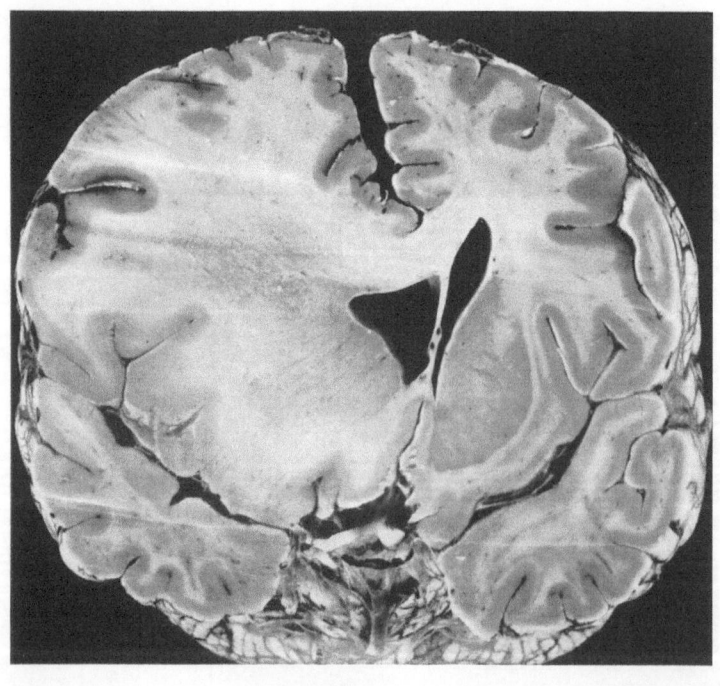

Fig. 230. Marked brain swelling in a case of fibrosarcoma (see Fig. 229)

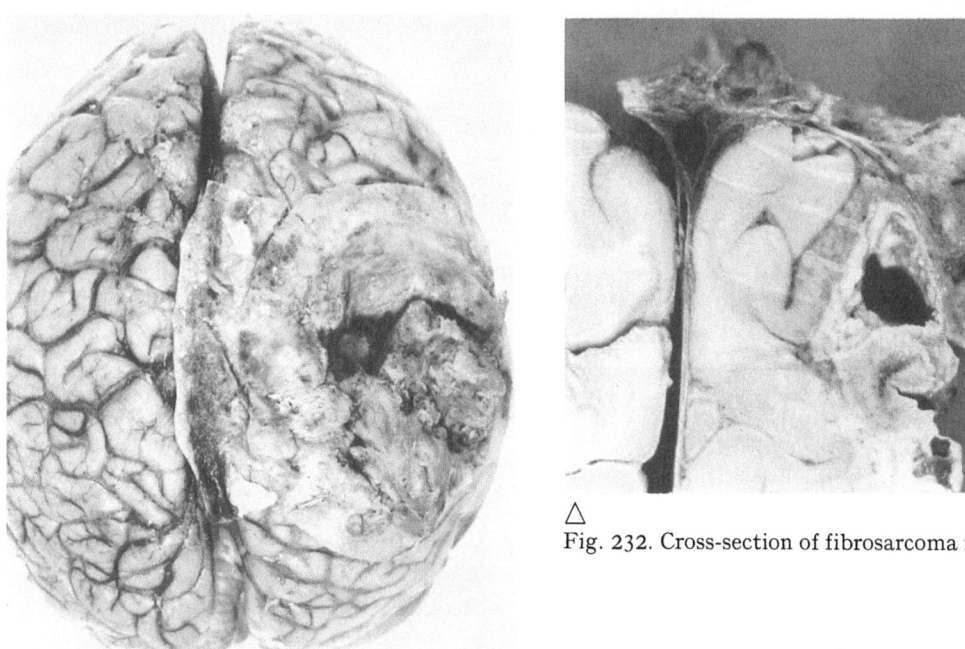

△
Fig. 232. Cross-section of fibrosarcoma in Fig. 231

Fig. 231. Annular fibrosarcomatous growth in the dural cicatrix from a craniotomy 6 years before for a cerebral extraventricular ependymoma. The patient had undergone extensive post-operative radiation therapy (approximately 8000 rad). At autopsy no sign of the primary ependymoma was found

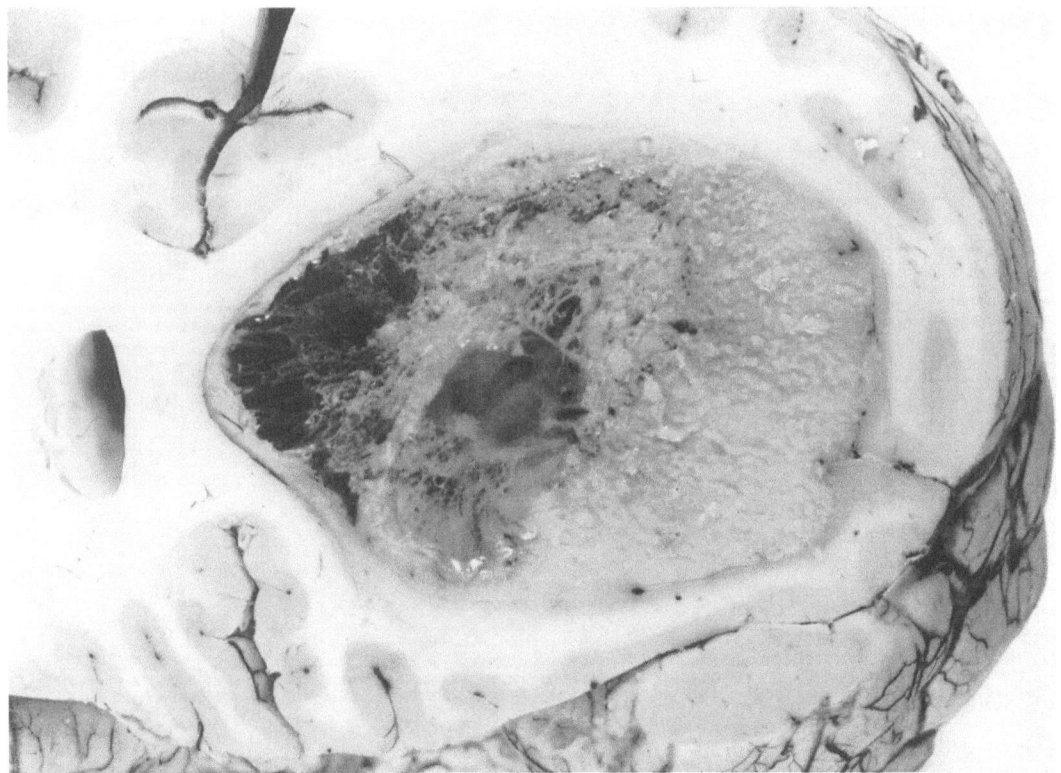

Fig. 233. Egg-sized, well-circumscribed monstrocellular sarcoma with formation of a large cyst. Note the cut surface which typically resembles asbestos

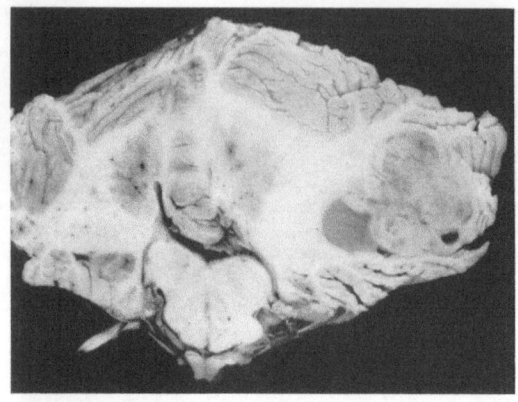

Fig. 234. Partly nodular and partly cystic monstrocellular sarcoma of the cerebellum simulating a metastasis

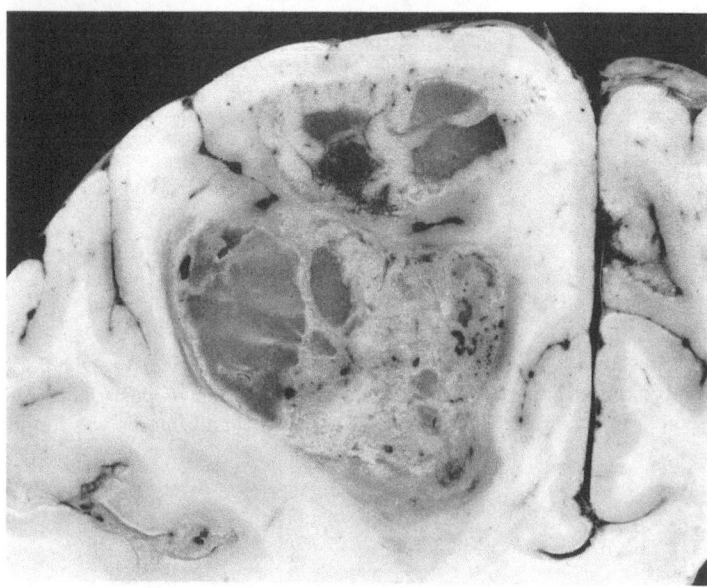

Fig. 235. Enormous, cystic monstrocellular sarcoma of the parietal lobe

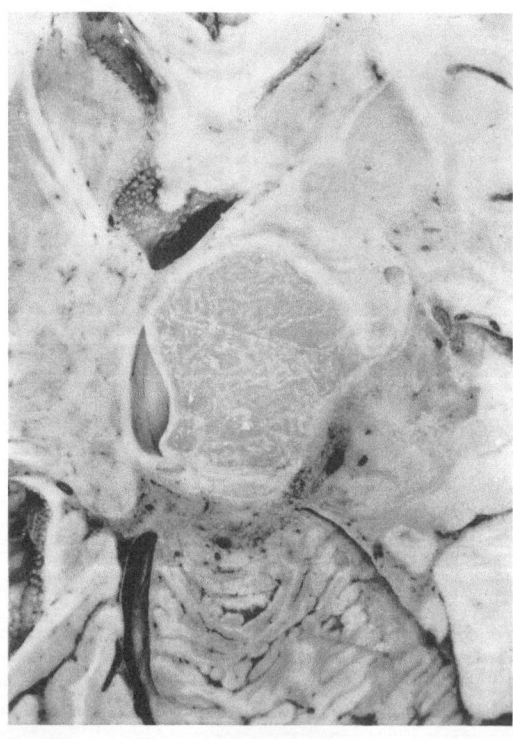

Fig. 236. Monstrocellular sarcoma of the thalamus which has extensively invaded the leptomeninges of the adjacent basal cisterns

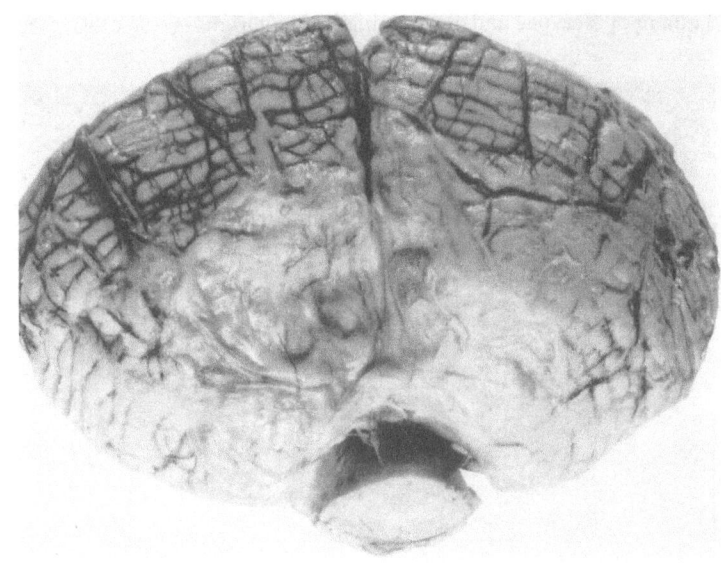

Fig. 237. Diffuse infiltration of the leptomeninges of the basal cisterns in a case of monstrocellular sarcoma

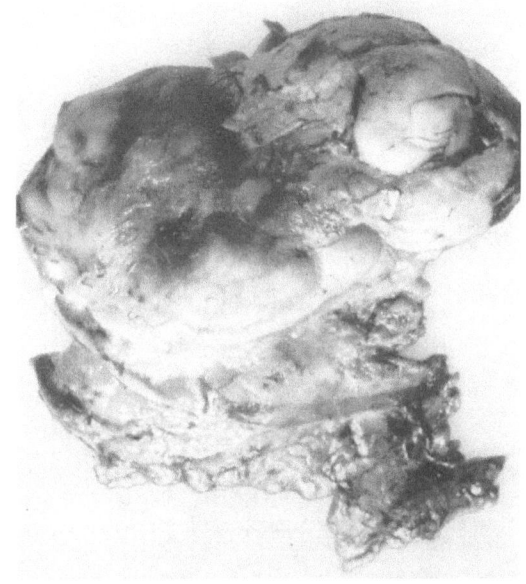

Fig. 238. Surgical specimen of a totally necrotic monstrocellular sarcoma. This necrosis was probably due to a primary ligation of the ipsilateral carotid and later massive irradiation

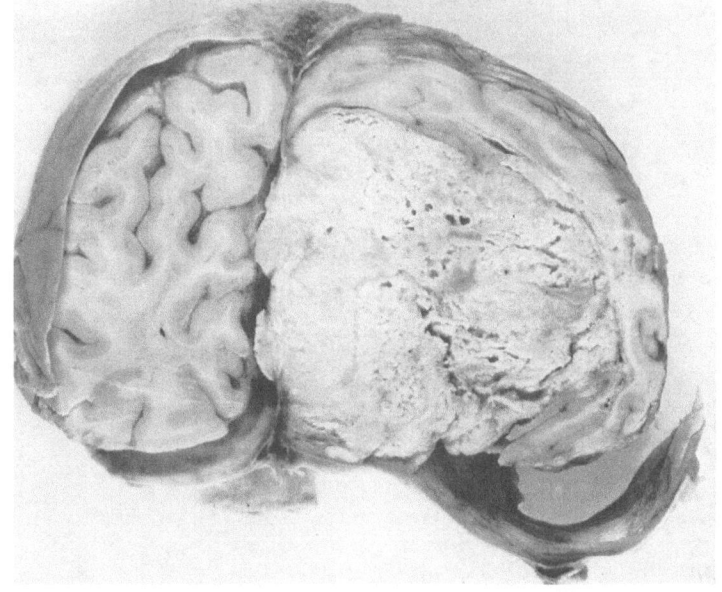

Fig. 239. Huge recurrent monstrocellular sarcoma of the right occipital lobe (c.f. Figs. 237, 238). The falx has been invaded and two small nodules may be seen on its opposite surface. The tumor is totally necrotic, probably secondary to massive repeated irradiation

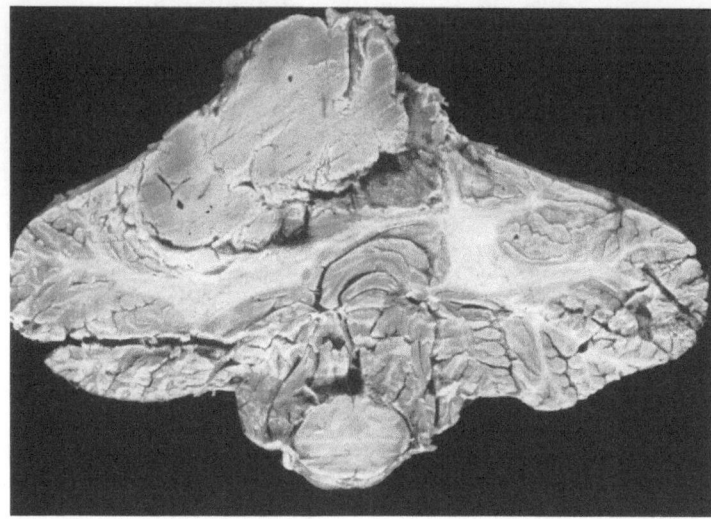

Fig. 240. Large so-called "cerebellar arachnoidal sarcoma" on the external surface of the cerebellar hemisphere

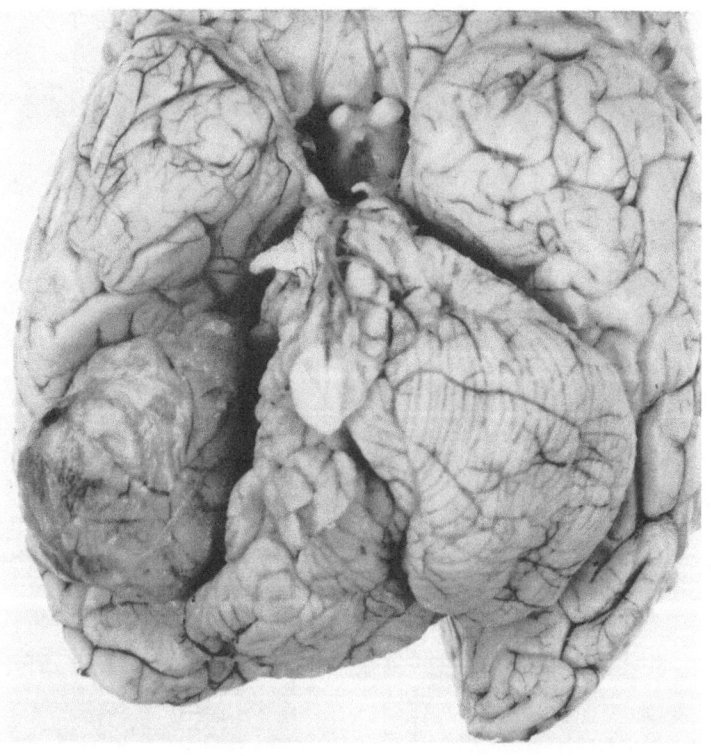

Fig. 241. So-called "cerebellar arachnoidal sarcoma" located in the right hemisphere and sharply demarcated from surrounding brain

1.2.7 Pineal and Pituitary Glands, Craniopharyngeal Duct

The Pinealomas (Germinomas, Embryonal Carcinomas)

Pinealomas lie, rather understandably, in the region of the quadrigeminal plate, except the few examples of true, so-called "ectopic" pinealomas.

They range in size from a hazelnut to a chestnut and grow mainly by expansion, but may infiltrate into the marginal zone. They often appear quite distinctly circumscribed. They compress adjacent anatomical structures, displacing the quadrigeminal plate downward (Figs. 242–245) and later pushing the posterior third of the corpus callosum and the deep central veins (which may well be compromised) upward; the thalami may be shoved to either side by the tumor, thereby gaining access to the caudal portion of the third ventricle. Finally, they may press the superior vermis downward and force themselves beneath the tentorium.

The so-called "ectopic" pinealomas commonly lie in the infundibular region (Fig. 242). There is still much discussion as to whether this particular type is a secondary consequence of the very common seeding of pinealomas within the cerebrospinal fluid stream (Fig. 242), or whether an embryonic rest may be the site of origin. Though this controversy is far from settled, metastases to the infundibular area are well known in medulloblastomas and various authors have shown that an ectopic ("infundibular") pinealoma implant would be perfectly consistent with the principles of general seeding to the third and lateral ventricles from the usual primary site. Ectopic pinealomas of the infundibulum commonly manifest themselves clinically with diabetes insipidus and visual signs.

The classification of the pineal tumors is still under discussion (teratomas, germinomas, dysgerminomas of the pineal region), because of some similarities with cells and architecture of the above-mentioned tumors.

The most common, anisomorphous ("two-cell type") pinealoma is a semimalignant tumor, yet highly sensitive to radiation. "Polymorphous" tumors with a higher malignancy rarely occur. Metastases via the spinal fluid pathways occur to the spinal cord and cauda equina. However, metastases to other portions of the body (lungs) have also been rarely de-scribed. In the same region a highly malignant variant occurs ("pineoblastoma"; Figs. 245, 246) which is very similar to the medulloblastomas (see p. 104ff.).

It is difficult to gain an accurate impression of their incidence. In our collection of 9000 cases they comprise 0.5%, in CUSHING's 0.7% (1932, 1935). However, the figures published by Japanese authors and shown to me during a visit to Japan range up to ten times higher in incidence. Patients with pineal tumors are predominantly males (33 males:15 females, i.e., almost 2:1 in our series). In our own review of 53 cases from the literature, only 9 cases were females. Pinealomas usually make their clinical appearance in the second and third decades, but some of them occur also in the first and fourth decades and even later.

The Pituitary Adenomas

By their intrasellar growth, the pituitary adenomas produce an expansion of the pituitary fossa, so that its dural and bony walls are laterally forced downward towards the sphenoid sinus (Fig. 254) and whereby the dura of the sella may be extremely thinned. Later, the *chromophobe* adenomas may extend upward well beyond the sella and compress the optic tract (Fig. 247) or the caudal portion of the chiasm, depending on the anatomical variations in the form and position of these structures. In still later stages, the chiasm may be displaced anteriorly, or more commonly pushed up and stretched over the tumor, while the carotid arteries are usually displaced laterally. After rupturing the diaphragma sella, the tumor may grow towards the floor of the third ventricle and may even occupy its lumen (Fig. 250). The chiasm, if sufficiently displaced, can be cut into by the overlying anterior communicating artery, while the constricting effect of the chiasm can produce an indentation or "waist" in the tumor itself. The larger adenomas may grow around both carotids or may extend anteriorly into the frontal fossa (Fig. 247) or laterally toward the temporal lobes (Fig. 248), while extension in the direction of the paranasal sinuses is usually less pronounced. There are exceptional cases where the suprasellar growth is so much more marked than the intrasellar component, that the chiasm is compressed without any gross change in the sella. On the other hand, the *eosinophilic* adenomas (Fig. 249) generally produce marked clinical (endocrine) changes before they reach the chiasm. Large, space-occupying tumors, therefore, usually belong to the chromophobe type (Fig. 251), while *basophilic* tumors are both extremely rare and rarely of any significant size or concern to the neurosurgeon. The pituitary adenomas appear well-encapsulated (Fig. 251) and range in size from that of a plum (Fig. 252) to that a child's fist (Fig. 250). Sometimes they are quite nodular (Figs. 253, 256). The eosinophilic adenomas, because of frequent hemorrhages into the tumor, often have a brownish color. The capsule of the tumor is quite tough, whereas its contents are commonly so soft that they can be removed with a surgical sucker. The adenomata grow into the brain purely by expansion and their capsule (Fig. 251) can be freely removed from the adjacent structures. Characteristic is the tendency toward degeneration of the tumor tissue which leads to the formation of smaller or larger cysts. This is very common in the chromophobe tumors, where almost the entire tumor can consist of a cyst. Very rare is an extension in the diploe of the base of the skull (Figs. 255, 256) from which the tumor surfaces by forming large nodules (Fig. 253). Space occupying pituitary adenomas comprised 6.6% of intracranial tumors in our collection of 9000 cases. In CUSHING's series (1932, 1935), because of the particular interest of the author, they occurred with a disproportionately high frequency of 17.8%. Of CUSHING's 338 cases, there were 260 chromophobe, 67 eosinophilic adenomas and 11 "adenocarcinomas". Of our patients with pituitary tumors, 336 were males and 260 females. Pituitary adenomas practically never occur under the age of 20 and tend to increase in frequency only in subsequent years. The peak of the age curve (see p. 46) lies around 37–55 years. The age incidence of the three types is roughly the same. Most of the adenomas are benign and only seldom show malignancy.

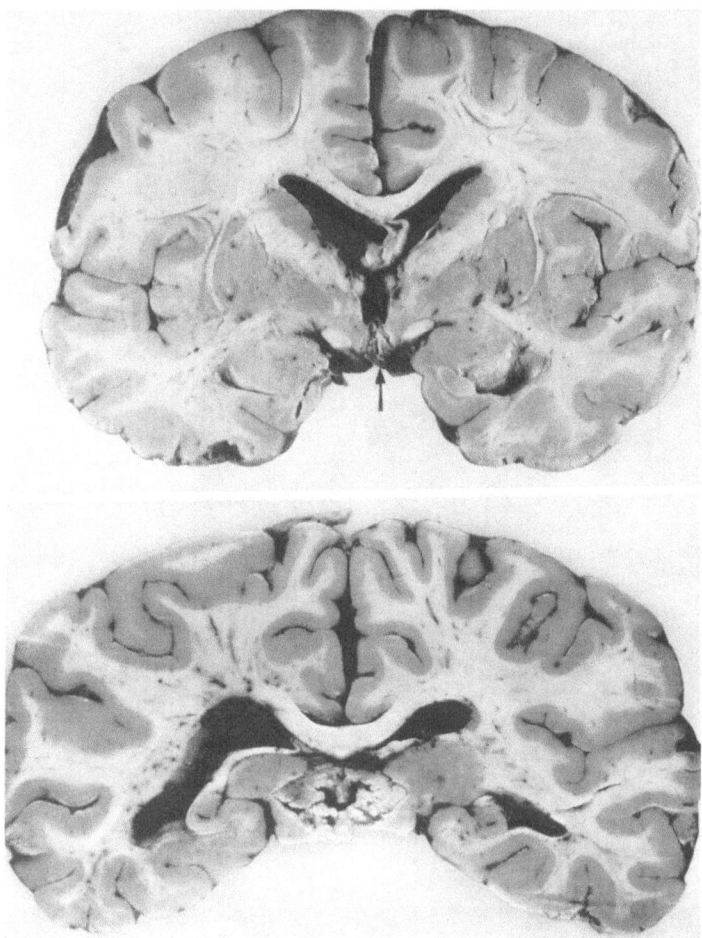

Fig. 242. Typical pinealoma with metastasis via the spinal fluid to the infundibular recess (arrow!)

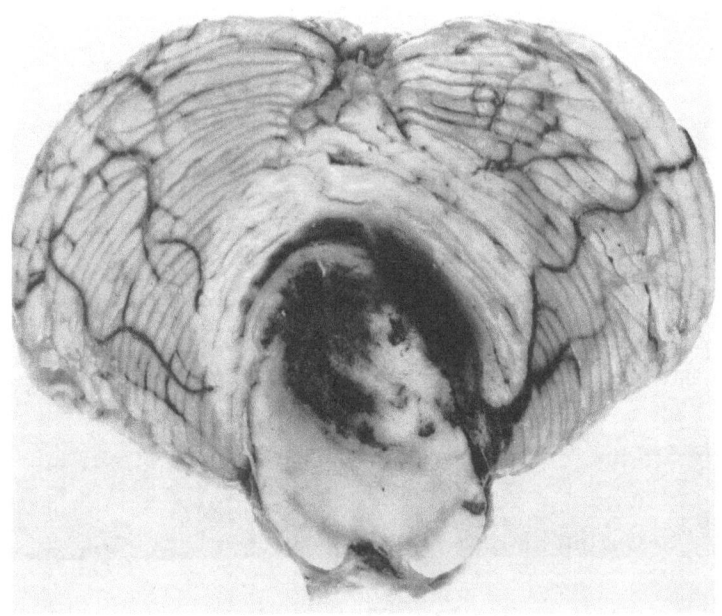

Fig. 243. Anisomorphous pinealoma with extension into the subtentorial brainstem. Note the hemorrhages into the tumor mass

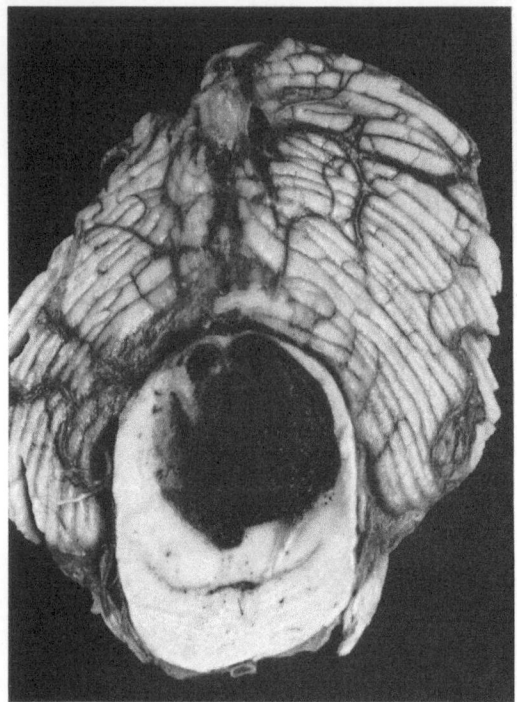

Fig. 244. Well-circumscribed anisomorphous pinealoma displacing midbrain and pons

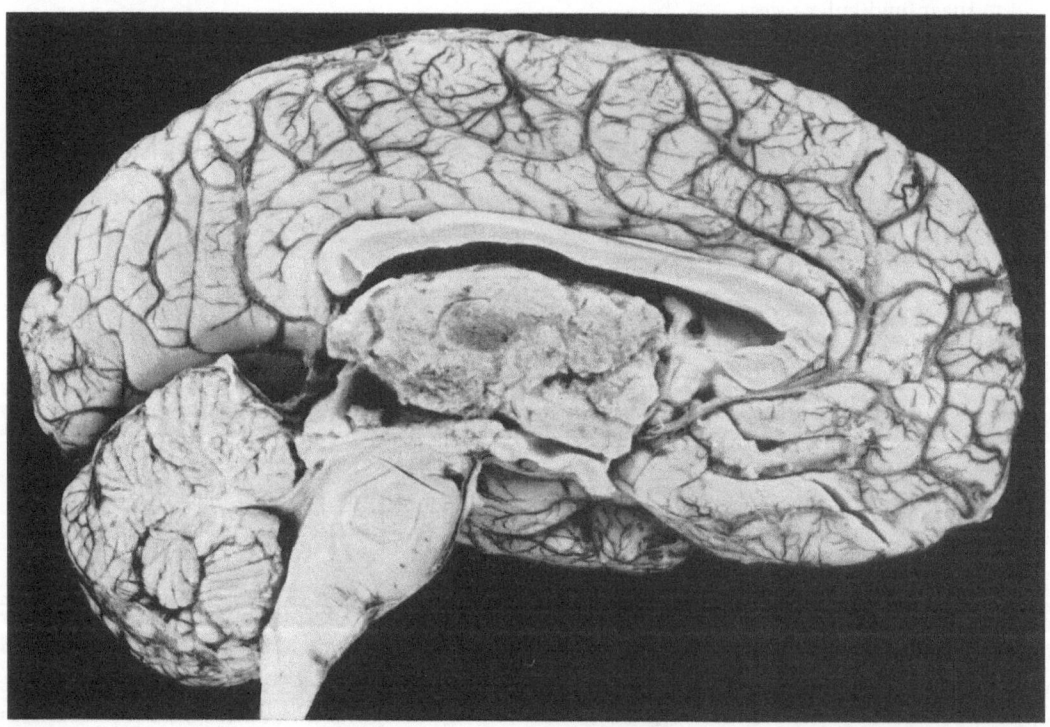

Fig. 245. Huge malignant pineoblastoma (similar to the medulloblastoma) in an 11 year old girl

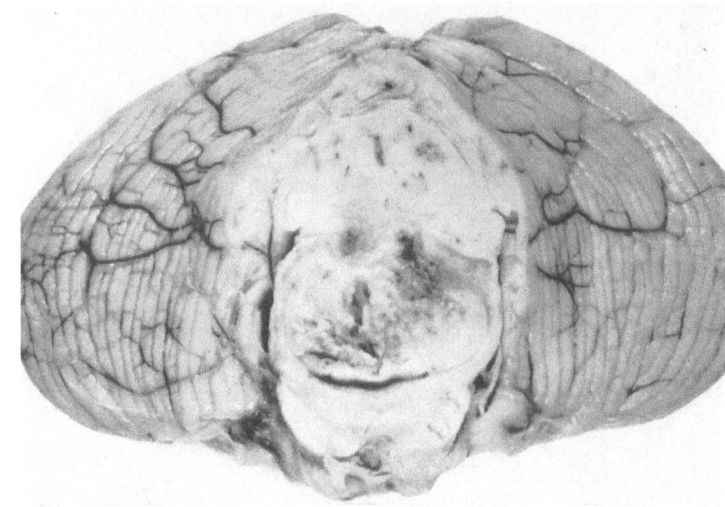

Fig. 246. Typical malignant pineoblastoma ("medullo-blastoma-like") which seems well-marginated, yet has histologically infiltrated the cerebellum

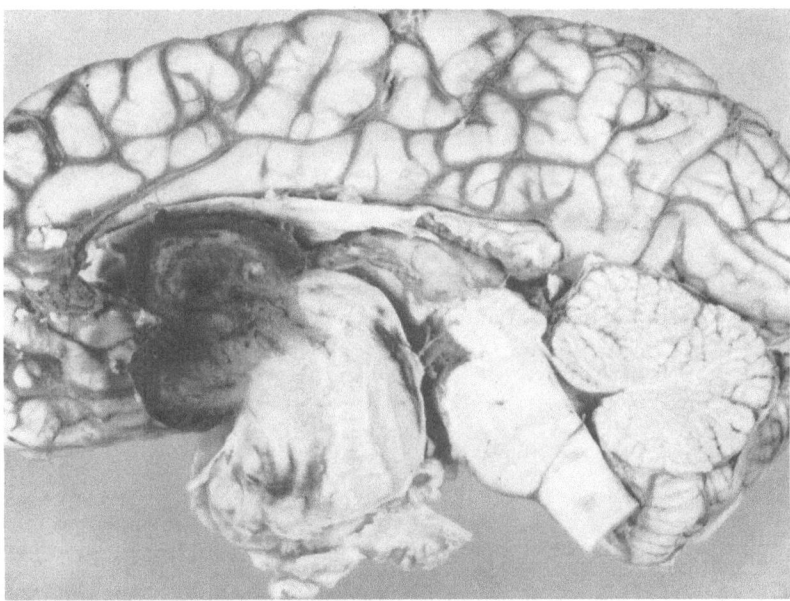

Fig. 247. Huge chromophobe adenoma which was surgically treated. Hemorrhages in the anterior portion of the tumor are noted secondary to surgery. An overt indentation in tumor substance by the chiasm is seen

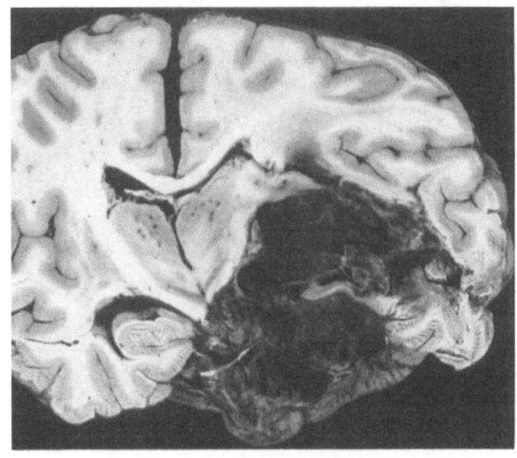

Fig. 248. Large pituitary chromophobe adenoma with hemorrhage formation which has extended predominantly into one temporal lobe

151

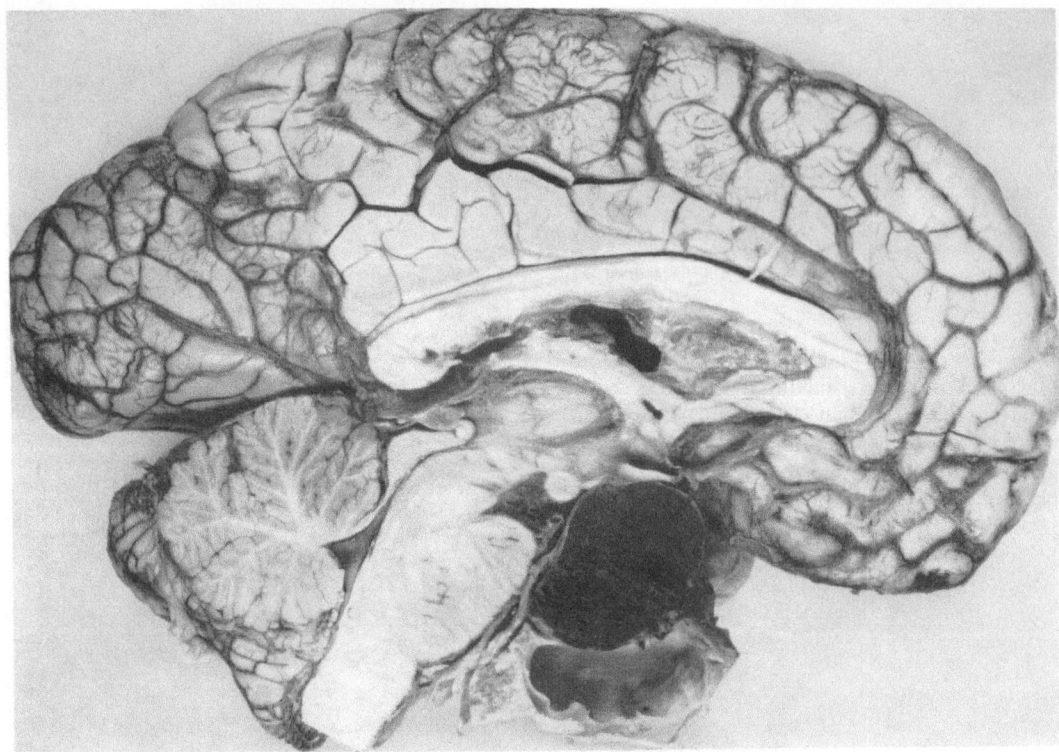

Fig. 249. Eosinophilic adenoma with diffuse intraparenchymatous hemorrhages. This lent a brownish-black color to the tumor at autopsy

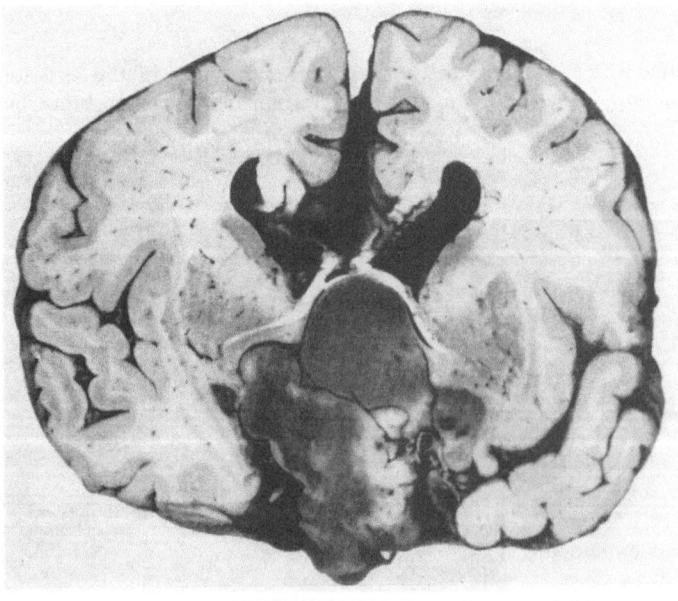

Fig. 250. Enormous chromophobe adenoma of pituitary which has extended mainly into the region of the third ventricle and has also impinged on both temporal lobes by way of nodular growth

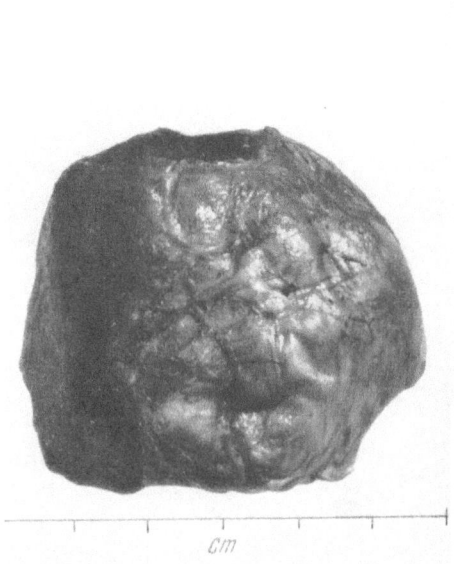

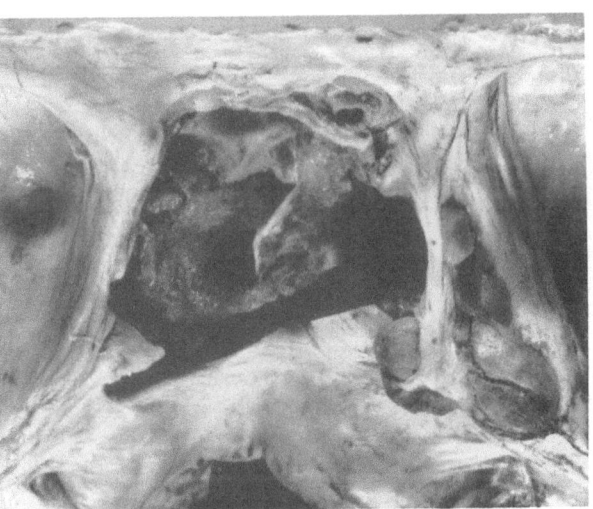

Fig. 251. Very large, well-encapsulated, cystic chromophobe adenoma, which was surgically removed

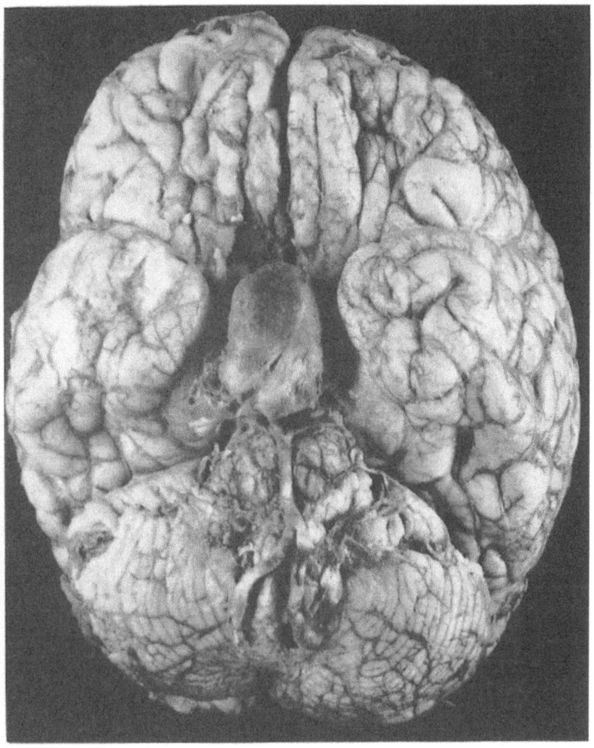

Fig. 252. Eosinophilic adenoma. Note the diffuse hemorrhages

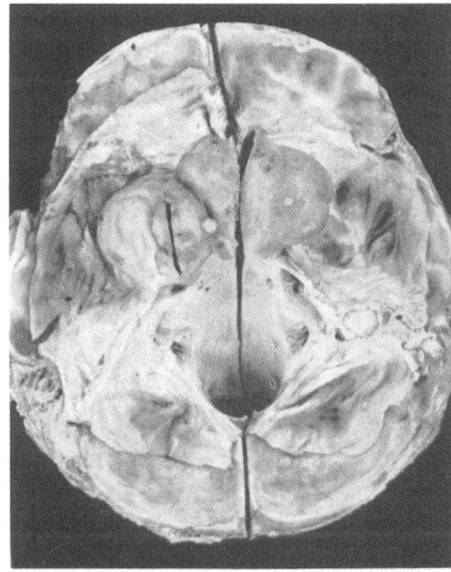

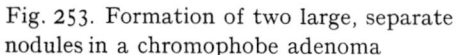

Fig. 253. Formation of two large, separate nodules in a chromophobe adenoma

Fig. 254. Subdural extension of a chromophobe adenoma which has penetrated the dura along perforating nerves and vessels and also partially infiltrated the brain substance (very rare!)

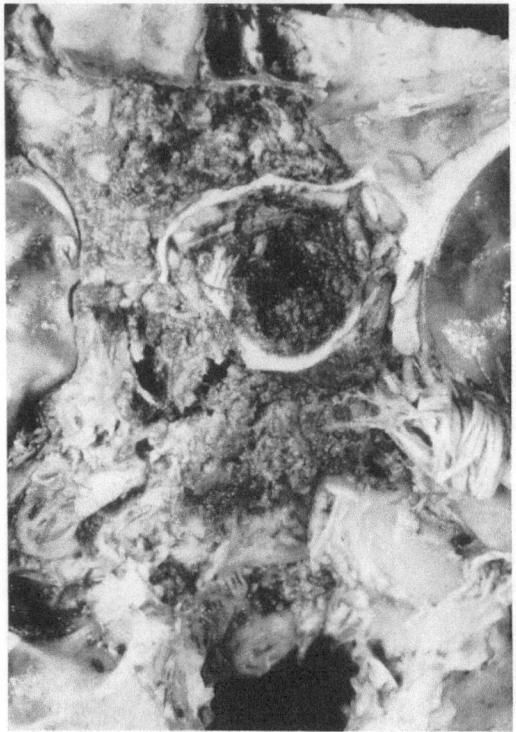

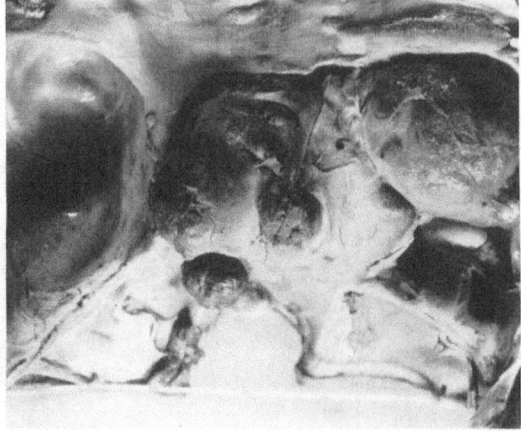

Fig. 255. Diffuse subdural growth of a chromophobe adenoma into the diploe of the base of the skull. The margins included the crista galli, the foramen magnum and both middle fossae

Fig. 256. Chromophobe pituitary adenoma with many nodules which are involving the dura at the base of the brain (c.f. Figs. 254, 255)

The Craniopharyngiomas (Hypophyseal Duct Tumors, Erdheim Tumors, Adamantinoma of Pituitary Region)

The craniopharyngiomas occur exclusively in the region of the sella, varying only in their relationship to the diaphragma sellae and in their direction of spread from this point. Thus, there are both intrasellar and suprasellar craniopharyngiomas (Fig. 257). At first, the intrasellar types are separated from the brain by the dura of the sella and the overlying arachnoid. As they grow, however, they push the diaphragma upward—generally breaking through it—and tend to bulge into the third ventricle (Fig. 258) from below. They may also extend into the interpeduncular fossa and in the direction of the pons (Fig. 259). They are well-encapsulated tumors, which grow purely by expansion. Their size varies from that of a peanut to that of a walnut (Figs. 258, 265) and at times may reach the size of a tennis-ball (Figs. 261–263). The tumor has a tough and tenacious consistency and can be rather hard in areas, particularly—as is so often the case—where calcification has occurred.

The suprasellar type originates in the arachnoid surrounding the pituitary stalk and adjacent cisterns and expands in the direction of the third ventricle (Fig. 257), whose place the tumor may eventually occupy (Fig. 260). The ventricular floor thus may become paper-thin in both the intra- and suprasellar types and may tear, so that the tumor capsule abuts directly against the ventricular wall and the adjacent structures. The relationship of the craniopharyngiomas to the chiasm may also vary. Some tumors displace it antero-superiorly, stretching it into a thin band; others, from the beginning, develop above the chiasm (Fig. 260) and force it downward; still others lie, so to speak, "in the lumen" of the third ventricle (Figs. 265, 266) and can scarcely be seen at the base of the brain. The matter of utmost concern for the neurosurgeon, however, is the fact that the capsule may be closely adherent to the optic nerve and chiasm, to the leptomeninges (where the vessels to the hypothalamus run, originating from the posterior communicating artery), and to the ventricular wall as a result of "scarring" secondary to reactive gliosis—a scar which sometime reaches the thickness of a few millimeters. This scarring

results from the fact that practically every craniopharyngioma forms cysts of degeneration (Figs. 258, 261, 264) filled with a cholesterol-containing fluid content which excites a marked inflammatory reaction within the adjacent structures as well as in the cerebrospinal fluid.

Depending on the extent of the degenerative changes, cyst size may vary considerably with some craniopharyngiomas (Fig. 258) being almost entirely cystic (only a small, cherry-sized solid part remaining) (Fig. 267). In fact, occasionally primary craniopharyngeal cysts are encountered that do not form a solid tumor at all. In most cases the cystic portion is situated anteriorly (with the solid part inferior) and is filled with a thick, brownish-yellow fluid (like motor oil) in which small glistening cholesterol crystals are suspended, the latter being type-specific for this tumor.

Also important is the tumor's relationship to the pituitary gland which will be compressed and flattened out against the floor of the pituitary fossa by the intrasellar type. The floor of the sella may be markedly eroded and its lateral walls (abutting on the cavernous sinus) extremely thinned. On the other hand, the suprasellar craniopharyngiomas often leave the hypophysis and the bony sella almost untouched.

Larger tumors can expand to either side and displace portions of the frontal (Fig. 261) or temporal lobes (Fig. 263) similar to the pituitary adenomas.

The craniopharyngiomas can definitely be considered tumors of childhood and adolescence, where they comprise the most common tumor in the region of the chiasm, but they do occur in adults as well (p. 47). CUSHING (1932, 1935) had two patients over 60 years of age and we have had similar experiences. In our series of 9000 cases they comprised 2.1% of all tumors, in CUSHING's 4.6%. There is a certain preponderance of the male sex with a ratio of around 3:2 (116 males and 69 females in our series).

Recurrences are likely if the tumor is not completely removed. However, the rate of growth is very slow. Metastases of true craniopharyngiomas are quite rare. Malignant degeneration has not been sufficiently documented yet.

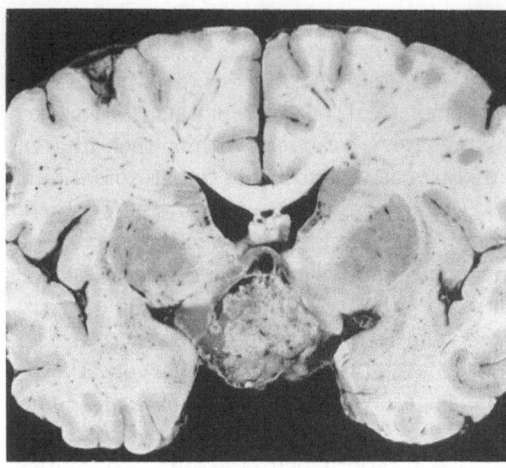

Fig. 257. Predominantly suprachiasmatic cranio-pharyngioma with only a moderate degree of cyst formation

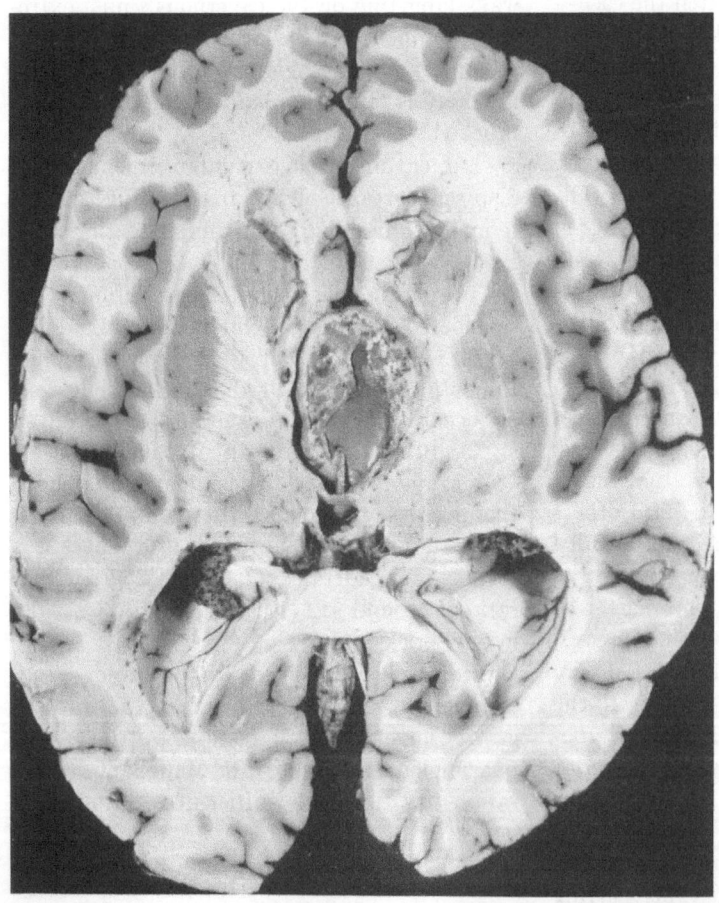

Fig. 258. Large craniopharyngioma, which has extended into the third ventricle with resultant obstructive hydrocephalus

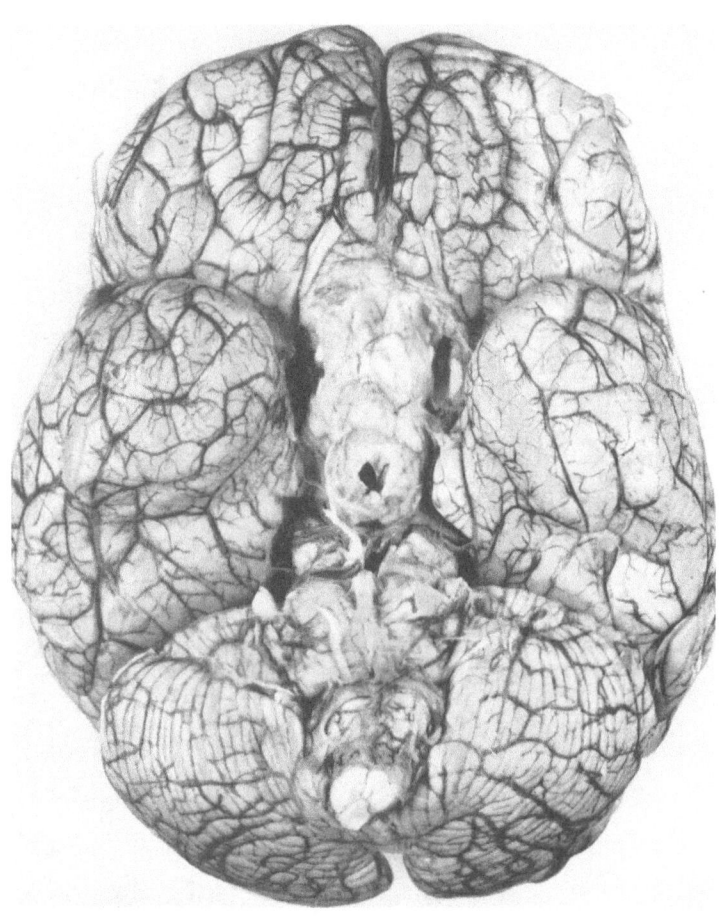

Fig. 259. Suprasellar extension of intrasellar craniopharyngioma. The chiasm was displaced superiorly and anteriorly. Both olfactory nerves were displaced laterally

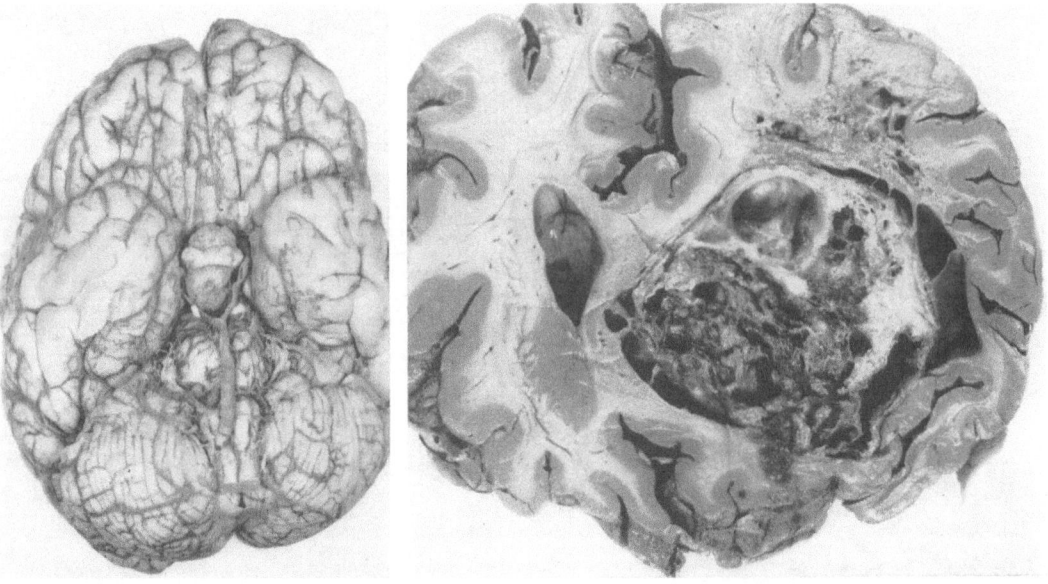

Fig. 260. Craniopharyngioma which arose in the parasellar and suprasellar regions

Fig. 261. Huge suprachiasmatic craniopharyngioma which has extended into the right frontal lobe. Cystic degeneration has taken place in the tumor. A second area of cyst formation in the white matter above the tumor was probably caused by edema

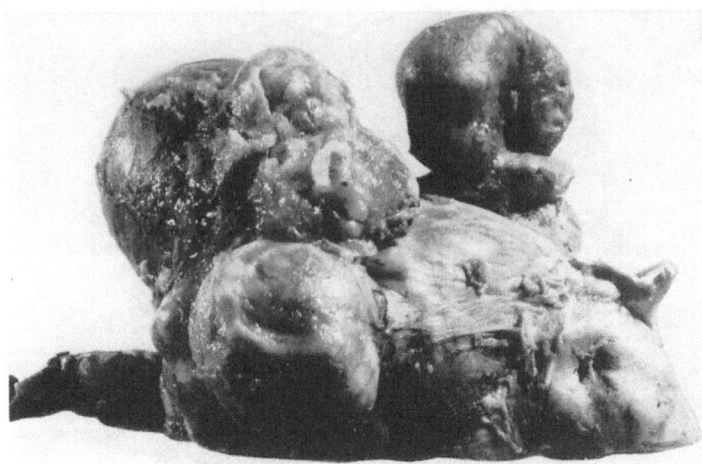

Fig. 262. The left half of the giant craniopharyngioma of Fig. 263 is seen here

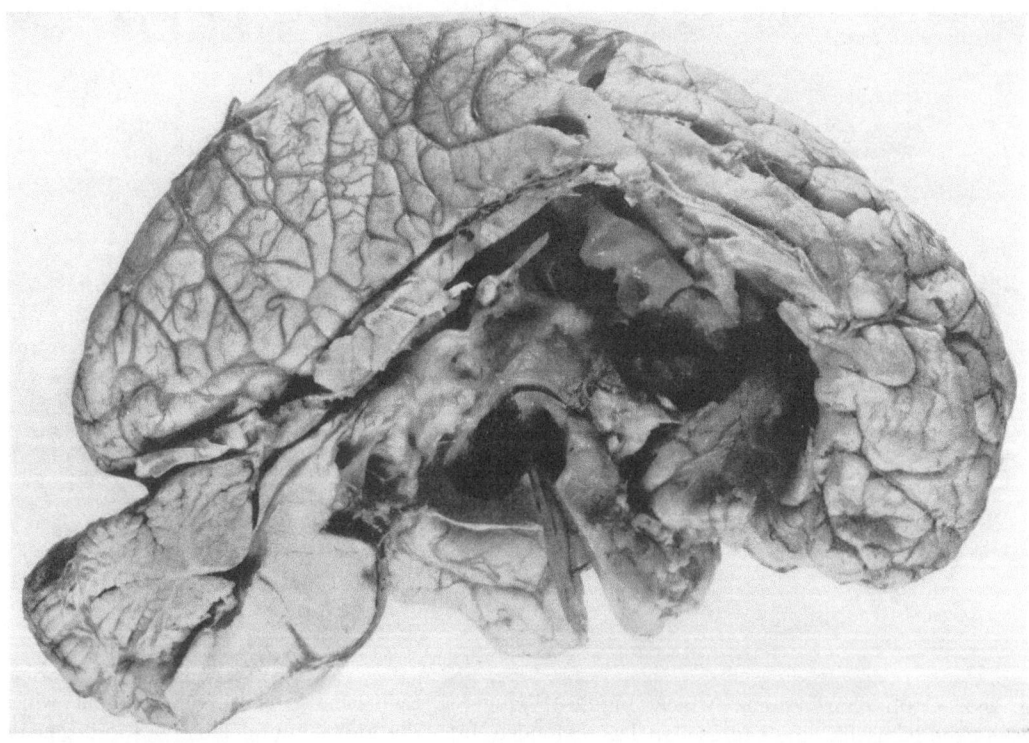

Fig. 263. Left hemisphere of a mental hospital patient (severe intellectual impairment). A fist-sized craniopharyngioma (see Fig. 262) was found at autopsy. The defect after tumor removal is shown above

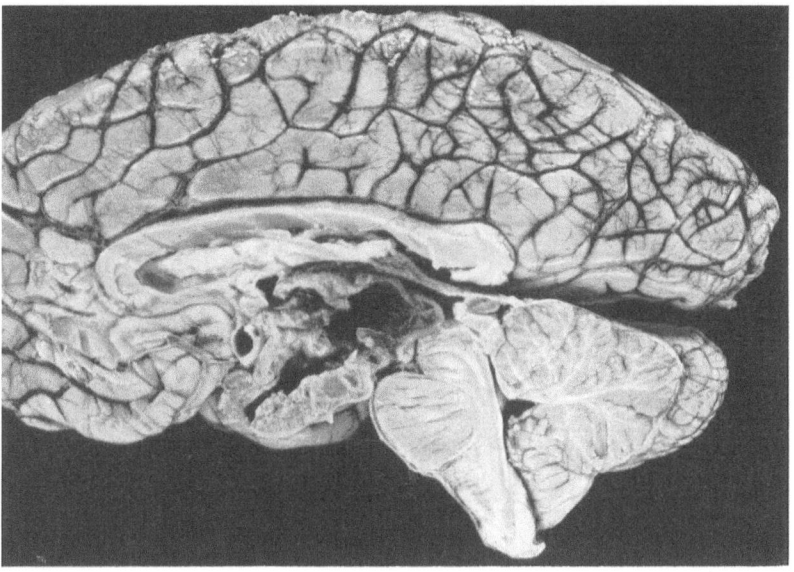

Fig. 264. Typical, partially cystic craniopharyngioma of large size, which has extended to the anterior border of the pons and the posterior portions of the third ventricle

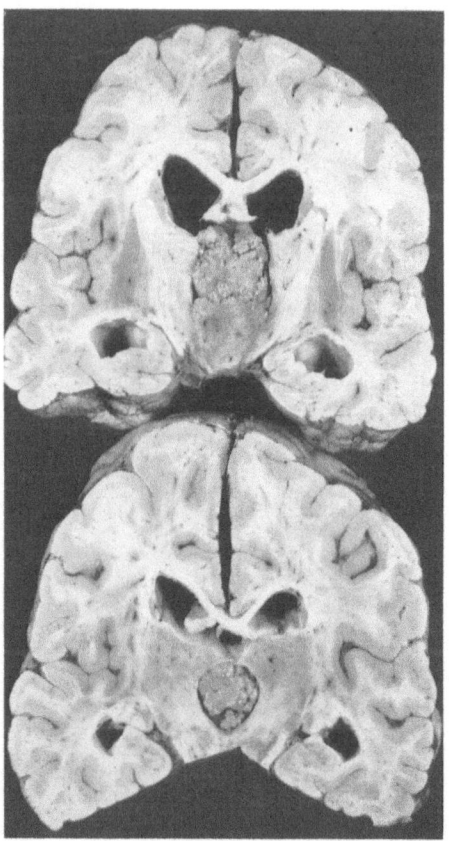

Fig. 265. Large intraventricular suprasellar craniopharyngioma in a 59 year old patient

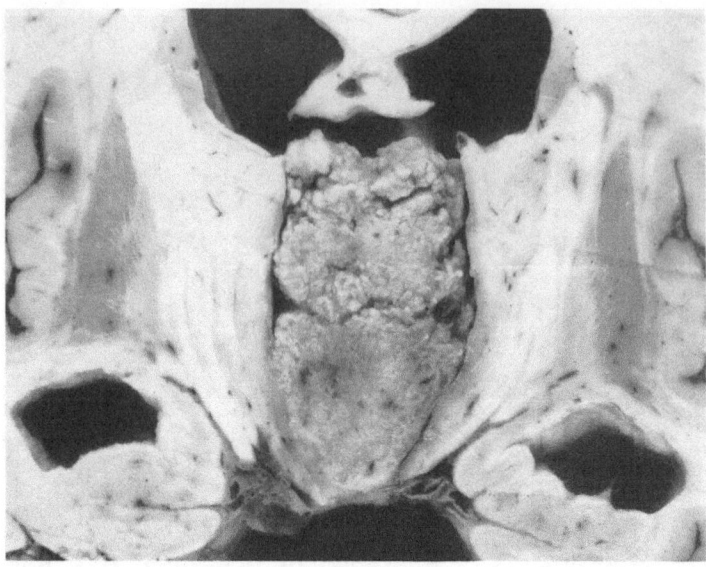

Fig. 266. Close-up view of Fig. 265

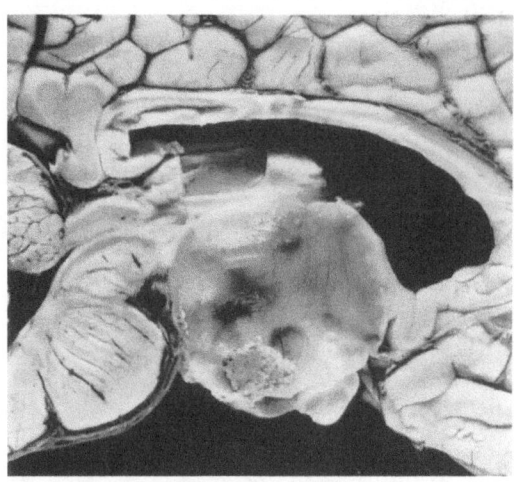

Fig. 267. Almost total cystic degeneration of a large craniopharyngioma. A mural nodule is seen at the base of the cyst

1.2.8 Paraganglia

The Glomus Jugulare Tumors
(Chemodectomas, Paragangliomas)

These tumors arise in the glomus jugulare but tend to invade the tympanic cavity of the middle ear quite early; in fact, the most common presentation is at the outer meatus acusticus. They may, however, extend into the region of the tip of the petrous bone or mastoid process and cause erosion of bone in these areas. They can surround the structures at the jugular foramen and extend extradurally into the posterior fossa; or, after causing much destruction in the neck near the foramen magnum, may invade the middle fossa. In even rarer cases invasion of the dura has occurred. Glomus tumors are very vascular and their presence can be demonstrated angiographically. The glomus tumors are seen between adolescence and senescence with a predilection for the fiftieth year. The tumor seems to grow slowly and there are no well-documented reports of metastases.

1.2.9 Dysembryogenetic
or Malformative Tumors

Teratomas, Epidermoids, Dermoids

Teratomas in the intracranial cavity vary in size from a pinhead to a child's fist.

They are nodular (Fig. 268) and encapsulated with a brownish-red color and have dark colored cysts on the surface. The cyst fluid may be yellow and clear, more commonly dark brown or greenish. They are usually hard, almost cartilage-like, and are occasionally calcified or criss-crossed by bony spicules. Their sites of predilection are the pineal region (almost half of the cases) and the hypophyseal region (about one fourth (Fig. 269), the remaining sites include cerebellum, spinal cord, lateral ventricles. The majority of these tumors are discovered in childhood or adolescence. In some instances malignancy has been noted.

The majority of teratomas grow extremely slowly and are benign; small ones may be found incidentally. The tumors in the mesencephalic and diencephalic regions are of neurosurgical importance. Our definition of teratomas, in contrast to other authors, corresponds to that of the general pathologist—i.e., formations from two ("teratoids") or three germ layers (true teratomas).

Epidermoids and Dermoids ("Pearly Tumor"). *Epidermoids* are space-occupying lesions containing a cholesteatomatous material with an external capsule made up of the three layers of the epidermis; they are, however, quite rare and are found in the arachnoidal spaces or in the diploë. The capsule consists of a delicate, transparent membrane (Fig. 270) through which one can see its pearly-white contents. The epidermoid may be firmly adherent to its surroundings because of a focal sterile meningitis and encephalitis produced by the irritative effect of the cholesteatomatous material.

When located in the ventricles (Fig. 271) or in the subarachnoid space at the base of the brain (Fig. 272), they are particularly prone to rupture and to extrude their contents into the cerebrospinal fluid, causing a marked chemical meningitis (Fig. 273).

Epidermoids preferentially occur at the following sites:

Cerebellopontine angle or parapontine (Fig. 272).

Chiasmal region or parapituitary.

Longitudinal fissure and anterior corpus callosum.

Around the quadrigeminal plate and posterior corpus callosum (Fig. 271).

Sylvian fissure.

Lateral ventricle.

Fourth ventricle and midline cerebellum.

Diploë of the skull.

Spinal cord.

The most frequent localizations are in the cerebellopontine angle (Fig. 272), in the supra- and parasellar regions, in the lateral and fourth ventricles, and in the quadrigeminal region (Fig. 271).

They are readily recognized by their whitish, shining, mother-of-pearl capsule (Fig. 270) and may be smooth, lobulated or knobby, with daughter nodules. The blood vessels run in the capsule. Upon sectioning, the contents consist of shining masses of friable, leafy material arranged in layers like onion-skin. The inside is occasionally soft.

161

The *dermoids* differ from the epidermoids in that they contain the accessory structures of skin: the dermis with hair follicles, hairs, sebaceous glands and sometimes sweat glands and their secretions.

The *dermoids* are particularly apt to lie around the pituitary, the pons, or along embryonic closure lines (Fig. 274). They are most common along the line of closure between the maxillae and the orbits (the embryonic naso-optic furrow) and may actually grow into one orbit; they are also encountered along the posterior fossa midline and in the sacral region. Neurosurgically, the most important dermoids are those of the neck (which penetrate all the way to the dorsal raphé of the cerebellum), those of the face (orbito-ethmoidal dermoids), and those in the region of the cauda equina. It is important to recognize that both dermoids and epidermoids can "melt" the adjacent parenchyma by setting up an inflammatory reaction; an epidermoid cyst of the fourth ventricle, for example, may have a broad connection with the cerebellopontine angle through the lateral recess, or an orbito-ethmoidal dermoid can dissect into the anterior horn of the lateral ventricle. The sizes of both der-

moids and epidermoids vary from that of a pinhead to that of an orange; however, the dermoids have a firm pod or shell and are generally filled with a greasy, soapy mass containing numerous short hairs.

The age curve of the epidermoids and dermoids shows a definite peak around the age of 40. In our material, it lies between 25 and 40 (the time of operation or autopsy); in the curve representing the age of onset of symptoms, however, the peak lies around the age of 15. These are, therefore, very slow-growing tumors. In CUSHING's material (1932, 1935) the epidermoids and dermoids comprised 0.7%; in our own series of 9000 cases, the epidermoids formed 1.5% and dermoids 0.1%. FINDEISEN and TÖNNIS (1937) found 48 cases of epidermoids among 5185 intracranial tumors—i.e., 0.9%. Dermoids are less frequent. The total number of epidermoids, dermoids and teratomas comprised 166 out of 9000 cases, i.e. 1.8% with an almost equal representation of both sexes (83 males versus 83 females). The epidermoids and dermoids are benign tumors. Carcinomatous degeneration occurs only in rare exceptions.

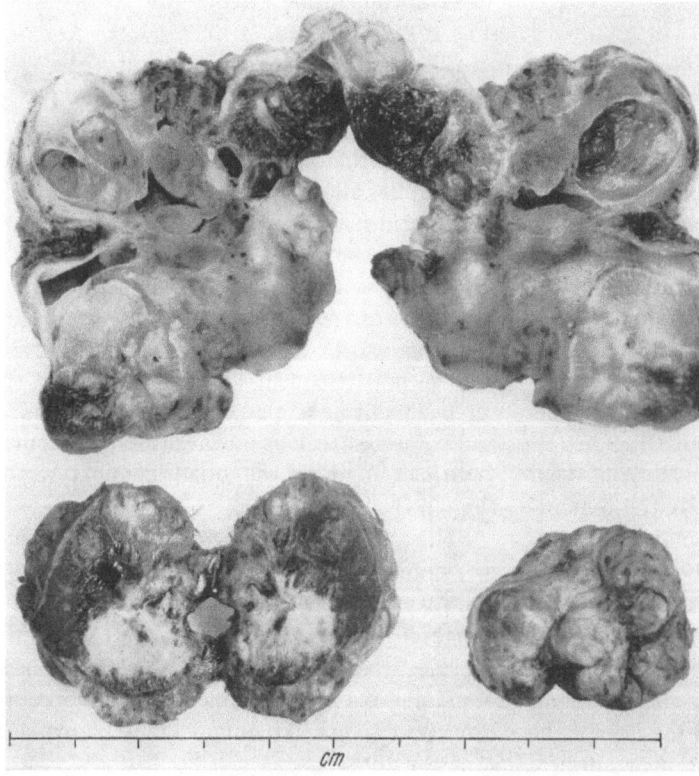

Fig. 268. *Above:* Huge, surgically-excised parasellar teratoma showing multiple small cysts. *Below:* Surgically removed teratoma of the pineal gland

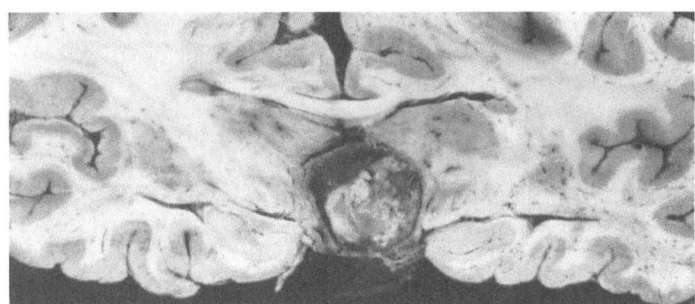

Fig. 269. Chestnut-sized teratoma of the chiasmatic region,
which was diagnosed as a
craniopharyngioma during
operation

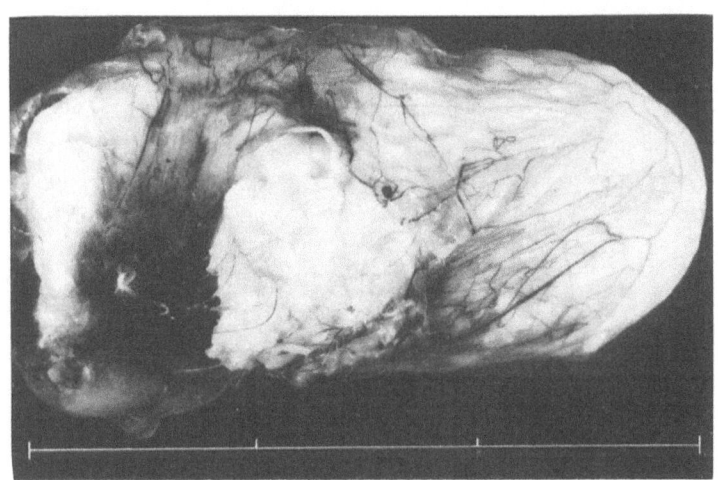

Fig. 270. Completely-excised
epidermoid demonstrating the
fine and delicate surface vessels of the capsule

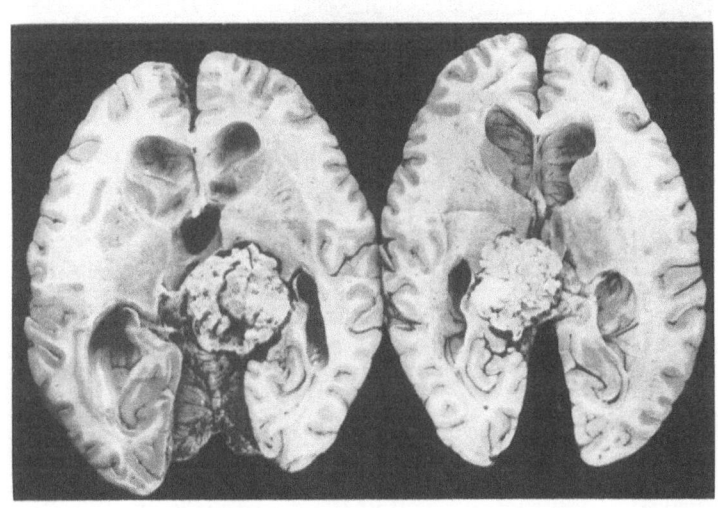

Fig. 271. Tangerine-sized epidermoid of the quadrigeminal
region which has ruptured into
the trigone

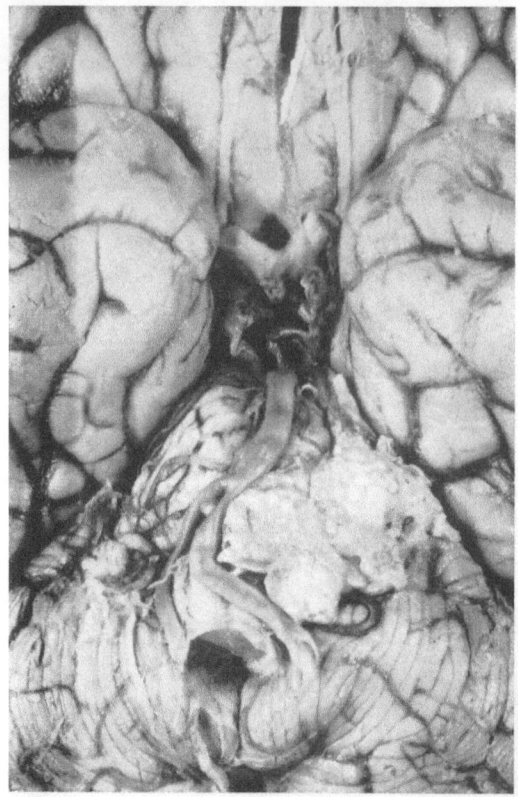

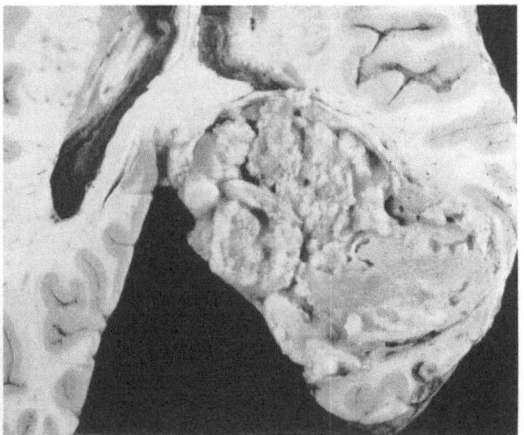

Fig. 272. Plaque-like epidermoid (cholesteatoma) in the left cerebellopontine angle with displacement of the pons and vertebro-basilar system

Fig. 273. Large epidermoid which originated in the falx and ruptured into the right medial occipital lobe. Note the contents of the cyst

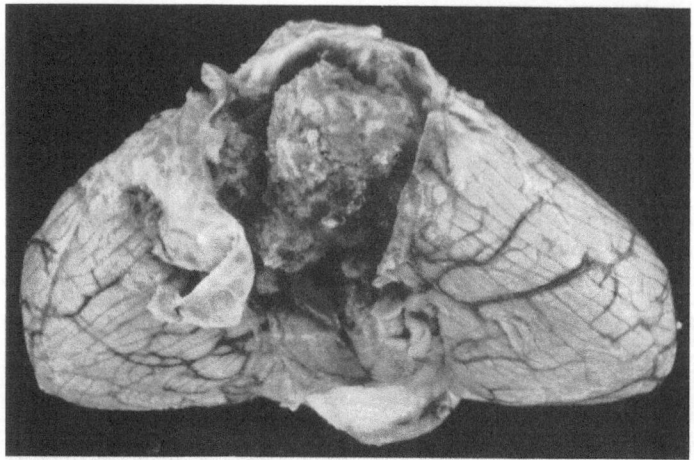

Fig. 274. Egg-sized dermoid cyst of the cerebellar midline which was partly calcified

1.2.10 Mesenchymal Tumors

The Chordomas

The chordomas are rare tumors (around 0.2% of our series) and vary in size from that of a little grain to that of a man's fist. In the pelvis they can attain the size of a child's head by developing antero-posteriorly. They are whitish-pink in color, translucent and gelatinous, or (after hemorrhages) brownish-red. Their surface is finely nodular or, occasionally, they may even be broken up into larger nodular segments. With rare exceptions chordomas are midline tumors occurring at the base of the skull—subsellar or on the clivus—from where they expand causing much bone destruction in the direction of the nasopharynx, the chiasm, or the foramen magnum (clivus chordomas). Spinal chordomas are found predominantly in the vicinity of the dens of the axis and in the sacrococcygeal region. The latter location and the clivus are most frequently involved. They are generally clinically present in the third and fourth decades, only the sacrococcygeal chordomas manifesting themselves earlier. Males are affected three times more frequently than females. Although they are usually slow-growing

and benign tumors, malignant degeneration occurs not unfrequently. They rarely metastasize.

The Chondromas

The chondromas are whitish-pink tumors (Fig. 275), hard and firm in consistency with a nodular surface. They firmly adhere to the dura or to the bone which they invade and may destroy. The chondromas which arise adjacent to the nervous system are similar to those elsewhere in the body and predominantly grow by expansion. They can produce bone and are often calcified.

Chondromas may arise from the dura of the falx, but most commonly occur in the dura at the base of the skull close to the foramen lacerum. They can also be found in the choroid plexus of the lateral ventricles or, occasionally in multiple sites on the spinal dura. In this latter location, however, they do not usually act as space-occupying lesions. Finally, they are also occasionally seen on the laminal arches. The chondromas are generally benign tumors, and in rare cases may show malignant features similar to those of the chondrosarcoma.

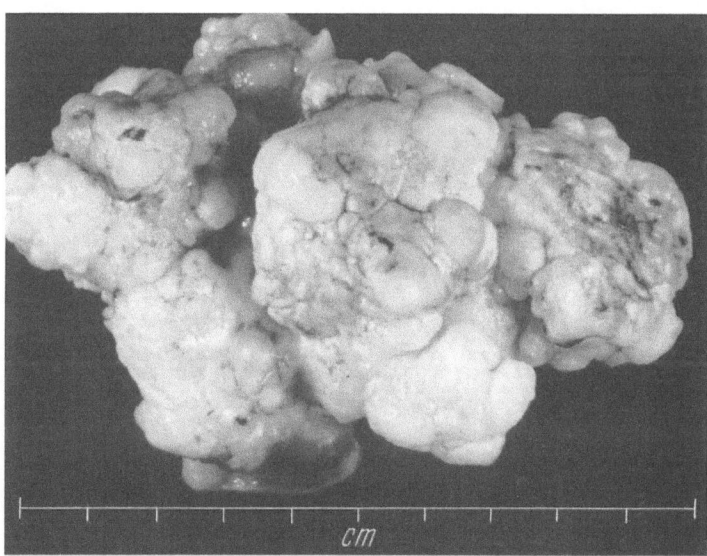

Fig. 275. Large surgically excised chondroma from the base of the skull

The Lipomas/Xanthomas

The lipomas are sharply circumscribed tumors of the arachnoidal spaces and are firmly attached to the adjacent nervous tissue, making removal difficult. They are similar to lipomas in other parts of the body. Lipomas occur predominantly in six places:

1. Above the corpus callosum—when all or a part of the corpus callosum is missing; they may take the form of a bean or appear as a plaque a few millimeters in thickness;

2. at the infundibulum as a pea-sized lesion;

3. on the quadrigeminal plate also as a pea-sized lesion;

4. attached to the choroid plexus of the lateral or third ventricles as a bean- to egg-sized tumor (Fig. 276);

5. in the other cisterns or over the convexity (rare);

6. alongside the spinal cord where they are found (a) in the lower thoracic region extending over a few segments, (b) drawn out over the whole spinal cord, or (c) in the region of the cauda equina. They usually lie dorsally in the region of the posterior columns.

The lipomas of the spinal cord are of special neurosurgical importance. The space-occupying lipomas manifest themselves in earlier decades of life than those which are encountered incidentally at autopsy. Although they are slow-growing, benign tumors, excision is difficult because of the penetration of the adjacent nervous tissues by strands of connective tissue and blood vessels. Recurrences are therefore common. Metastases are unknown.

Xanthomas are tumors, which arise by transformation and infiltration of mesodermal cells with special lipids. They occur particularly in the choroid plexuses.

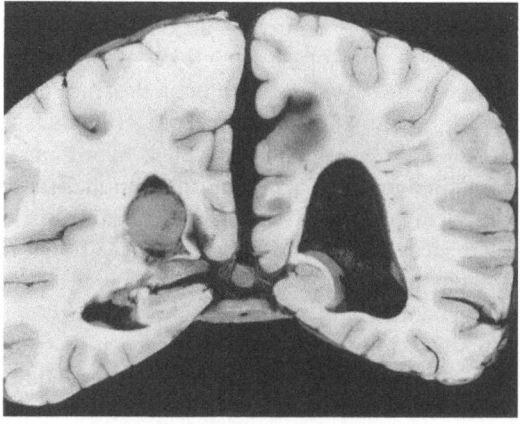

Fig. 276. Cherry-sized lipoma of the chorioid plexus of the left trigone

1.2.11 Epithelial Tumors

Cylindromas, Cylindromatous Epitheliomas, Adenoid Cystic Carcinomas, Cylindromatous Epitheliomas, Adenoid Cystic Carcinomas

These rare epithelial tumors of "cylindromatous" architecture occur at the base of the cranium in two sites. Beginning as "nasopharyngeal" tumors, in the first instance, they force their way from the nasopharynx through the crista galli, displacing the frontoorbital part of the frontal lobes upward like an olfactory groove meningioma (Fig. 277). However, the cylindroma may be distinguished by the bone destruction which is always seen at the base of the tumor as well as by a corresponding change in the radiologic appearance of the ethmoidal and sphenoid sinuses.

More commonly, however, they expand posteriorly (Fig. 278) in the direction of the Gasserian ganglion, which they usually invade, and impinge as well on the base of the temporal lobe. Here they resemble the neurinomas macroscopically and some regressive changes accompanied by the formation of smaller cysts are usual. Not only do the cylindromas tend to recur—total removal is almost impossible—but some of them undergo malignant degeneration and may even metastasize to other organs. More malignant tumors (true squamous cell carcinomas, lymphosarcomas, reticulum-cell sarcomas), the so-called "nasopharyngeal fibromas", and many other types are found in the same location.

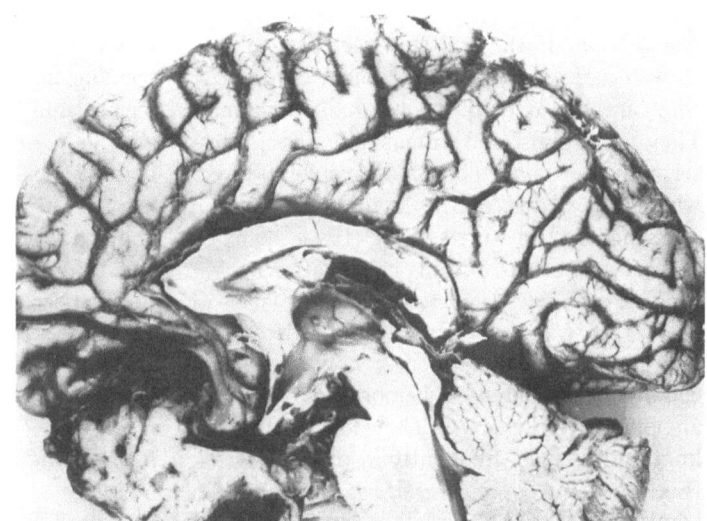

Fig. 277. Cylindroma (cylindromatous epithelioma) which has extended in the midline from the ethmoid sinus into the anterior fossa. It resembles an olfactory groove meningioma

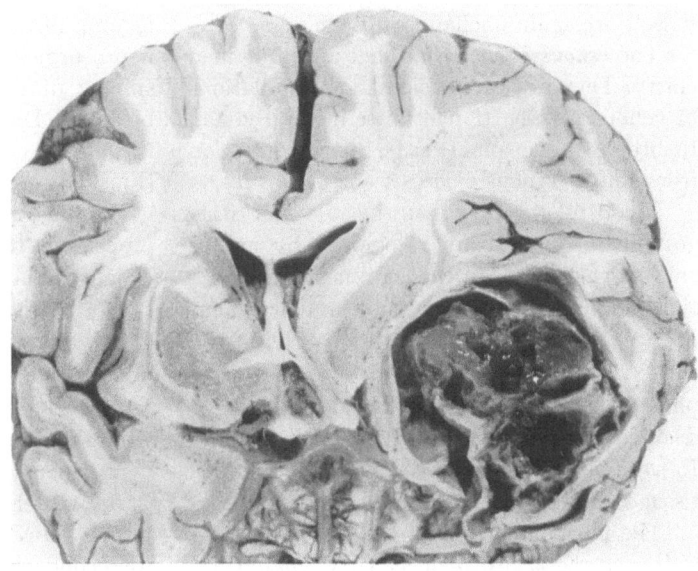

Fig. 278. Massive cystic cylindroma (cylindromatous epithelioma) originating from the region of the tip of the petrous bone which has ruptured into the temporal lobe

167

1.2.12 Vascular Structures of CNS: Non-Neoplastic Processes

Malformations/Angiomas and Aneurysms

Angiomas are frequently non-space-occupying lesions, but are included in this atlas because they can and often do produce a mass effect either through hemorrhage or reactive changes. A modern classification must include:

cavernous angiomas,
capillary angiomas,
venous angiomas,
capillary and venous angiomas (Sturge-Weber's disease),
arteriovenous angiomas (A.V. malformations).

It should be noted that the *cavernous angioma* occurs in the skull and vertebral column as well as in the brain and spinal cord. Still, they are not one of the common angiomas. They are a bluish-red, tumor-like mass of vessels which does not possess a capsule and over which the vessels of the leptomeninges cross unchanged. The surrounding tissue can be scarred and often contains calcifications.

The *capillary angiomas* (telangiectasias) of the CNS are usually small and are discovered only incidentally. They are, however, quite commonly a source of hemorrhage ("microangiomas?") (Fig. 279). They form a tangled knot and lie most frequently in the brain stem (Fig. 280), but probably also occur over the hemispheres. The overlying leptomeningeal vessels are again unchanged.

The *venous angiomas* are not a well-defined entity. They are varicocele-like accumulations of venous masses (for instance in the Sylvian fissure, over the spinal cord). Some distinction from simple venous varices seems necessary.

The *capillary and venous angiomas* of Sturge-Weber's disease are recognized by an increased vascularity of the leptomeninges and a sinusoid network of venous and capillary channels, no thicker than matches, overlying the cortex. The brain parenchyma becomes atrophic, scarred, and grossly calcified, probably as secondary sequelae of the disturbed circulation. In some instances heterotopias of the nervous tissue may also be encountered (see p. 139).

The most important of the CNS angiomas is the *arteriovenous angioma* (A.V. malforma-

tion or arteriovenous aneurysm). These lesions have been subjected to close scrutiny since their functional and morphological aspects are well-suited for analysis by angiography. They usually consist of a well-circumscribed network of arteries and veins (some of them as thick as half a centimeter) which are connected in part by large fistulous vessels of "intermediate" wall structure and in part by a capillary network. Arteriovenous angiomas may vary in size (from 2–6 cm in diameter; Fig. 281) and predominantly involve the cerebral cortex, where an overlying cluster of tangled cortical vessels—often in the form of a plexus—marks the site of the lesion. This is generally well-circumscribed and may lie superficially on the surface of the cortex, within the lateral ventricle, or be buried in the brain substance (Fig. 282). These angiomas consist of congeries of blood vessels in which vascular channels of varying size (often markedly dilated), filled with bright red or bluish-red blood, alternate and loop around one another. Such lesions manifest themselves most commonly between the ages of 18 and 30 years and account for about 1.5% of the larger neurosurgical series. The number of male patients is twice that of the females. Probably a significant percentage of the cases of "varicosis spinalis" really belong to this arteriovenous angioma group.

Aneurysms and Varices

The pathological "aneurysmic" dilatation of arteries in the brain and spinal cord is of great neurosurgical importance because of the possibility of rupture and diffuse subarachnoid bleeding. Distinction must be made between the more circumscribed "berry" aneurysm (Figs. 283, 284) and the longer (Figs. 285, 286) "fusiform" type. These terms correspond appropriately to the appearance of the aneurysm which is either a sack-like appendage ("berry") (Fig. 287) attached to the artery or a "fusiform" dilatation of the vessel itself (Fig. 285). Aneurysms are elastic in consistency or hard if they are thrombosed (Fig. 288). The inside is often filled with laminated thrombi (Fig. 288). Berry aneurysms are most apt to occur where blood vessels branch (usually at the distal carina between two branches) (Fig. 283) and are secondary to congenital defects in the vessel wall. Their sites of preference are well-known on the basis of a large number of cases and they are found most commonly on the anterior communicating (Figs. 291, 292), posterior communicating, middle cerebral (Figs. 293, 295), and internal carotid arteries (Figs. 288–290) as well as on the vertebro-basilar system (Figs. 283–287). On the carotid, distinction is made between infra- (Figs. 289, 290) and supraclinoid aneurysms (Figs. 288, 294), the latter group being more common. The site and extension of a hemorrhage from a ruptured aneurysm is very typical and is usually diagnostic (Figs. 296–298). Arterial aneurysms usually appear after the age of 30 and are significantly more frequent than the "venous varicoses" which are supposed to consist of an accumulation of varicose enlarged veins in a network. From here, there is a gradual transition to the true varices—i.e., phlebectasias. It is often difficult to know where to draw the line between these two rare venous abnormalities, although the decision may be facilitated by angiography. True phlebectasias may occur near the superior sagittal sinus in the form of an enlarged Pacchionian granulation or near the great vein of Galen.

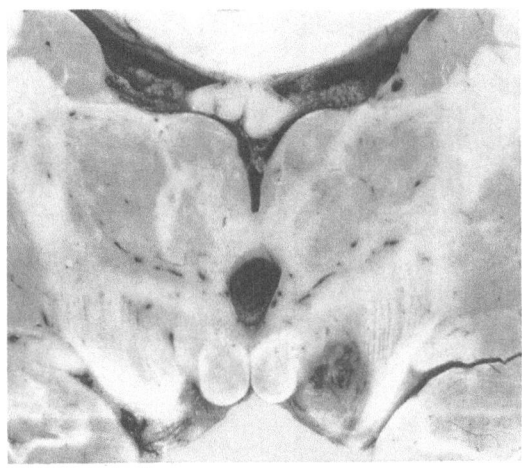

Fig. 279. Pea-sized capillary angioma in the cerebral peduncle (incidental finding)

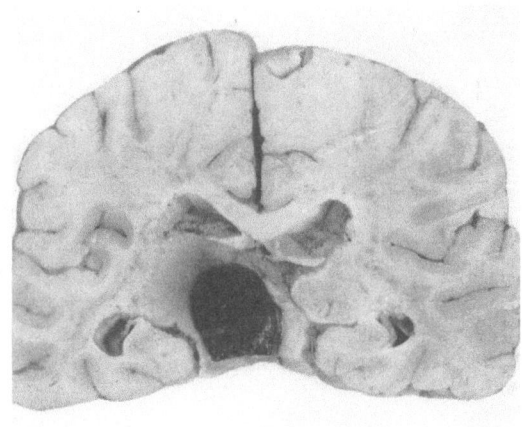

Fig. 280. Cherry-sized, fatal mass-hemorrhage from a capillary angioma of the left peduncle (c.f. Fig. 279)

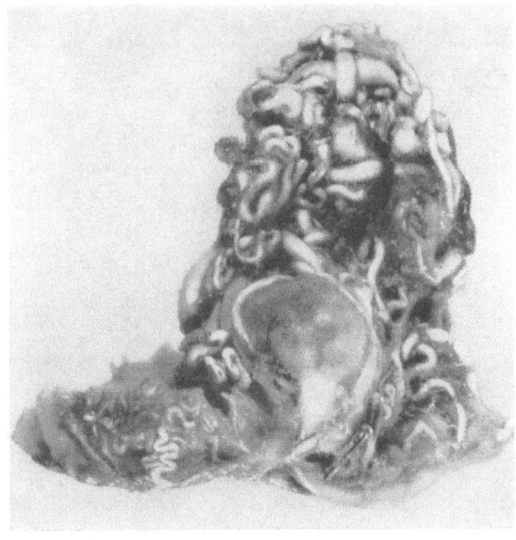

Fig. 281. Large arteriovenous angioma (AVM) surgically removed from the parietooccipital region. The angioma was injected with contrast medium post-operatively

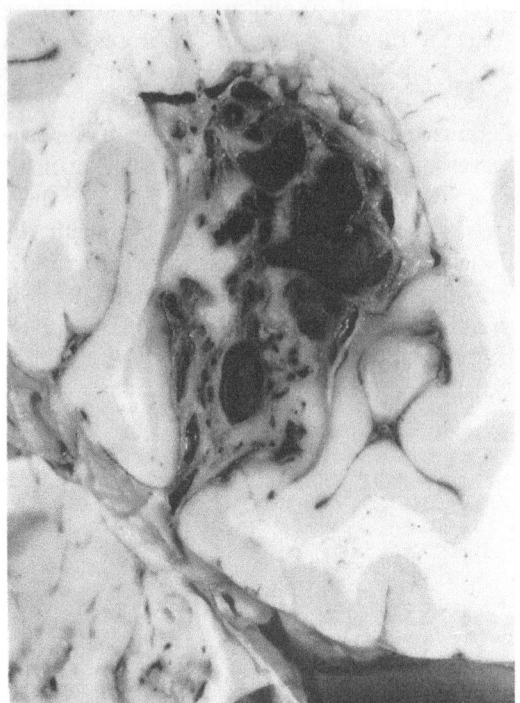

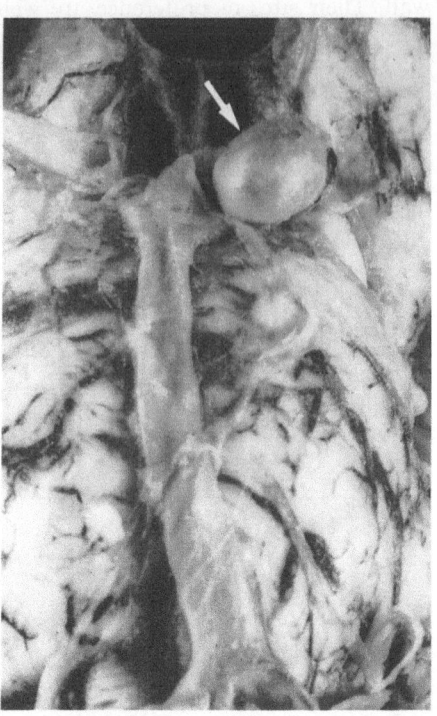

Fig. 282. A large arteriovenous angioma (AVM) of the medial occipital lobe

Fig. 283. Bean-sized aneurysm of the posterior cerebral artery (arrow!)

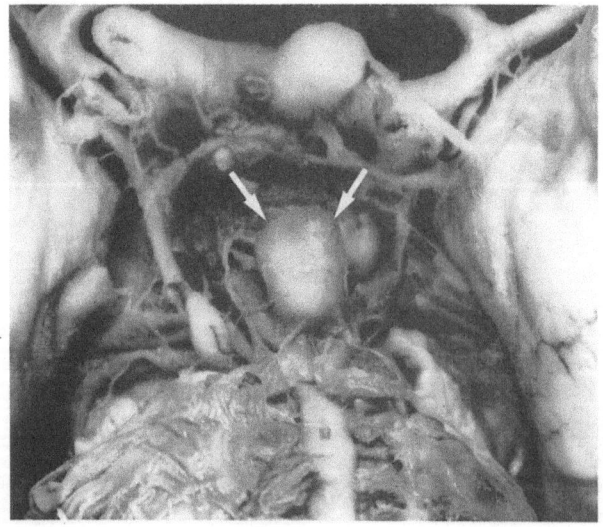

Fig. 284. Bean-sized aneurysm at the bifurcation of the basilar artery into the posterior cerebral arteries (arrows!)

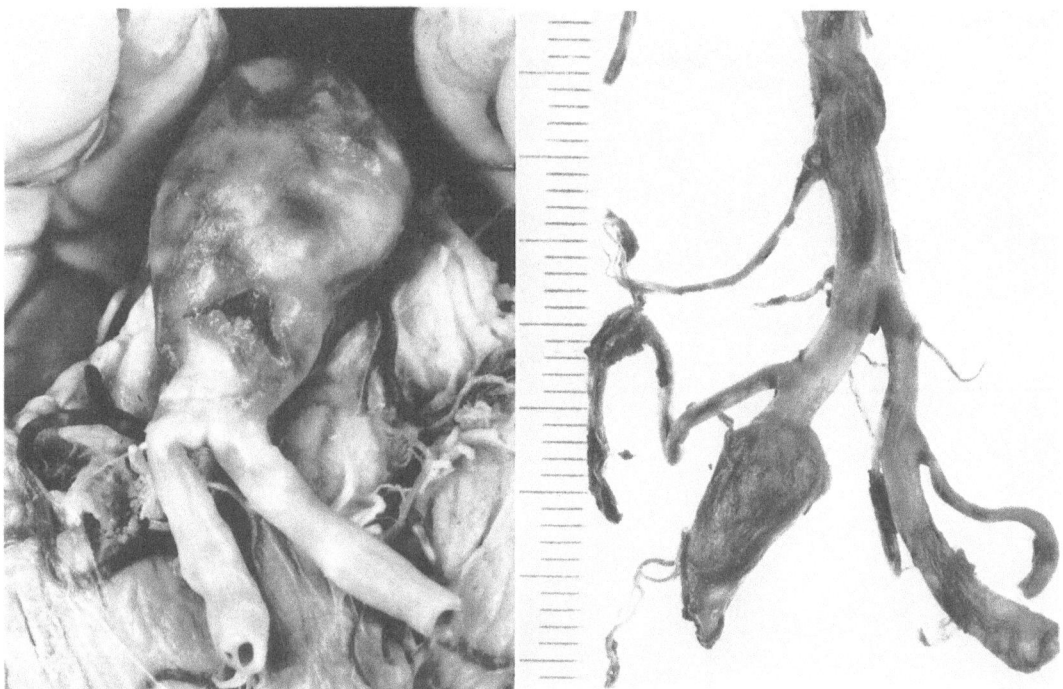

Fig. 285. Enormous fusiform aneurysm of the basilar artery which had ruptured

Fig. 286. Bean-sized aneurysm of the left vertebral artery

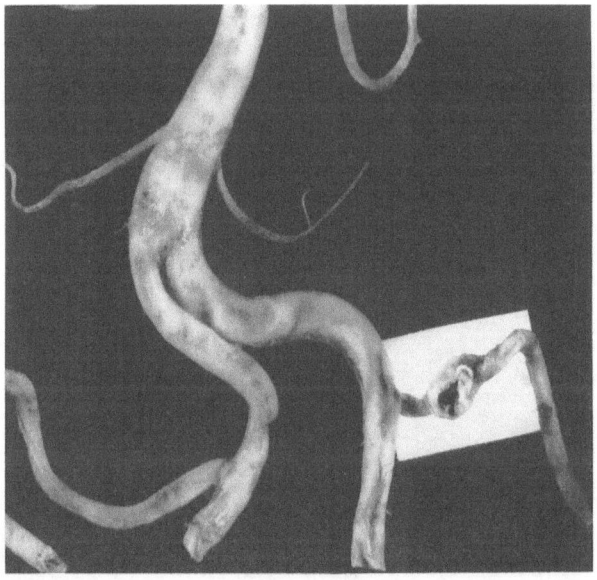

Fig. 287. Small ruptured aneurysm of the left posterior inferior cerebellar artery

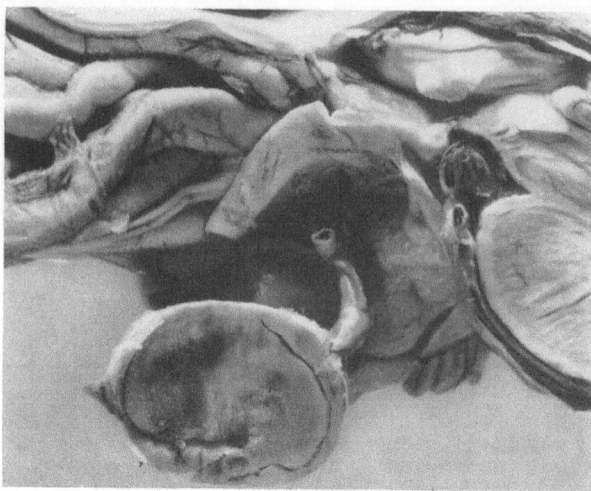

Fig. 288. Chestnut-sized supraclinoid aneurysm of the internal carotid artery which is completely thrombosed

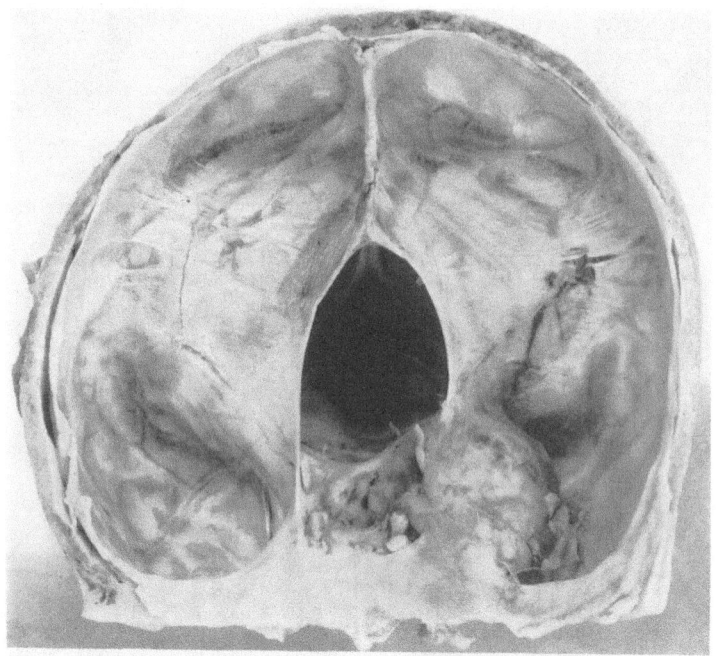

Fig. 289. Huge infraclinoid aneurysm of the left carotid artery (c.f. Fig. 290)

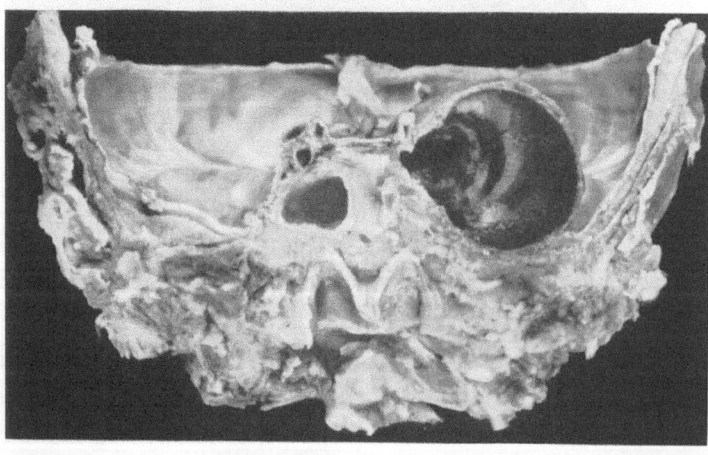

Fig. 290. Cross-section through the aneurysm shown in Fig. 289, which better demonstrates its size and location

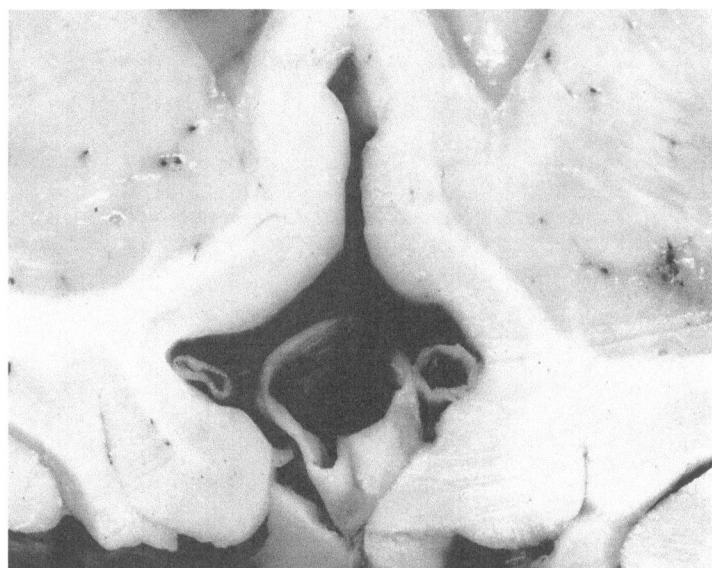

Fig. 291. Cross-section through a cherry-sized aneurysm of the anterior communicating artery

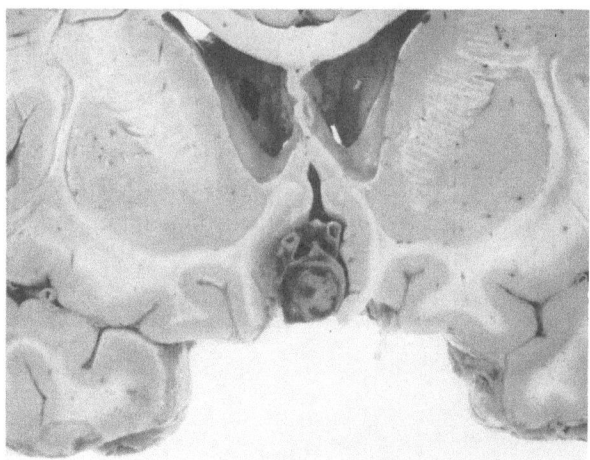

Fig. 292. Cherry-sized berry aneurysm of the anterior communicating artery

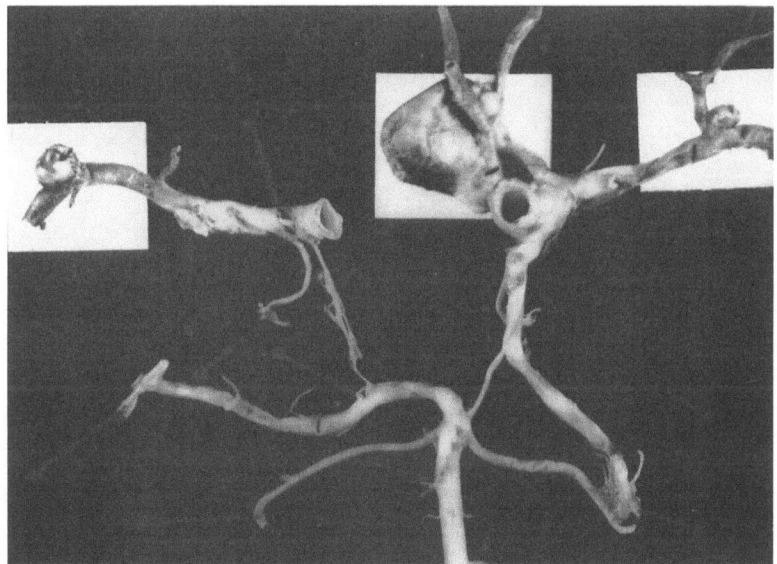

Fig. 293. Berry aneurysms of the anterior communicating artery and both middle cerebral arteries

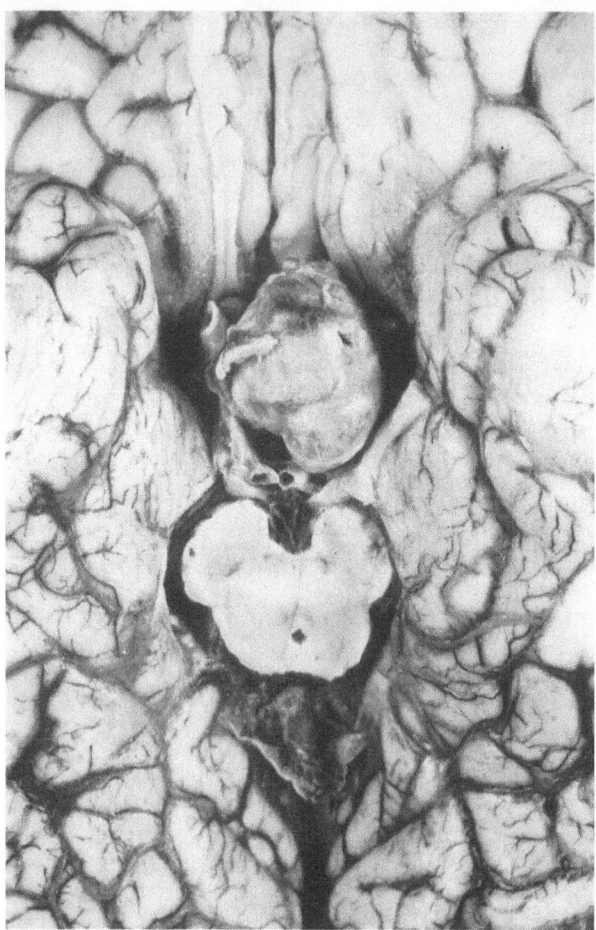

Fig. 294. Large supraclinoid aneurysm of the left carotid artery. These may have a mass effect similar to a chiasmatic tumor

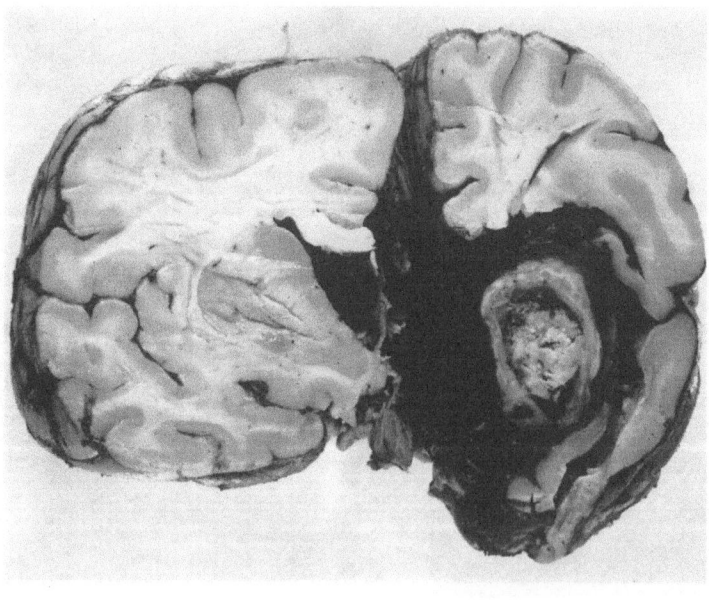

Fig. 295. Cross section through a huge thrombosed aneurysm of the left middle cerebral artery

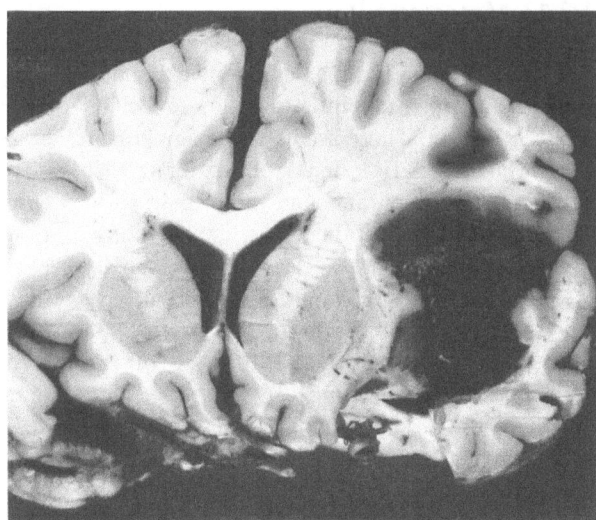

Fig. 296. Typical site of hemorrhage in case of ruptured saccular aneurysm of the middle cerebral artery

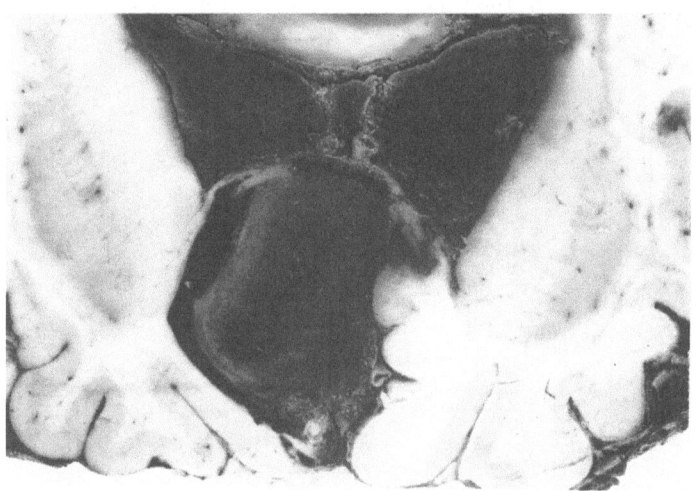

Fig. 297. Hemorrhage in ruptured aneurysm of the anterior communicating artery

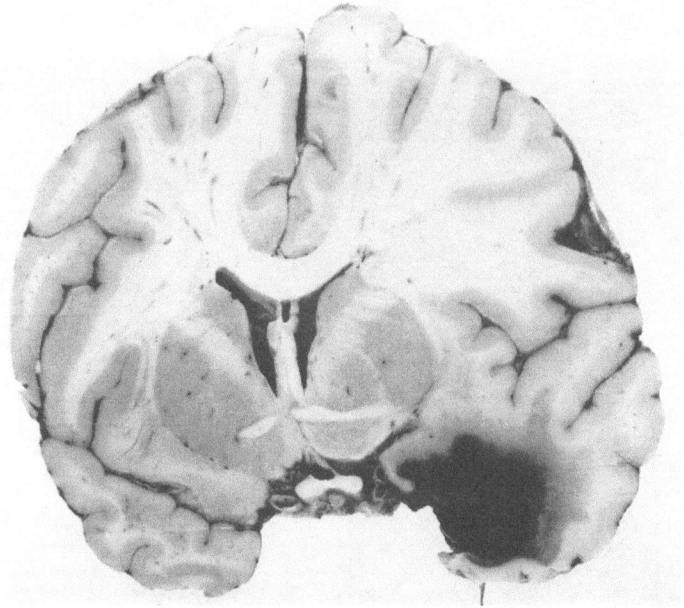

Fig. 298. Hemorrhage in ruptured aneurysm of the posterior communicating artery

1.2.13 Metastatic Tumors

In some cases, brain metastases of body tumors are operated intentionally, in others unintentionally. There seems to be agreement that if the metastatic lesion is solitary (or at least is thought to be solitary) and the primary process sufficiently contained—as, for instance, in some hypernephromas (clear cell carcinomas) of the kidney—no contraindication for surgery exists. Any part of the brain can be the site of a metastatic tumor, and the size of the metastasis is rarely indicative of the high degree of the accompanying intracranial pressure. In fact, metastases share the dubious distinction with the glioblastoma of provoking more associated brain edema and brain swelling Figs. 299, 300) than any other tumor (see

p. 202 ff.). Many metastases are either dural implants or so firmly attached to the dura (Fig. 301) that they are often initially misinterpreted at operation as meningiomas (Fig. 308). Metastases may be sharply delineated (Figs. 300, 303, 307) or diffuse (Fig. 302) or soft or hard (Figs. 307, 308); degeneration with the formation of cysts and hemorrhages may occur, particularly in hypernephromas and melanoblastomas (Fig. 306). The most common source for metastases to the brain is lung cancer (bronchogenic carcinoma) with an incidence ranging from 15 to 35%, followed by hypernephromas, and in women, breast carcinomas. Sarcomas metastasize even more readily than carcinomas. The peak of the age curve lies around 45–70 years. In our collection of 9000 cases 636 were metastases, i.e. 7.1%.

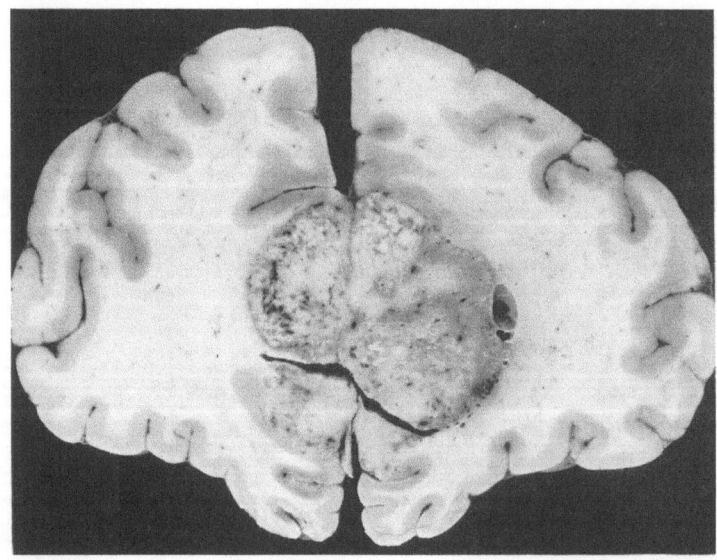

Fig. 299. Large metastasis of breast carcinoma mimicing an anterior bilateral falx meningioma

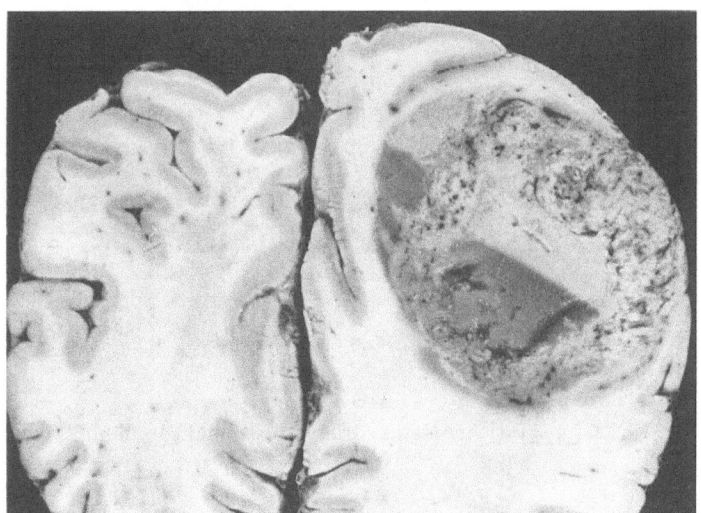

Fig. 300. Large frontolateral metastasis

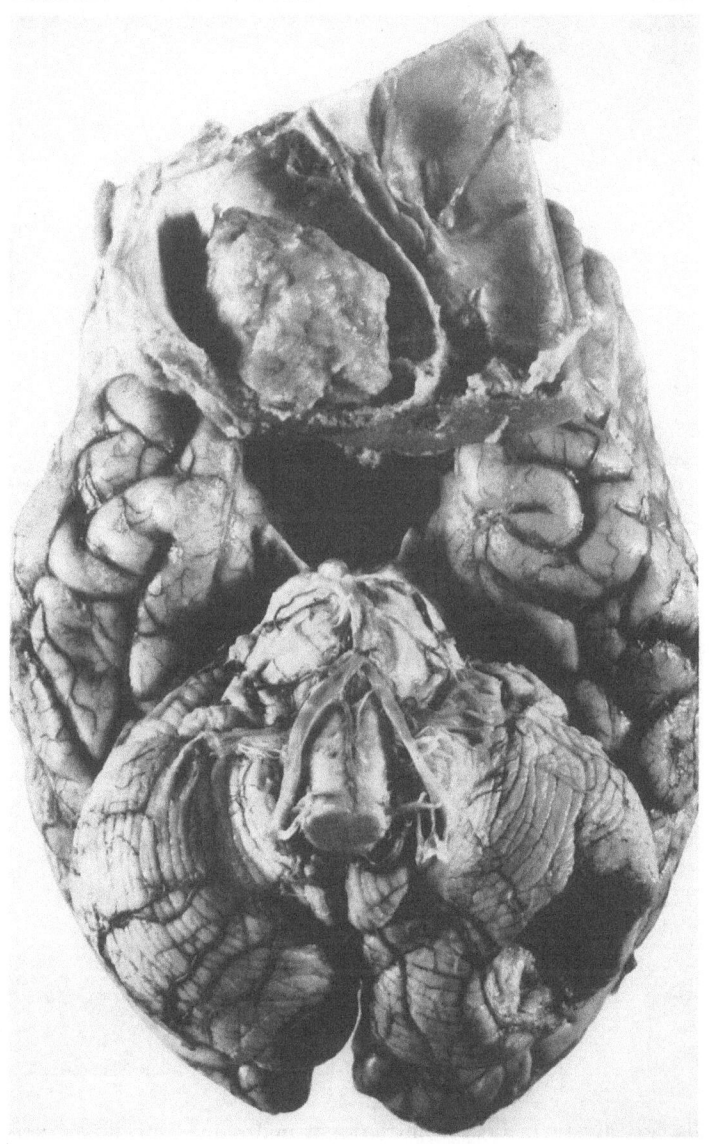

Fig. 301. Solitary metastasis of an adenocarcinoma into the left cerebellar hemisphere which was so firmly attached to the overlying dura and bone (above!) that at autopsy it was unavoidably displaced from its bed (below!)

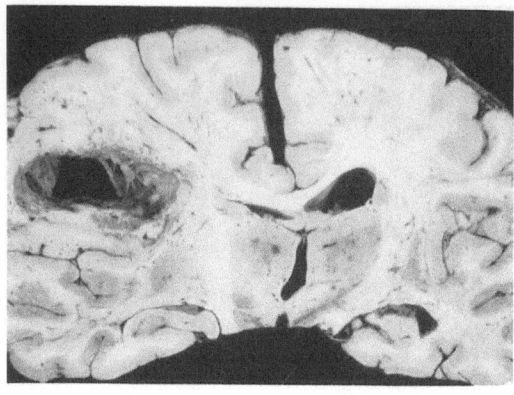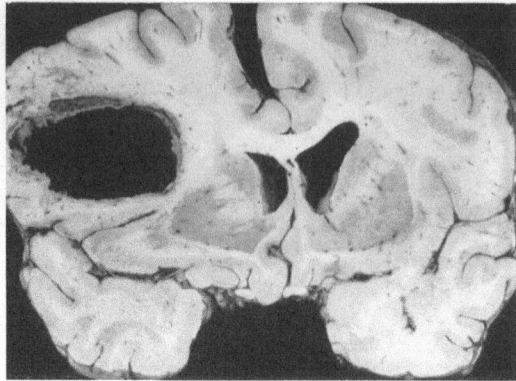

Fig. 302. Large cystic metastasis from a bronchial carcinoma (oat-cell)

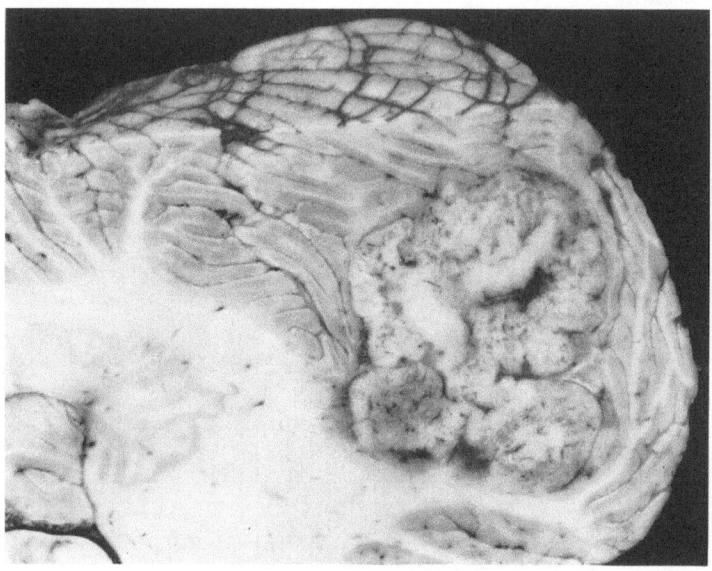

Fig. 303. Nodular scallopped metastasis in the cerebellar hemisphere

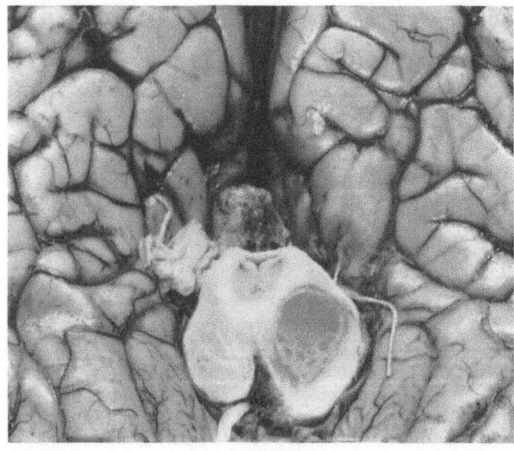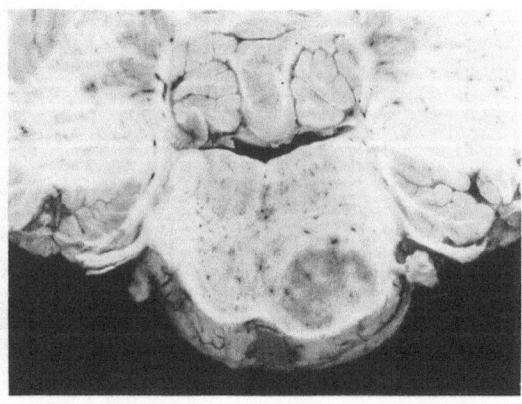

Fig. 304. Cystic metastasis in the right midbrain

Fig. 305. Cystic pontine metastasis in a case with multiple seeding from a bronchogenic carcinoma

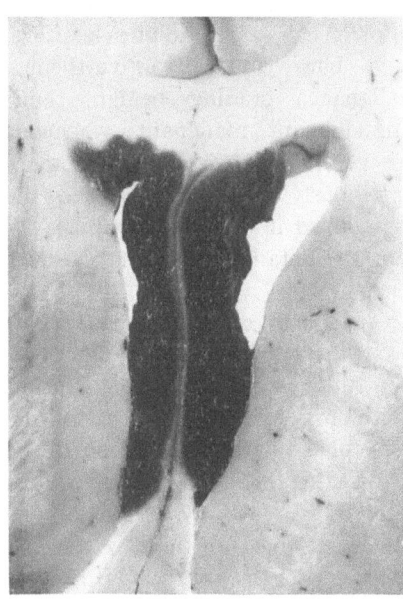

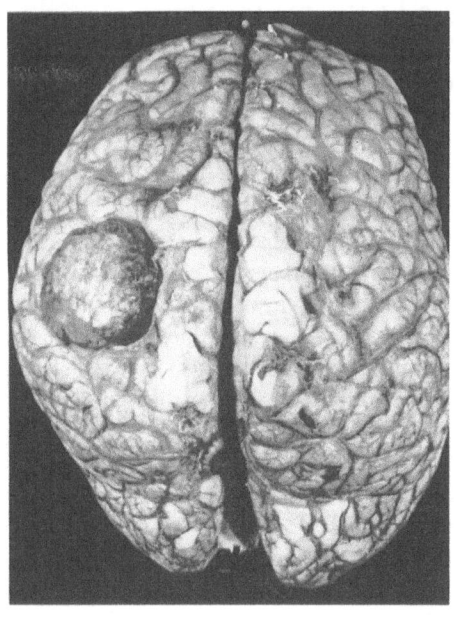

Fig. 306. Curious seeding of a malignant melanoma under the ependyma of the septum pellucidum and corpus callosum

Fig. 307. Nodular, sharply-demarcated, firm metastasis of a squamous-cell carcinoma to the left parietal lobe

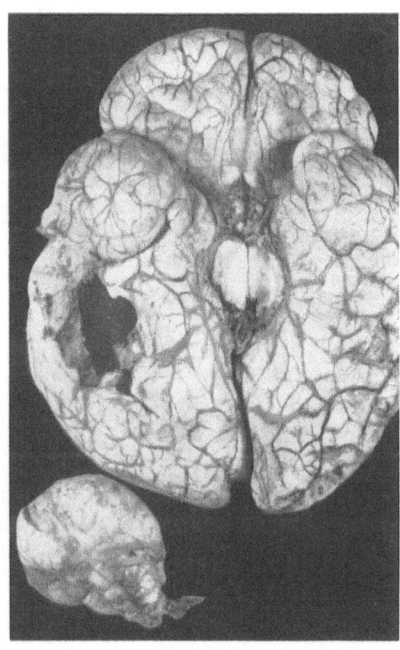

Fig. 308. Nodular metastasis which was easily shelled from its bed in the base of the temporal lobe

1.2.14 Unclassified Tumors, Multiple Tumors, Odd Space-Occupying Masses

The neurosurgeon will receive *"unclassified tumor"* as the diagnosis for at least a few of the specimens he submits for neuropathological classification. There are two main reasons for this situation—insufficient specimen and atypical tumor. Sometimes, only a very small biopsy specimen or some debris from the aspiration needle or sucker flask are available. In such cases the neuropathologist is often able to establish the neoplastic nature of the specimen, but not able to render a specific diagnosis of the tumor type. The certainty of a histological classification is in many ways proportional to the amount and the quality of the material submitted for study. On the other hand, despite sufficient material, the histologic picture may not fit into an existing classification, regardless of the terminology that has been adopted (Figs. 309–316). In no instance have we tried to force such cases into our classification. We have, however, tried to give them a specific malignanca grading—benign, semibenign, semimalignant, malignant—whenever possible (see p. 34, 35). On occasion, tumors which had previously been unclassified are subsequently assembled into a new grouping, although the precise details of its origins may yet remain unclear.

Multiple tumors of different nature (Fig. 317) occur and are not infrequently described in the literature. A common combination of various tumors exists in the hamartoblastomatoses (phakomatoses) as in von Recklinghausen's disease (1882).

Various *other space-occupying* masses are not mentioned here, because they are uncommon or of no neurosurgical interest. However, one may occasionally encounter the situation of "delayed" radionecrosis (Figs. 318, 319) "growing"—i.e., acting as a space-occupying process (Fig. 320).

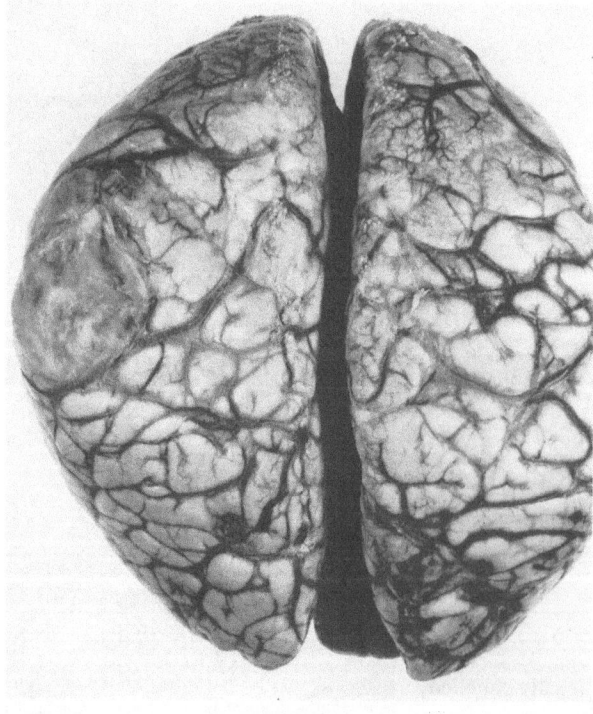

Fig. 309. Mandarin-sized tumor of the left frontoparietal region which presented on the cortical surface as a mushroom-like mass. Note the demarcation from adjacent brain

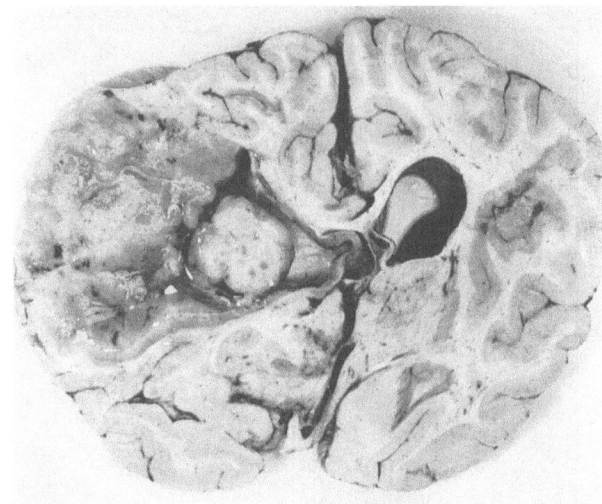

Fig. 310. Huge, mostly cystic, malignant tumor of the left cerebral hemisphere in a child. It was located at the outer ventricular wall resembling a typical ependymoma (c.f. Fig. 64). Histologically unclassified

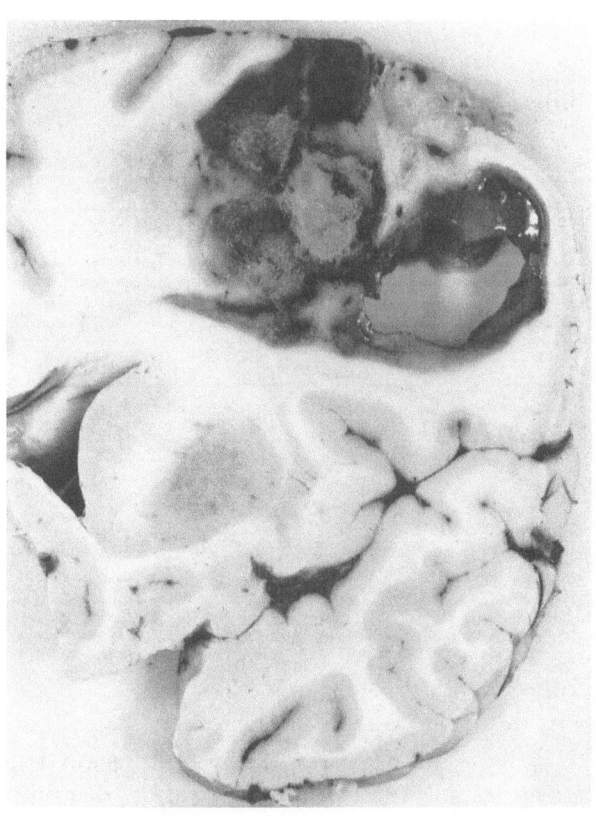

Fig. 311. Apple-sized, glassy tumor in the left fronto-parietal region which is well-demarcated from adjacent brain. A cyst is seen in the depth. Histologically unclassified

181

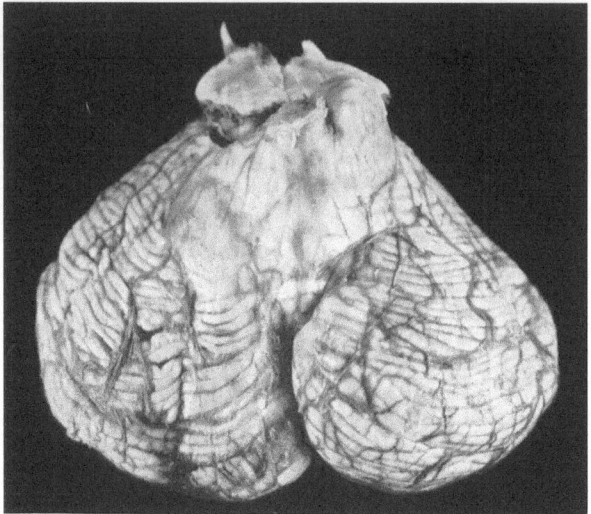

Fig. 312. Another large nodular malignant tumor in the upper vermis, which was histologically unclassifiable

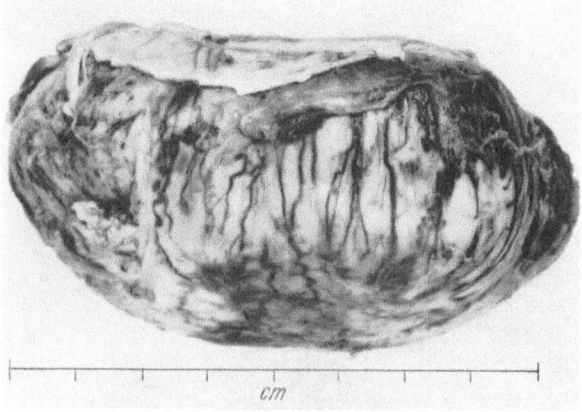

Fig. 313. Encapsulated tumor firmly attached to the dura. Histologically, the tumor contained astrocyte-like cells but could not be exactly classified

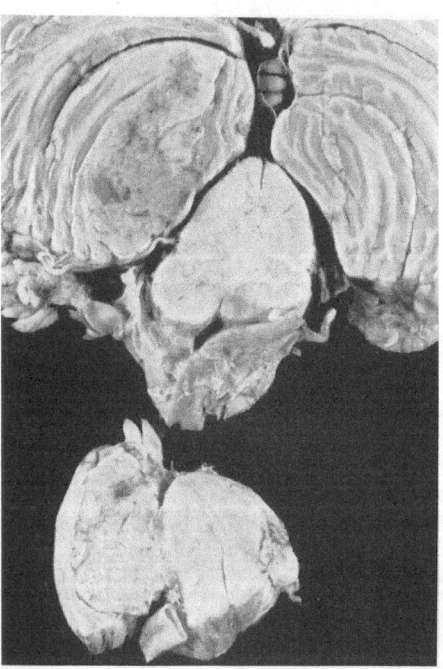

Fig. 314. Unclassified tumor of the left cerebellar tonsil. Histologically it resembled most closely a polar spongioblastoma with signs of malignant degeneration

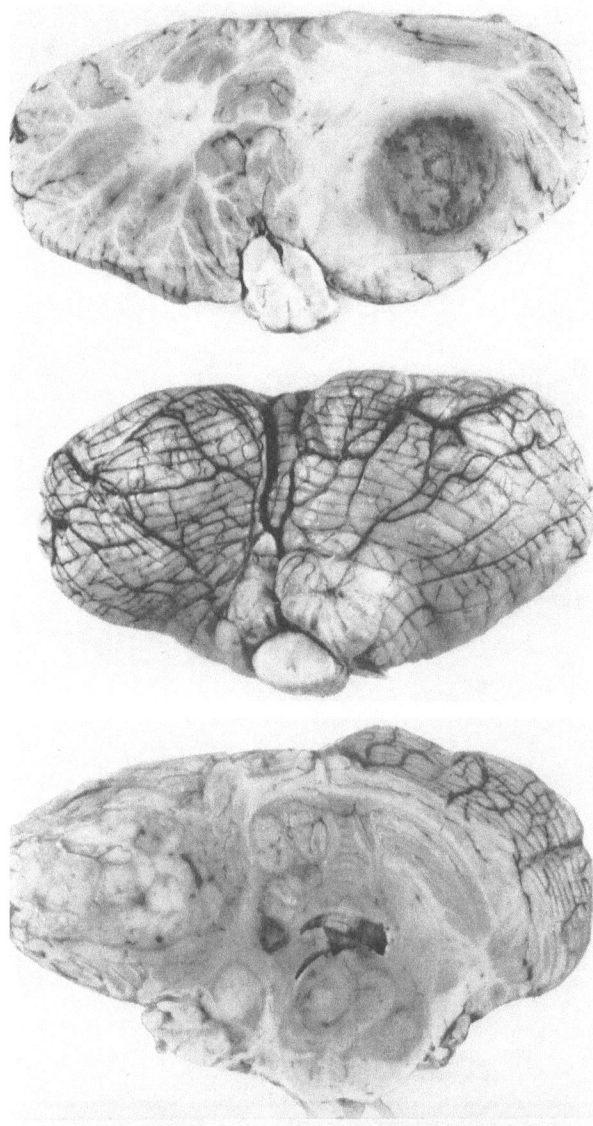

Fig. 315. Walnut-sized, necrotic, malignant tumor in the right cerebellar hemisphere associated with marked perifocal edema. Histologically unclassified

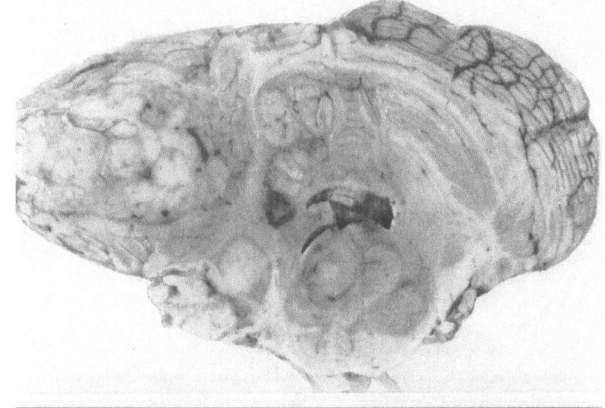

Fig. 316. Nodular cerebellar tumor, which could not be classified

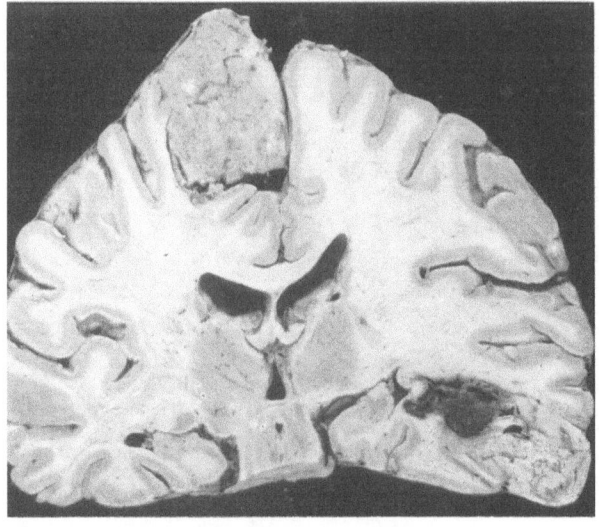

Fig. 317. Simultaneous, co-existing, unrelated tumors in a 65 year old female. A parasagittal meningioma (of the middle third of the sinus) is apparent on the right and a monstrocellular sarcoma of the temporal lobe may be seen on the left

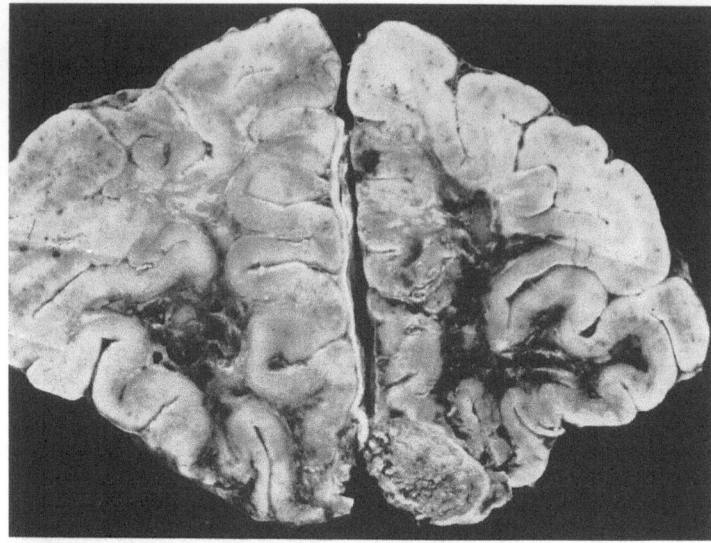

Fig. 318. Delayed radionecrosis: Complete destruction of frontal white matter with scar formation. Excellent preservation of the cortex (see Fig. 319)

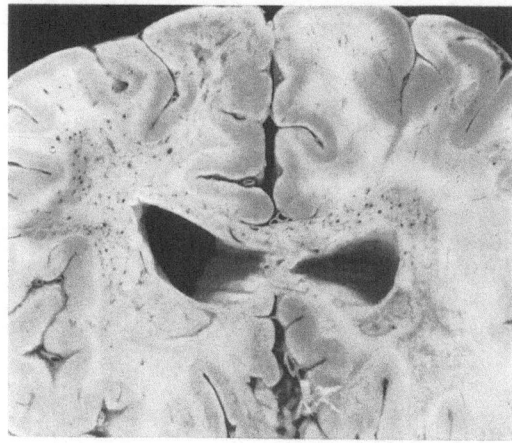

Fig. 319. Another more posterior section of the same case depicting an earlier stage of necrosis in the white matter (self-perpetuating process?) adjacent to the previous section. Five years postirradiation of an olfactory meningioma

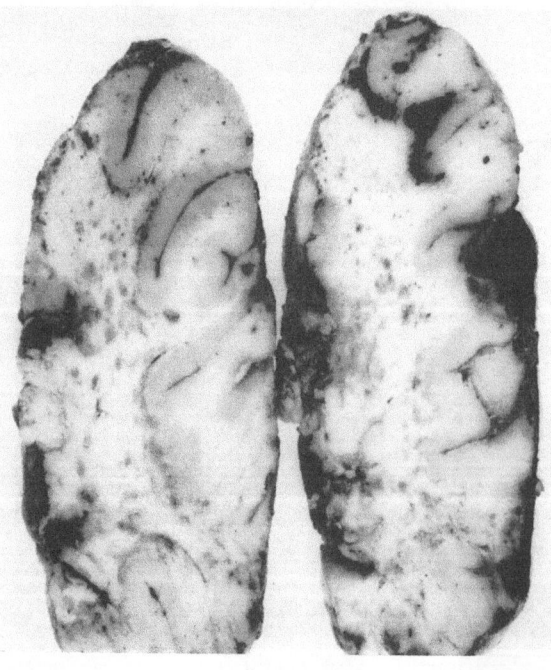

Fig. 320. Mass effect secondary to delayed radionecrosis

1.2.15 Parasites

Despite the great numbers of parasites, cysticercosis and echinococcal infestations (Fig. 322) are responsible for most of the cerebral mass lesions encountered, and they still constitute a significant neurosurgical problem. Other parasites (schistosomiasis, paragoniomiasis, coccidiosis, etc.) form only granulomatous reactions.

Cysticercosis is usually a systematic parasitosis with involvement of the brain being only one manifestation of a generalized disorder. The cysticerci usually settle diffusely throughout the brain (Fig. 323) and infest the leptomeninges as well, especially in the cisterns. Here they may assume a "racemose" form, often being bunched together like a cluster of grapes (Fig. 321) or like pearls in a necklace. They are firmly attached to the neighboring tissue in which they induce an inflammatory reaction. Sometimes they float freely in the CSF. Cysticerci are also occasionally observed in the narrower parts of the fourth ventricle or aqueduct. To the naked eye they appear as floppy, grey-red vesicles the size of lentils or beans (Fig. 321) and are filled with a clear or cloudy fluid. This watery fluid contains either the larvae themselves or whitish crumbly masses. They may be the cause of a communicating or non-communicating hydrocephalus due to blocking the foramina or the arachnoidal and cysternal passages. When they present in a diffuse intra-parenchymatous distribution they produce a diffuse "swelling" of the brain and increased intracranial pressure (Fig. 323). Rarely, a single cysticercus in the Rolandi fissure (convulsions!) may be amenable to surgical therapy.

The *echinococci* may be multilocular, but are more frequently unilocular. They consist of smooth-walled cysts ranging in size from a cherry to a goose-egg or a tennis ball, with daughter vesicles lying either inside the cyst (Fig. 322), adjacent to it, or floating free. In the rarer multiloculated form the gelatinous vesicles are compressed and the membrane wrinkled up. The cerebral white matter and the cerebellum are said to be most commonly affected. Echinococcal infestation near the vertebral column may lead to an invasion of the epidural space of the vertebral canal (Fig. 322). They increase in incidence in the middle decades, although the cerebral forms occur in younger patients as well.

In *trichinosis*, the cyst wall is often calcified and visible on x-rays, and occasionally there may be granulomatous zones around the trichinella—but this is hardly of neurosurgical importance.

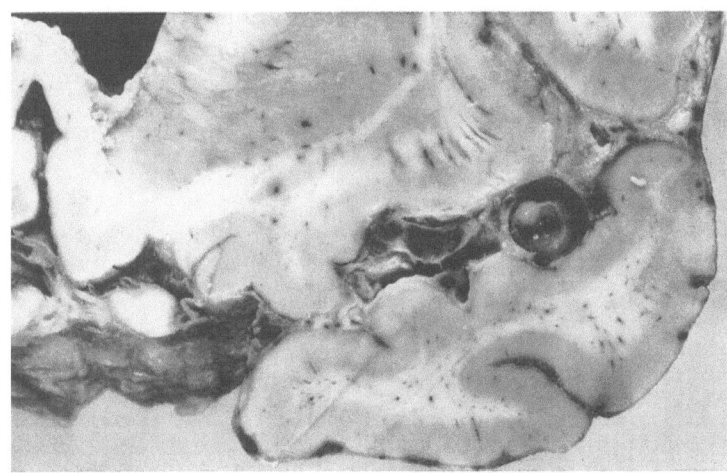

Fig. 321. Multiple cysticerci in the cistern of the Sylvian fissure giving rise to a chronic inflammatory reaction (racemose type of cysticerci)

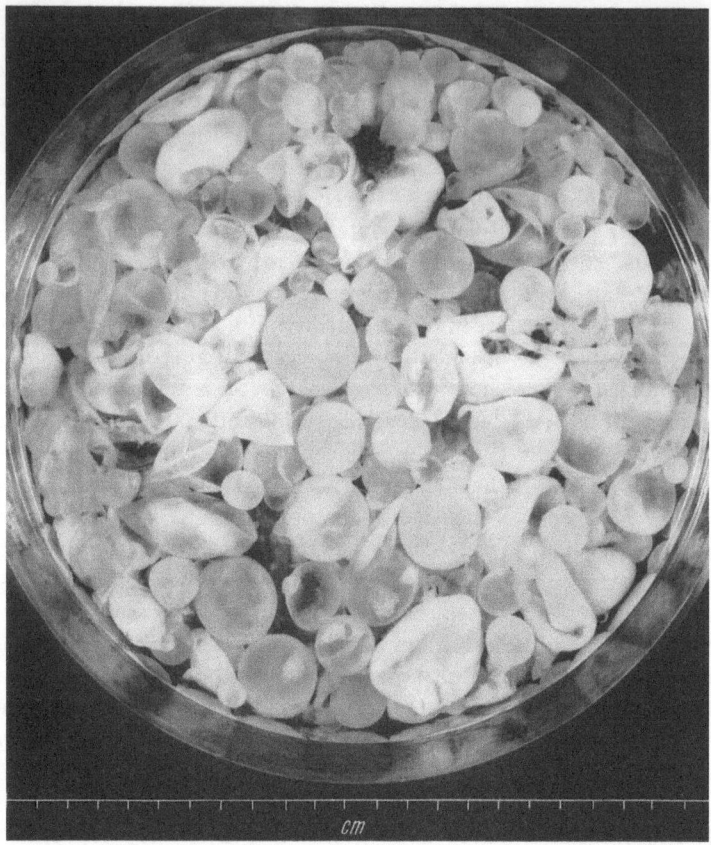

Fig. 322. Multiple echinococci which were removed at operation from the spinal epidural space and its adjacent areas

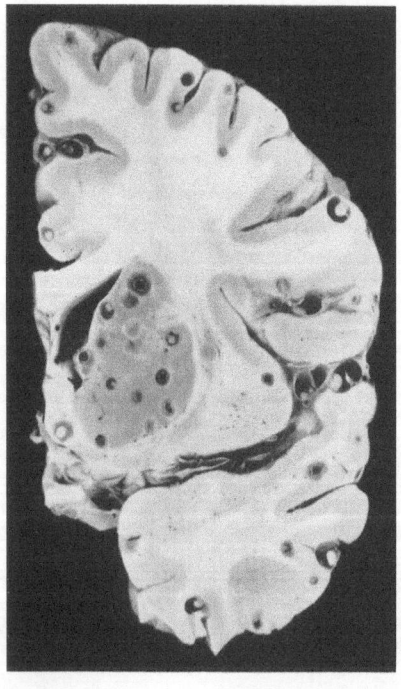

Fig. 323. Frontal section of brain with hundreds of cysticerci

1.2.16 Inflammatory and Post-inflammatory Processes

Granulomas, Arachnoiditis, Arachnoidal Cysts

Granulomas of the brain are becoming rare as syphilis and tuberculosis—the main sources of such lesions—are decreasing in incidence.

Tuberculomas consist of a hard, brittle tissue which may be either caseous or necrotic, but are occasionally soft and filled with tuberculous pus so that they cannot be distinguished from an abscess (Fig. 324). Since tuberculous meningitis or miliary tuberculosis of the meninges is rarely evident at surgery, the characteristic caseous consistency of the tumor's central portion is frequently the only indicator of the correct diagnosis. On occasion, they are completely calcified. The surface is at times coarsely nodular or lobulated (Fig. 325), and may even be multilocular with only small tissue bridges connecting individual tuberculomas.

Gummas (luetic granulomas, syphiloma) are also very rare nowadays. They are circumscribed lesions, more difficult to separate from the brain than the tuberculoma, and are usually softer and more elastic (almost "rubbery") because of the number of reticulin and elastic fibers found in the central necrotic parts. Here, there may be a jelly-like infiltration of the adjacent leptomeninges, with the appearance of a circumscribed chronic meningitis. There is no site of predilection, although they are said to occur frequently in the hypothalamic region.

Other granulomas, such as those seen in *actinomycosis* of the CNS, have always been very rare as have the *Hodgkin's granulomas*. The *eosinophilic granuloma* on the other hand, is frequently seen in the calvarium, and is most common in the frontal bone, where they infiltrate neither the dura nor the brain. *Fungus* infections (torula, blastomycosis, and the yeast granulomas) seem to be occurring with greater frequency since the use of steroids and the immuno-suppressive drugs has become so widespread.

Arachnoiditis and Arachnoidal Cysts. Following acute or subacute leptomeningeal infections (probably even some transmitted transplacentally), a chronic reaction in the arachnoid may occur. This is particularly marked in the cisterns and may lead to a blockage of the CSF pathways (Fig. 331) and to the formation of arachnoidal cysts (Fig. 326). Such cysts are almost exclusively located in the region of the large cisterns (Fig. 329). Of particular importance here are those cases occurring in the cistern of the Sylvian fissure (Figs. 327, 328), the cisterna supracallosa, the prepeduncular, crural and ambient cisterns, and the cisterna magna. All the basal cisterns may be involved with widespread adhesions as well as cysts (Figs. 329, 330), and rings of adhesions are particularly prone to close off the chiasmatic and prepeduncular, crural and ambient cisterns, the cerebellomedullary and pontocerebellar cisterns and the cisterna magna (Figs. 329, 330) thus effectively obstructing the normal flow of CSF over the hemispheres, leading to a communicating hydrocephalus (see p. 210). In the region of the chiasm (Fig. 326), cicatrical arachnoiditis is said to be of particular importance, while in the spinal cord a posttraumatic etiology of a similar cicatrical arachnoiditis, with formation of small cysts, has been observed. In the mesencephalic region large cysts may displace the tectum and block the aqueduct (see Fig. 332). The largest cysts are usually found in the Sylvian fissure and most are "congenital" (Figs. 327, 328). Some cases in this area appear to have been caused by developmental malformation, and they show different histological features. Enormous cysts are also seen in the cisterna magna, frequently resulting in hydrocephalus (Figs. 329, 330). The larger arachnoidal cysts reach the size of a chestnut or a man's fist (Figs. 328, 330, 334) and are usually filled with a clear watery fluid. However, the afore-mentioned developmental cysts may contain a milky fluid. Arachnoidal cysts not only produce a corresponding displacement of the brain substance and ventricles, but can also lead to a prominent bulge of the over-lying cranium (Fig. 334), which is apparent on the plain skull x-rays. This is most commonly seen over the Sylvian fissure. Porencephalic cysts have to be distinguished from the congenital cystic formations or those which follow arachnoiditis (Fig. 335).

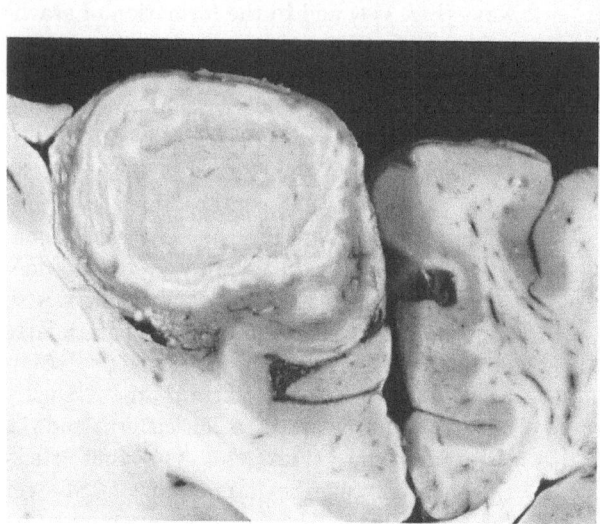

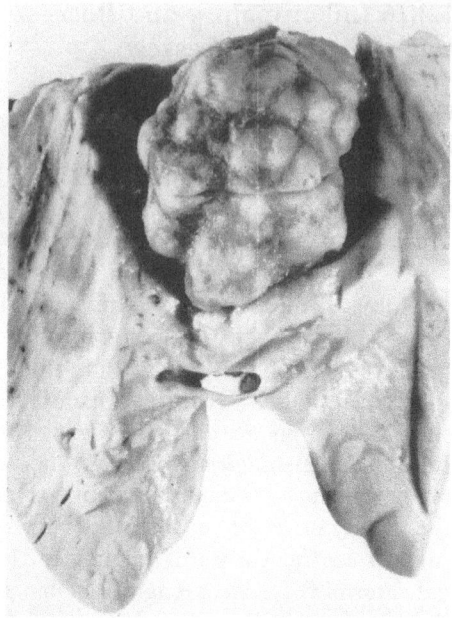

Fig. 324. Parasagittal, parietal tuberculoma in a case where multiple areas were involved. They were caseous and liquefied and at operation were believed to be abscesses

Fig. 325. Chestnut-sized tuberculoma of the midbrain which also compromises the third ventricle

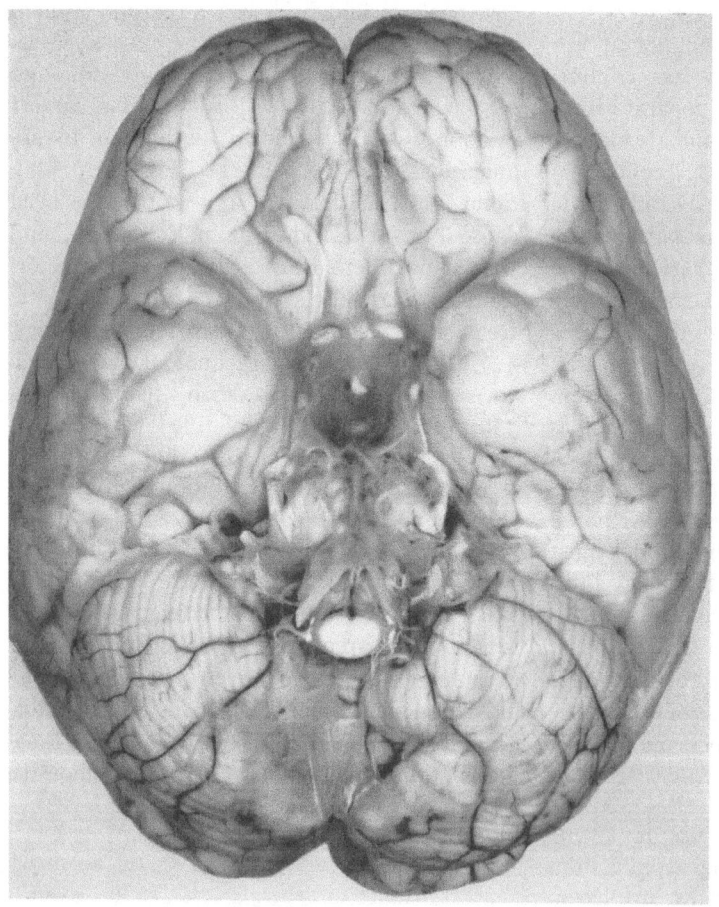

Fig. 326. Network of arachnoidal cysts consisting of multiple fluid-containing compartments of the basal cisterns. The floor of the 3rd ventricle is elevated

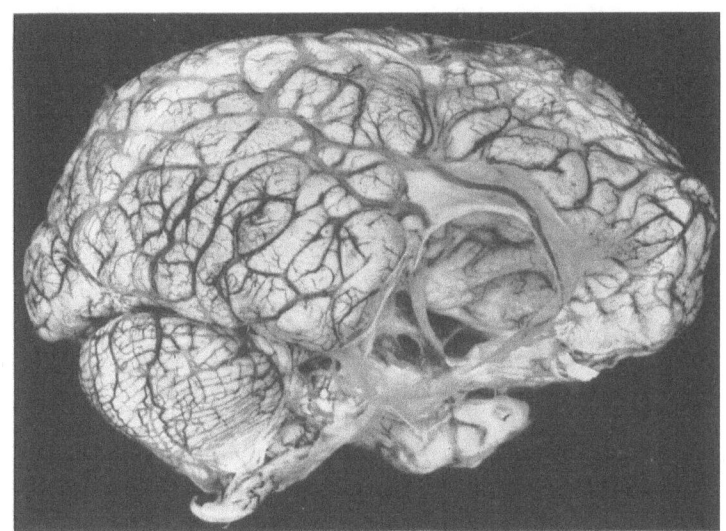

Fig. 327. Apple-sized cyst of the right Sylvian fissure of unknown etiology (incidental finding)

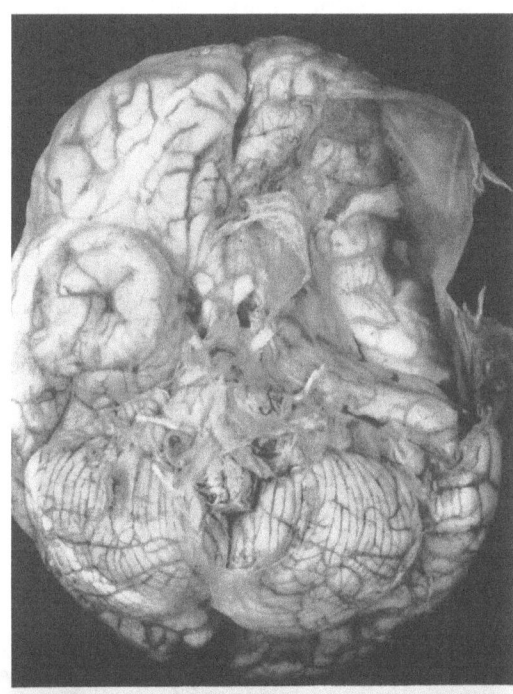

Fig. 328. Large, congenital arachnoidal cyst in the Sylvian fissure. An overlying, post-traumatic, chronic subdural hematoma was evacuated without benefit because of the mass effect of the unrecognized cyst. (DANDY reported a similar case in his book on Brain Surgery)

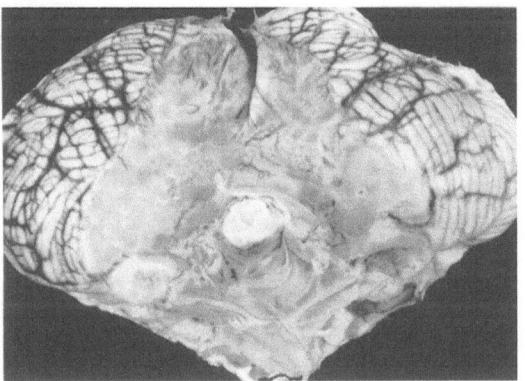

Fig. 329. Extensive formation of arachnoidal cysts in the cisterna magna and the adjacent basal cisterns. The foramen of Magendi was obstructed, resulting in a massive hydrocephalus

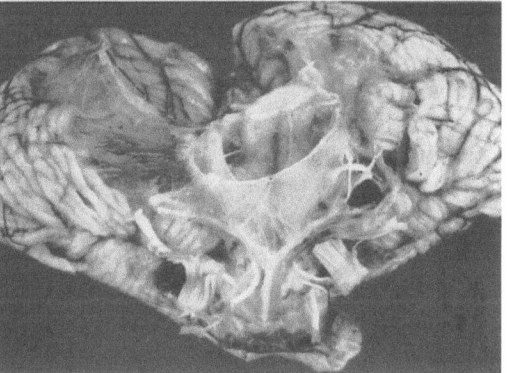

Fig. 330. Huge network of cysts located in the cisterna magna and cerebellopontine angle associated with extensive atrophy of the displaced brain tissue

189

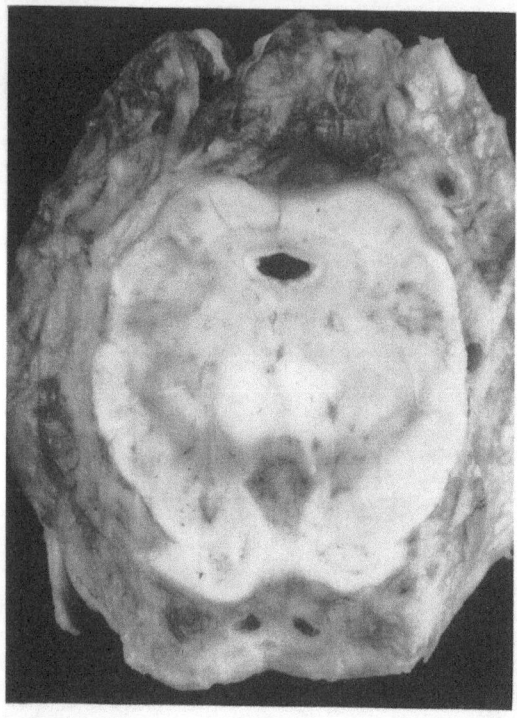

Fig. 331. Complete obliteration of the crural, ambient and basal cisterns in a case of tuberculous meningitis in the early days of streptomycin therapy. Scar tissue prevented the spinal fluid from access to the Pacchionian granulations and thus a communicating form of hydrocephalus resulted. The aqueduct was dilated and showed extensive tuberculous ependymitis

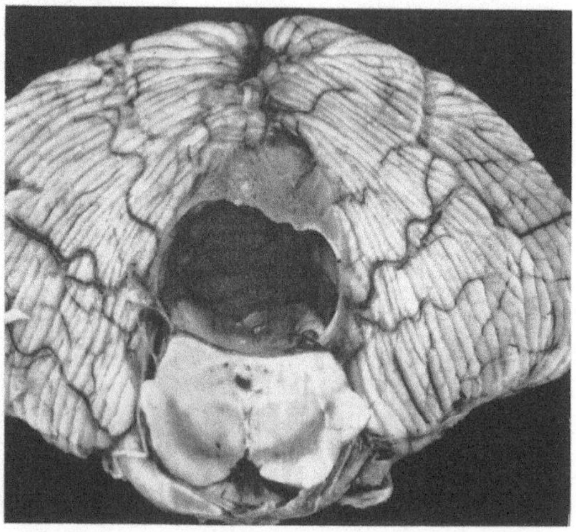

Fig. 332. Large encapsulated cyst in the quadrigeminal cistern overlying the mesencephalon which acted as a space-occupying lesion

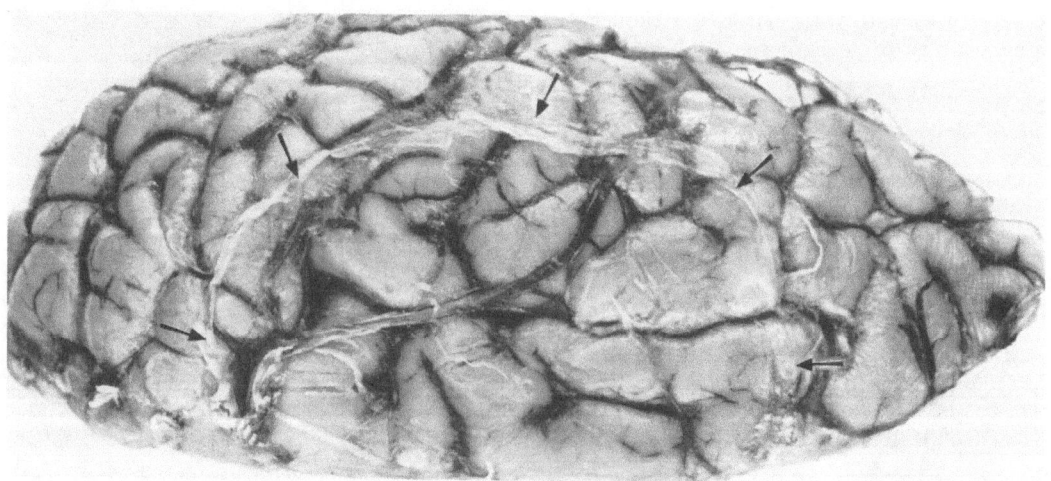

Fig. 333. Large parasagittal arachnoidal cyst (arrows!) with expansion of the overlying bone (c.f. Fig. 334)

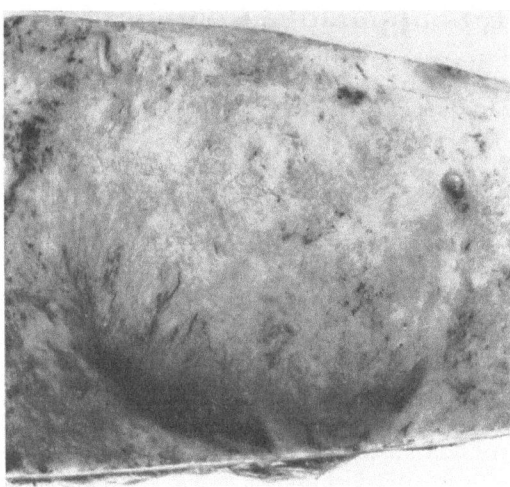

Fig. 334. Crater-like impression of the vault resulting from the parasagittal arachnoidal cyst of Fig. 333

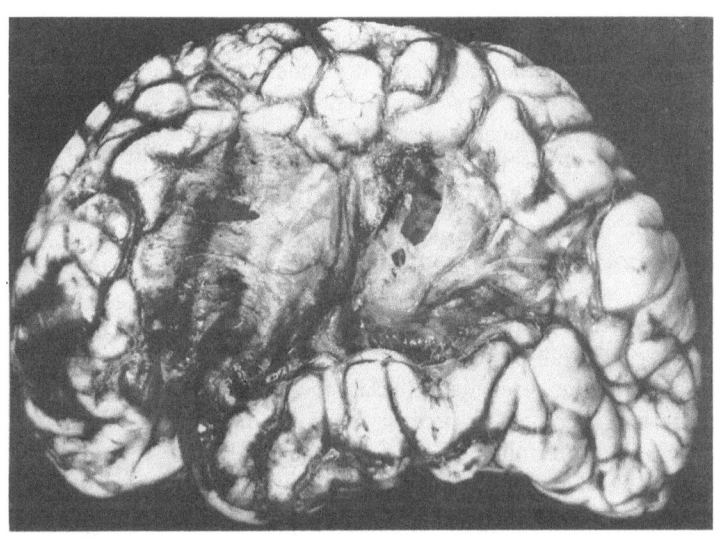

Fig. 335. For differential diagnosis: Porencephaly—Surgical specimen of a left hemisphere (hemispherectomy). Note the cyst in the area of supply of the middle cerebral artery consequent to a suspected congenital infarction

1.3 Suppurative Complications

Brain Abscess

A brain abscess may be a fresh and ill-defined inflammatory phlegmon (Fig. 336), or it may be well-encapsulated (Fig. 337). This depends upon its location, the nature and the virulence of the infecting organism, previous antibiotic treatment, and upon the patient's general resistance. A brain abscess may result from extension of an adjacent infection, as those of rhinogenous (Figs. 336–338) and otogenous origins, or it may be secondary to an extracranial infection of the scalp or skull. Abscesses may also be of "embolic" origin, following an infection elsewhere in the body, and then are often multiple (Figs. 339, 340).

Otogenous abscesses arise in the temporal lobe or in the cerebellum (basal, medial and posterior). Cerebellar abscesses may be more diffuse and interfoliar, or large and "central". *Rhinogenous* abscesses involve the medial and basal parts of the frontal lobes and are either solitary or multiple. *Extradural intracranial* abscesses may follow osteomyelitis of the skull and septic infections of the sinuses or mastoiditis.

Subdural Abscess or Empyema. Subdural abscess or empyema may be either rhinogenous or otogenous, following paranasal sinus diseases or inflammatory processes of the ear. Gross accumulations of pus may be localized or more diffusely spread over the convexity of the hemisphere, about its base, or over the cerebellum in the posterior fossa.

A peripituitary empyema after sphenoid sinusitis or septic thrombosis of the cavernous sinus is very rare. Since the advent of the antibiotic era post-traumatic infections of subdural clots are also rare.

A complicating thrombosis of the cerebral veins (Fig. 359) may arise on occasion and can result in occlusion of the venous sinuses.

Metastatic abscess of the brain often follows suppurative lesions of the thorax, infectious endocarditis, pyelophlebitis, or occasionally furunculosis of the skin. They may be multiple.

Post-traumatic abscesses after infections of open brain wounds still occur, but the disastrous consequences of these lesions, so prominent in World War II, are now rarely seen. However, such situations do occasionally arise in unusual or neglected cases, leading to subcortical abscesses. This is most often secondary to insufficient débridement of open wounds; but even when adequately handled, infection of a missile tract or even abscess formation around an inaccessible missile may occur.

Post-Infectious Empyema of the Ventricles. When abscesses rupture secondarily into the ventricles (Fig. 338) or when a communication has been created by the primary lesion, ventricular empyemas arise which may secondarily block the narrow parts of the ventricular system—the aqueduct or the foramina of Magendi and Luschka—leading to a secondary obstructive hydrocephalus. However, such rupture almost invariably leads to death.

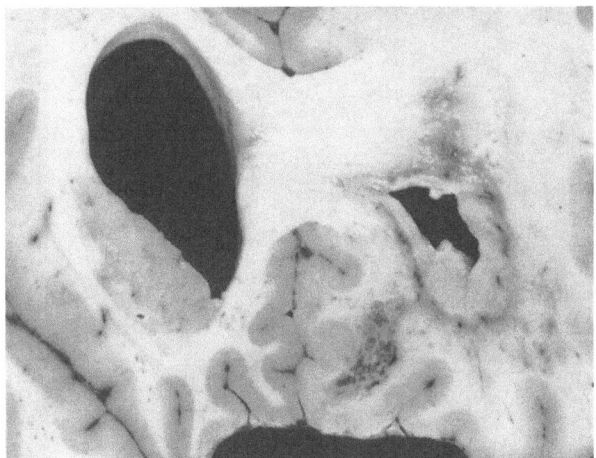

Fig. 336. Posterior extension of a fronto-basal abscess with rupture into the frontal horn

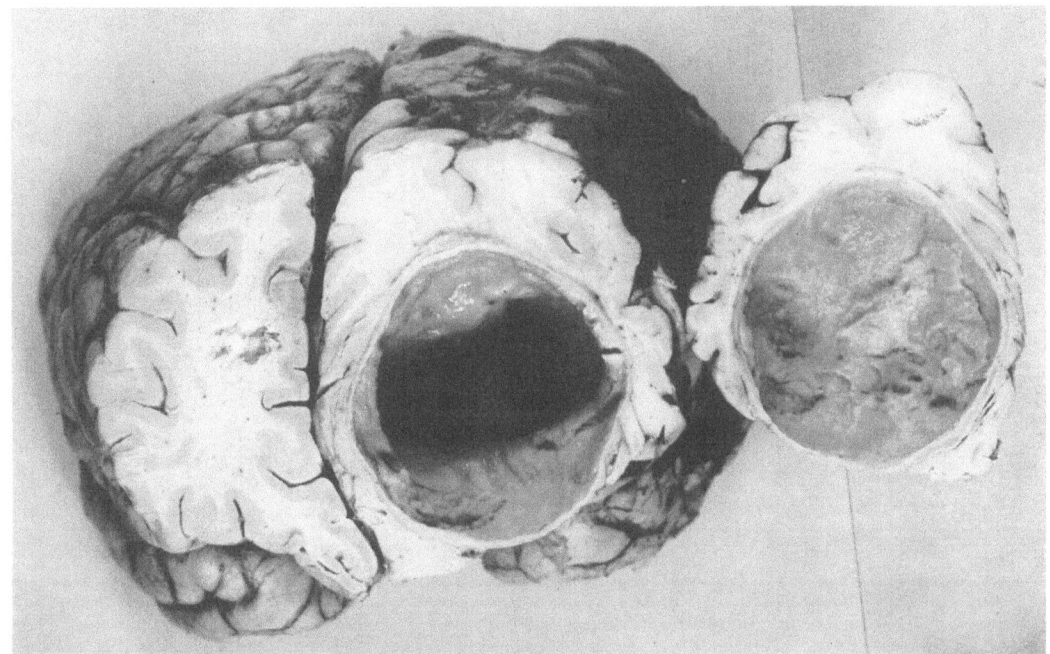

Fig. 337. Chronic, encapsulated frontobasal abscess secondary to a frontal sinusitis

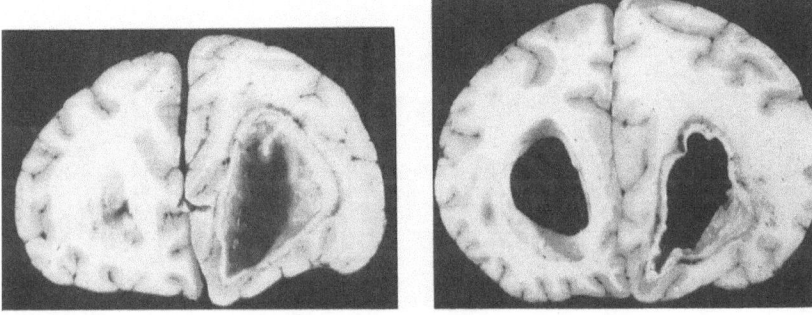

Fig. 338. Large frontobasal abscess secondary to infection of the right frontal sinus

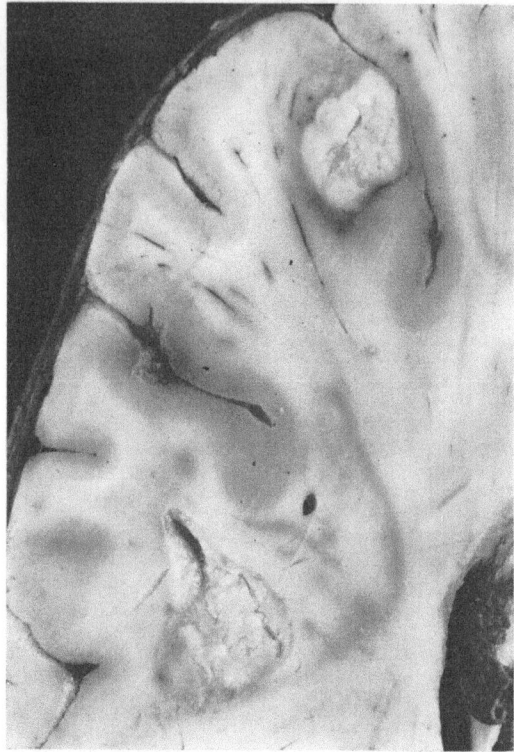 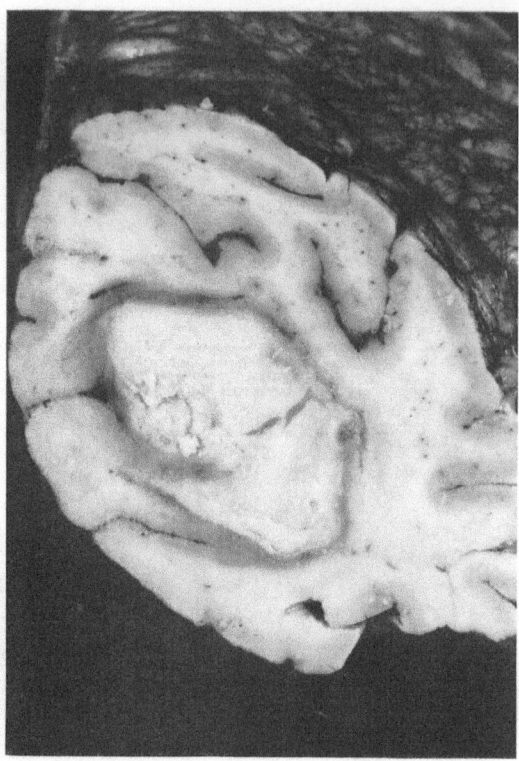

Fig. 339. Multiple small abscesses in the occipital lobe

Fig. 340. Case of multiple abscesses: this lesion involved the occipital lobe

194

1.4 Hemorrhages (Subarachnoid, Epidural, Subdural, Cerebral) and Infarcts

Neurosurgical procedures influence the course of intracranial hemorrhages: (1) by eradication of the source of hemorrhage in many cases and (2) by removing the blood clot which is space-occupying and the source of secondary perifocal edema at the same time. Indication for surgery may therefore give insight to pathogenesis and will be discussed in some detail.

The following classification may serve as a basis for discussion.

Hemorrhages Mainly Due to Localized Causes: Trauma:

a) Epidural hematoma. In the majority of cases this follows a traumatic lesion of the middle meningeal artery and, rarely, venous oozing in the presence of decreased intracranial pressure may be possible. The site and extension of epidural bleeding can be explained by the anatomical fixation of the dura to the skull; therefore, the localization is different from that of the freely spreading typical subdural hematoma, whose predilection for the free subdural fronto-temporo-parietal space is well known. Epidural hemorrhage may, on the other hand, be more limited to frontal (Figs. 341–343), temporal or occipitoparietal regions (Fig. 344) depending on the site of the fracture interrupting a branch of the middle meningeal artery. A second etiology, which becomes apparent after surgery, is secondary to venous oozing into the epidural space and is related to the preceding surgical flap in as much as venous pressures could hardly be expected to effect a separation of dura from bone in the natural state.

b) Subdural hematoma including acute, subacute, and chronic encapsulated hemorrhages can spread more easily than the epidural ones because of the open subdural space. Their site of predilection is the area of confluence of the three great lobes—that is, over the fronto-temporo-parietal region (Fig. 345). This fact may be explained by the mechanical advantage of displacing brain substance at this particular point, inasmuch as such lateral shifts are determined to a large extent by local resistance of brain tissue to compression or deformation by a hematoma—i.e., the relative ease of forcing brain matter beneath the fixed dural septae, the degree of fixation of brain to skull (pituitary stalk, vessels, nerves) particularly at the base, and finally the inherent properties of the brain itself (great fasciculi of the white matter). These facets may in turn be influenced by both CSF and intra-arterial pressures. Such shifts (Figs. 16, 17) are often of great diagnostic significance in these and other space-occupying lesions by virtue of the characteristic distortions they produce radiologically and on echoencephalograms. These may be absent, however, when the hematomas are bilateral.

The acute subdural hematoma usually is associated with extensive brain trauma, but may stem from a solitary laceration of a major arterial vessel (Fig. 346) usually on the surface of the brain (as in our own case of a man aged 56). Here, if diagnosed early enough, and if this is the sole lesion, surgical evacuation should not be difficult. The site of predilection of the acute subdural hematoma corresponds to that of the subacute and chronic types. A second etiology for an acute subdural accumulation of blood may follow when the intracranial pressure is reduced below normal—as, for instance, following the evacuation of a subdural hematoma when a recurrence occurs—or, even more significantly, when shunting of the CSF causes the pressure to drop in the subdural space.

In the pathogenesis of the chronic subdural we distinguish between two types: (1) a primary degenerative process of the dura in the old-age group, called the true "pachymeningitis" or "pachymeningosis" of Virchow, and (2) the post-traumatic subdural hematoma which may also become encapsulated and is more common in younger people. Macroscopically, in their final stages they both seem to be very similar; microscopically, degenerative changes and/or lymphoid infiltration are seen in the dura of the first type, whereas in the traumatic form the dura is unchanged or only secondarily affected.

The development of an encapsulated hematoma commences with a small blood film underneath (Fig. 348) the dura. This becomes organized and forms capillaries, in the fashion of a cavernous angioma, which are fragile and which may break and form small blood clots. These blood clots, in turn, attract cerebrospinal fluid by osmosis according to the postulates of Gardner, who defined the inner membrane of the hematoma as an osmotically-active membrane. Thus, small hematomas may grow in size by taking up cerebrospinal fluid. Other vessels in the granulating tissue are torn, new blood is added, the osmotic pressure is increased, cerebrospinal fluid is absorbed, and the cycle repeated; hematomas grow in size and unite, forming a bigger blood clot. At a certain stage it becomes too large for the available subdural space, even though this space may be enlarged through atrophy of the aged brain. Finally, the point of maximum compensation is reached, intracranial pressure begins to rise, and neurological symptoms appear.

This working hypothesis can be adopted not only for the post-traumatic form of subdural hematoma but also for pachymeningosis as well, if it is presumed that the initial blood in the subdural space is not due to traumatic rupture of bridging veins but results from oozing of the internal or "endothelial" surface of the degenerated dura. In the majority of cases a flat brownish granulating layer remains on the inner side of the dura. In this case trauma usually induces a space-occupying hemorrhage into this granulation tissue. Thus, the thin primary blood film in the subdural space, which is later transformed into a thin granulation layer on the inside of the dura of one or of both hemispheres, may be of dual etiology: rupture of the bridging veins (traumatic) or oozing from the inside of the degenerated dura. Trauma may be regarded as the main cause in the younger age group, whereas in older patients pachymeningosis—

i.e., a primary degenerative process in the dura—may be considered as the primary cause, and the formation of the hematoma by minor trauma as a secondary cause.

c) Subarachnoid hemorrhage. Traumatic subarachnoid hemorrhage is usually associated with simultaneous subdural hemorrhage, whereas subarachnoid hemorrhage from berry-aneurysms and angiomas (see p. 168) tends to invade and destroy the surrounding brain tissue. Hemorrhage from ruptured saccular aneurysms penetrates into the neighboring brain in regions which are typical for the origin of the aneurysm involved. Thus, we see a bilateral penetration of blood into the base of the medial frontal (Fig. 297) lobes from ruptured aneurysms of the anterior communicating artery. In those of the posterior communicating artery rupture (Fig. 298) may occur into the temporal horn, and finally hemorrhage within the Sylvian fissure may break into the adjacent frontal and temporal lobes in aneurysms of the middle cerebral artery (Fig. 296).

d) Intracerebral hemorrhage (contusion and laceration of deep vessels in the white matter). Post-traumatic intracerebral hemorrhage is usually subcortical and may be readily detected and attacked surgically in the acute phase. Moreover, it may be found as a special form in the old-age group—the so-called "Schwarzacher Markblutung"—but details of the pathogenesis of this type are not yet quite clear (Fig. 347). The little traumatic pericapillary hemorrhage in contusion may extend and magnify the significance of the local lesion by perifocal edema. Hemorrhages into the mesencephalon and the pons are usually (Fig. 349) the consequence of an "axial shift" of the brain stem. This may be the direct effect of acute acceleration/deceleration phenomena or, more commonly, a consequence of an "axial shift" of the brain stem following subacute mass displacements in space-occupying lesions within the supratentorial space. In either case, tearing of the finer ramifications of the arteries and veins ensues resulting in periarterial or perivenous hemorrhages in the terminal regions of the vessels, as shown by postmortem injection techniques. Mass hemorrhages may also follow anticoagulation or fibrinolytic therapy and may be amenable to surgical therapy (Fig. 350).

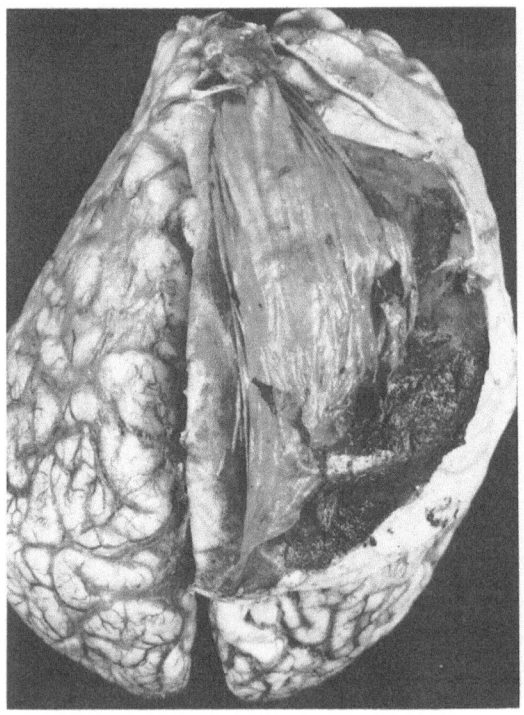

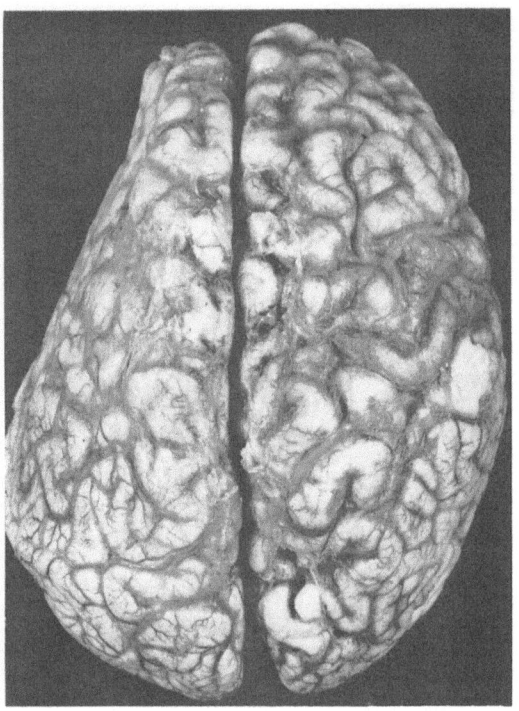

Fig. 341. Marked depression of the anterior left hemisphere by an extensive epidural hematoma

Fig. 342. Frontoparietal depression of the hemisphere and marked displacement to the right (see Fig. 341)

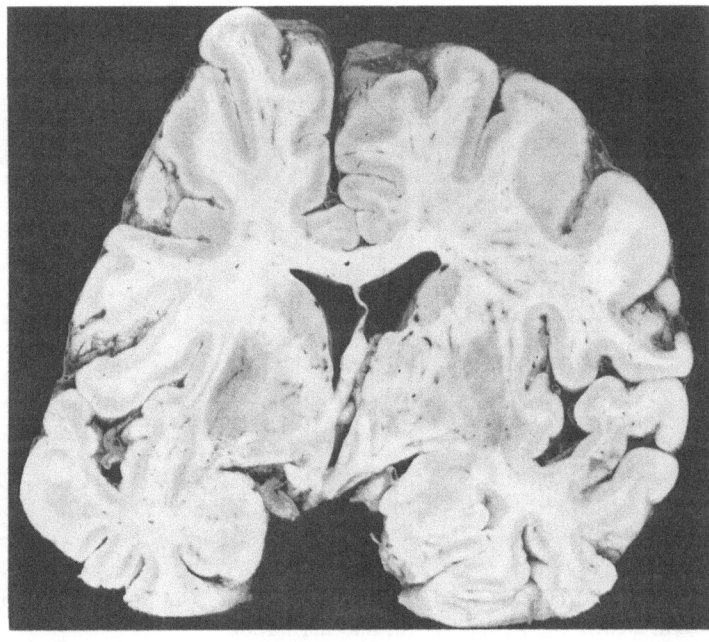

Fig. 343. Frontal section of the previous case. Note the lateral shift

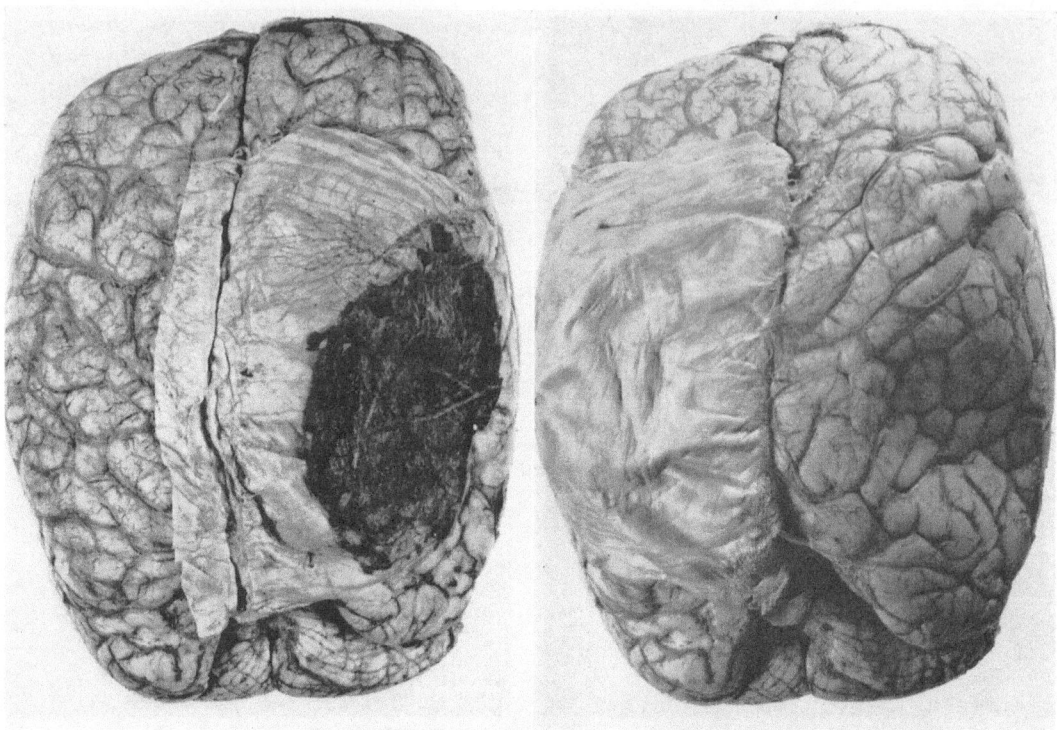

Fig. 344. Large epidural hematoma overlying the parietal lobe

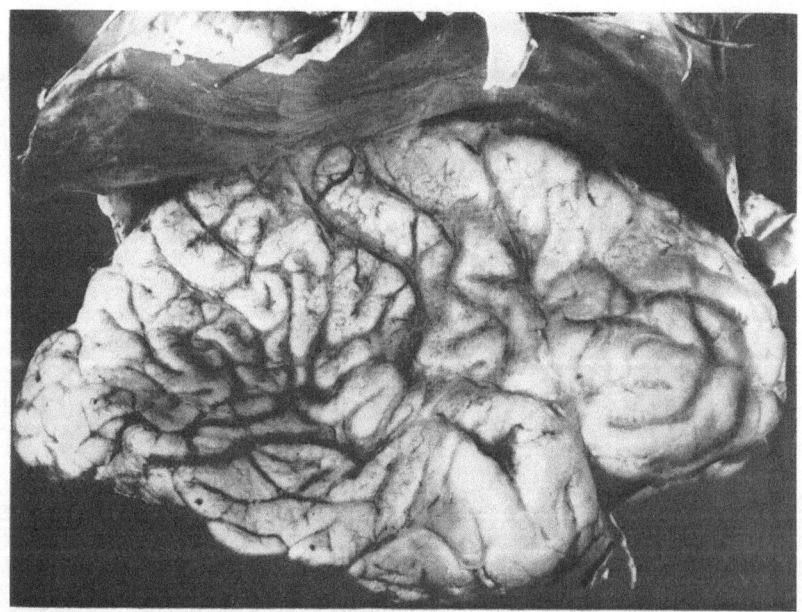

Fig. 345. Old chronic subdural hematoma. Note the impression left by the lesion in the underlying brain. Death due to mass effect and herniation

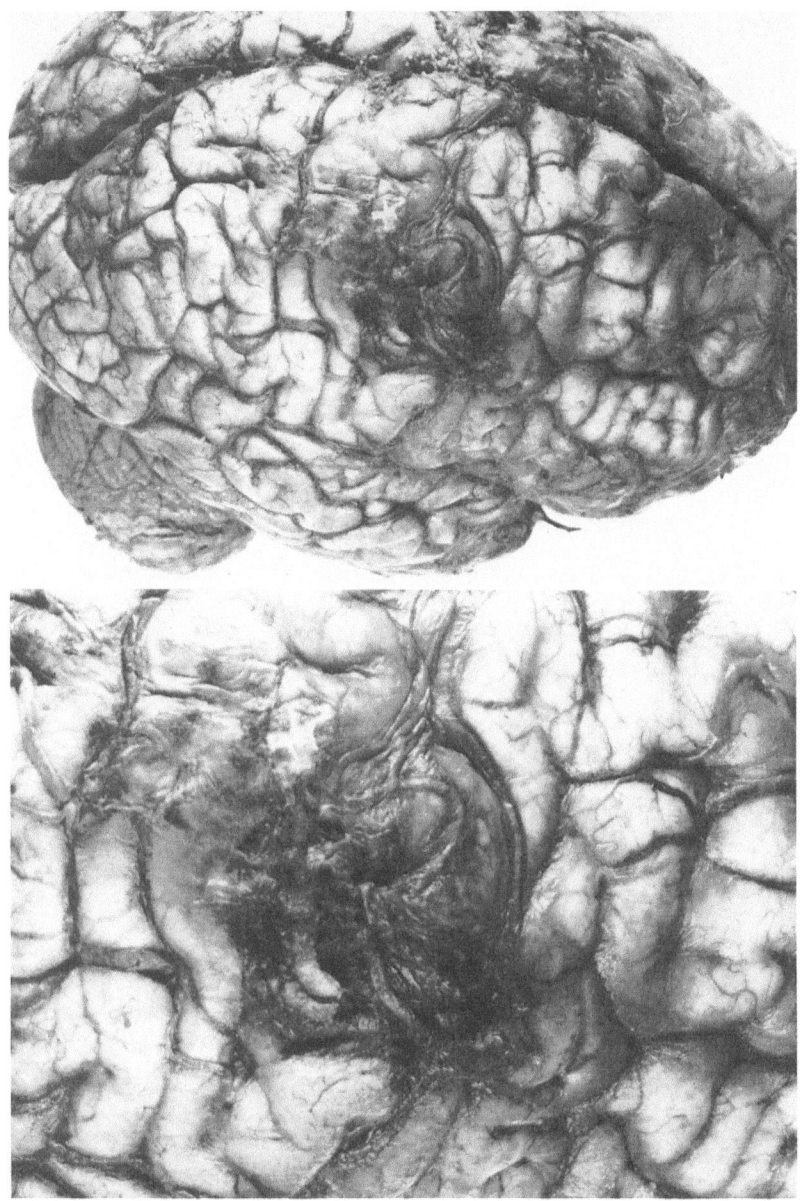

Fig. 346. Traumatic laceration of cortical arteries giving rise to acute subdural hematoma without much damage to underlying brain (rare!)

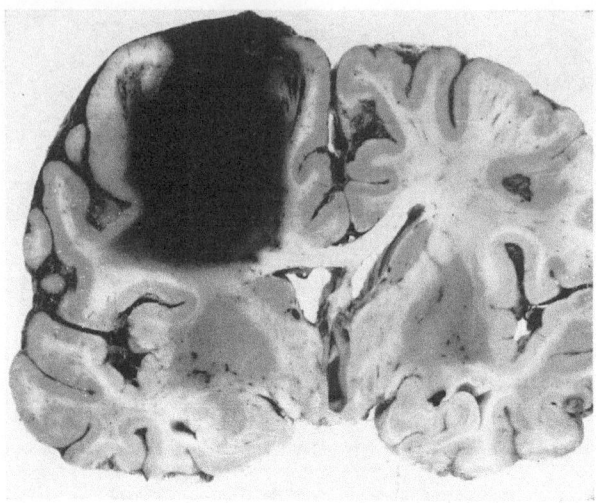

Fig. 347. Atypical subcortical hemorrhage. No relationship to the striatal arteries, no "microangioma"

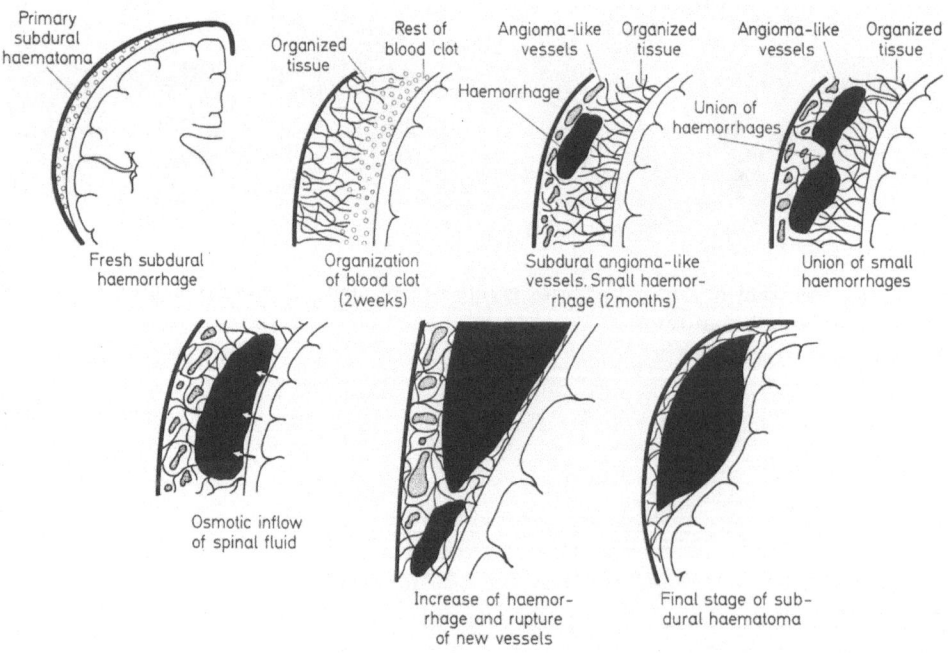

Fig. 348. Various stages of the pathogenesis of the capsulated subdural hematoma

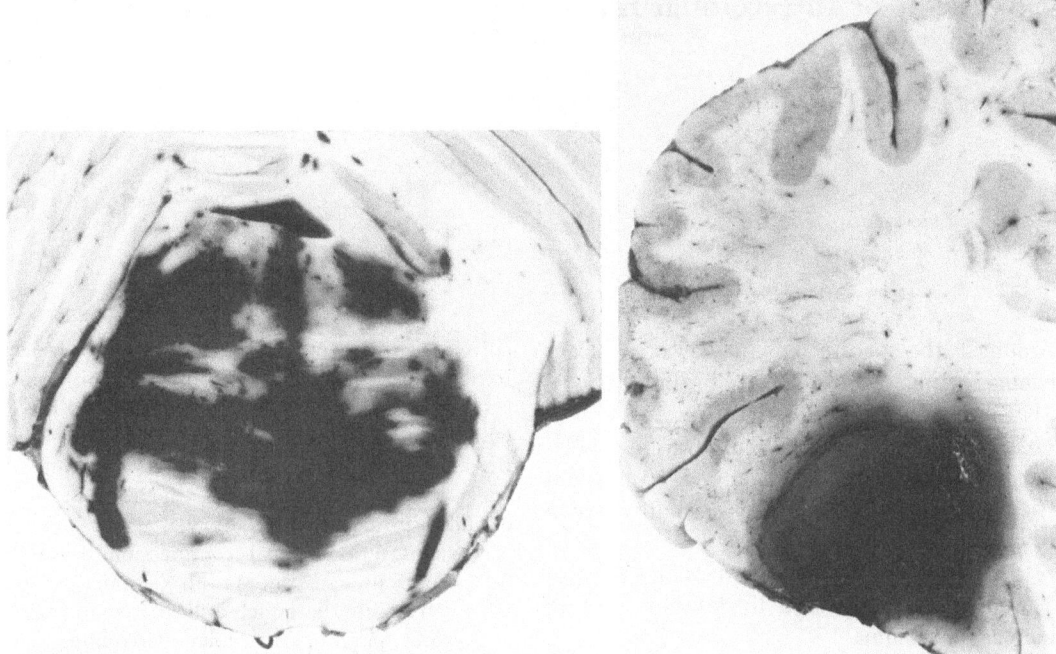

Fig. 349. Typical hemorrhages around bulbar veins and arteries following marked "axial shift" in a supratentorial tumor with gross brain edema. Similar hemorrhages were called hemorrhages of Duret-Berner in the older literature

Fig. 350. Mass hemorrhage in the "watershed" zone following fibrinolytic therapy (streptokinase) for thrombosis of a middle cerebral artery with infarction, which is apparent above the hemorrhage

1.5 Extra- or Intracellular Edema (Brain Edema and Brain Swelling)

Amongst the space-occupying factors, "brain edema" (Figs. 351–356) and "brain swelling" play prominent roles. The resulting increase in volume can cause clinical deterioration by elevating the intracranial pressure, as well as aid the process of localization of a smaller lesion in neuroradiology.

In English speaking countries the term of "swelling" is often used to describe only an increase in volume.

There has been much discussion on whether the old German school's separation of brain "edema" and "swelling" into two distinct entities has still any bearing for neurosurgery or neuropathology. Yet the facts remain that: (1) a gross distinction is possible—in brain edema the fluid runs out of the cut surface and the blood in the vessels smears, whereas in brain swelling the cut surface is dry and sticky and cross sections of the vessels remain visible; (2) distinction is also possible by microscopic examination and in ultrastructural pictures where fluid is noted in edema between the cell membranes in the interstitial spaces (*inter*cellular edema), whereas in brain swelling the increase in volume is within the cells (*intra*cellular edema); (3) there are also pathologic

correlates which may be cited—in a generalized toxic process (such as TET intoxication) *intra*cellular volume may increase (brain "swelling"), while a corresponding increase in the *inter*cellular fluid is never seen. Conversely, in a variety of other pathological processes—such as trauma, circulatory disturbances of venous or arterial origin, infarctions, local compression, localized inflammations, restricted intoxications (diphtheria toxin, for example), and microembolism—a clear-cut, partly perivascular (perivenous, pericapillary) and partly diffuse interstitial *inter*cellular edema can be produced. (4) And finally, employment of certain indicators with differential permeabilities as regards the blood-brain barrier (Evans blue, peroxyde, etc.) has clearly demonstrated two distinct lesions which correspond respectively to the old terms of brain edema and brain swelling (see Table 8).

Our knowledge of the morphology and pathogenesis of brain swelling and edema is still rather incomplete. However, on the basis of the above explanation it seems certain to us that these two conditions are different and that they can either exist separately, or one following the other, or else they may be mixed.

Table 8. Types of "brain edema" according to pathogenesis and localization

	Pathogenesis	Lesion in man	Localization
Intracellular edema	Metabolic or toxic lesions of parenchyma	Schizophrenia Internal and external intoxications	White matter Cortex
Extracellular edema	Metabolic or toxic lesions of vasculature	1. Mass hemorrhage 2. Infarct 3. Traumatic necrosis 4. Toxic { necrosis / necrobiosis 5. Infections: Purulent abscess, Encephalitis, Meningitis etc. 6. Intracerebral tumor	White matter more than cortex (perifocal) Propagation along the myelin bundles and pathways of white matter

However, in order to follow the accepted English terminology, I shall use the terms *"intra- or extracellular edema"*.

Primary intracellular edema is most easily demonstrated in the cortex, affecting astrocytes and neurons, and in the myelin sheaths of the white matter. Primary extracellular brain edema, on the other hand, has a particular preference for the white matter. Here, however, the myelin may also "secondarily" undergo an "intracellular" uptake of edema fluid and thus become at the end an intracellular edema as well. Both processes have a distinct mass effect and both can lead to a marked abnormality of the neural tissues with either atrophy (particularly of the white matter) or, in acute and particularly heavy extracellular edema, even "edema necrosis". These two lesions are common sequelae of different pathological processes:

1. *Intra*cellular brain edema ("dry" edema):
   a) Primary, generalized intracellular brain edema such as occurs in association with many general medical conditions, with psychiatric diseases (for instance, catatonia and schizophrenia), and with intoxications.
   b) Primary, focal (collateral) intracellular brain edema, such as occurs around malignant tumors (Fig. 351).
   c) Secondary intracellular brain edema, such as follows intercellular presence of edema fluid in the interstitial tissues (Figs. 352, 356).

2. *Extra*cellular brain edema ("wet" edema):
   a) Extracellular edema of a mechanical, hemodynamic origin (transudate)—as, for example, from obstruction of the venous outflow, thrombosis of veins and sinuses (Figs. 357–359) or in cases of compression. This condition is predominantly found in the cortex and in the edema fluid has a low protein content.
   b) Extracellular edema of a predominantly reactive or "chemical" origin (exudate). This arises from disturbances in the metabolism of the tissue, such as abnormalities of pH, and tends to occur in the vicinity of necrosis (Fig. 356), infarcts (Fig. 360a, b), hemorrhage, or inflammation (Figs. 353, 354). It has a predominantly peri-

capillary and peri-venous location and the protein content of the fluid is apt to show varying degrees of elevation, being highest around abscesses or phlegmons (Fig. 354). This type of edema includes that edema occurring in the white matter around veins in the para-infectious encephalitides, and also that edema as seen in fat embolism.
   c) Tumors with a predominantly expansive growth pattern may show secondary circulatory disturbances with necrosis of the adjacent tissues leading to intra- and extracellular edema and more necrosis. Such a reaction may be seen in the meningiomas (Fig. 212) and also in the acoustic neurinomas where pressure atrophy and post-edematous softenings occur in the adjacent pons. The occlusion of a sinus—particularly the right transverse sinus—can lead to an enormous increase in volume of the hemisphere secondary to a sterile edema.

As a rule of the thumb one can assume that in two-thirds of the cases the right sinus transversus drains the brain mantle and in this case the left drains the system of the vena magna Galeni. The reverse pattern is encountered in about 10% of the cases. In only 10% does a "complete" and equal mixing of the drained blood take place in the Torcular Herophili. In the remainder, different types of patterns are found.

The same can happen in large abscesses where an entire hemisphere may be "drowned" in a perifocal, protein-rich, extracellular edematous infectious exudation (Fig. 353).

After trauma—as in the diffuse concussive injuries—generalized edema may occur, reaching its greatest intensity around the third day. Local contusions or surgical wounds (Fig. 356) concurrent hemorrhages may produce a perifocal edema and thus add to the total effect of the primary lesion. Traumatic sinus occlusions are also implicated on occasion.

A similar increase in volume may be seen in the malignant tumors as well, where a small glioblastoma or metastasis can lead to an enormous swelling of the adjacent white matter—in this instance by *intra*cellular edema—with mass movements away from the side of the lesion.

Pseudotumor Cerebri (Nonne)

The term "pseudotumor cerebri" denotes an increase in volume of the brain substance which is not caused by any of the usual factors increasing intracranial pressure (see p. 2). It is characterized by an increase in interstitial fluid (brain edema, see p. 202) caused by a number of now detectable factors, both of mechanical and systemic nature. These include obstruction of the jugular veins, thrombosis of the sinuses (particularly of the right transverse sinus), and some less well-defined hormonal and metabolic processes. Abrupt cessation of prolonged steroid therapy (corticosteroids in children, contraceptive drugs in young women) has been incriminated in this regard, as have many other diverse factors.

However, in the majority of cases with this obscure condition, the true etiology of the intracranial hypertension remains to be elucidated.

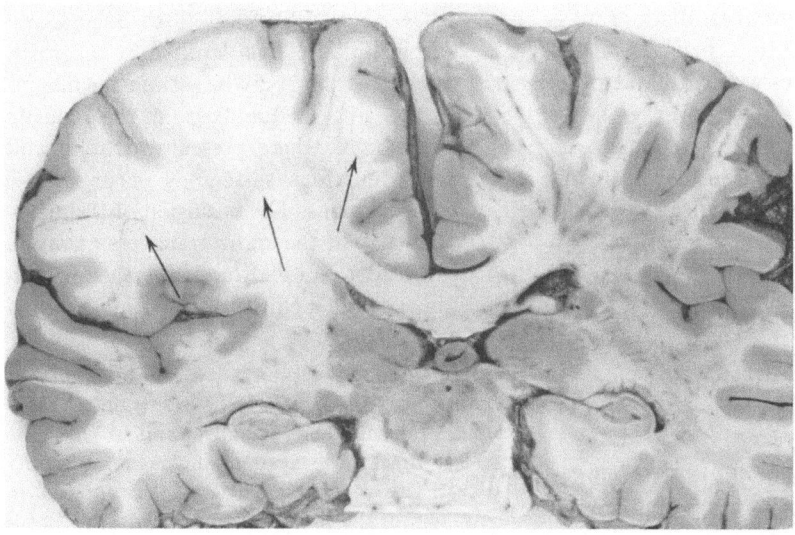

Fig. 351. Extensive posterior brain-swelling in a glioblastoma (arrows!). Sub-falceal herniation at this level is difficult because of the close approximation of the falx to the corpus callosum posteriorly

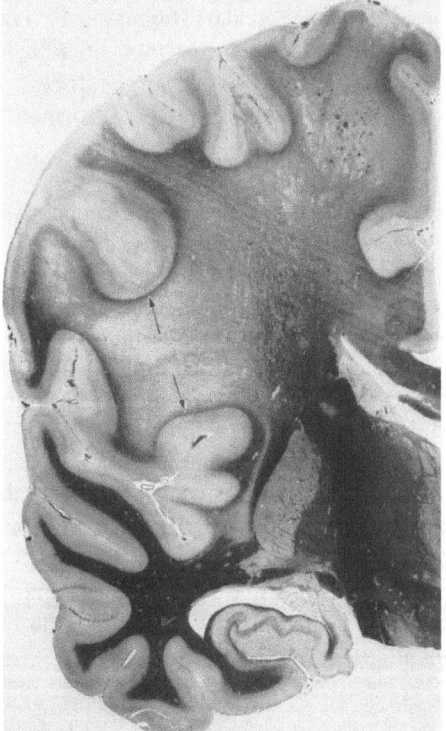

Fig. 352. Extensive edema in the white matter of the parietal lobe secondary to infected gunshot wound. The U-fibers stand out clearly against the edema (arrows!). Death 25 days post trauma. Myelin-stain

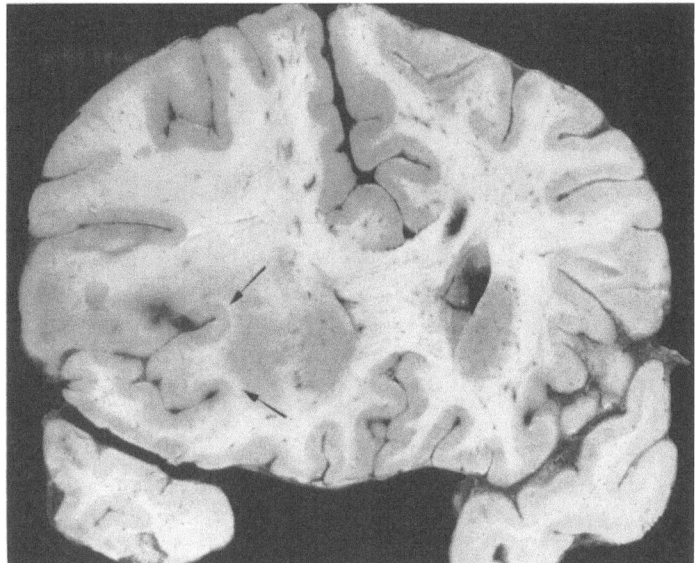

Fig. 353. Extensive edema in a case of a pea-sized metastasis from a bronchial carcinoma into the frontal operculum. Small hemorrhagic tracks are noted secondary to needle punctures. The U-fibers (arrows!) are now quite well demarcated within their edematous surroundings

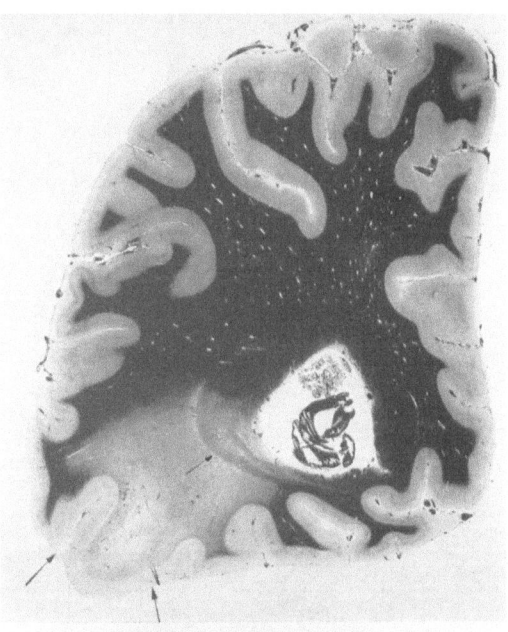

Fig. 354. Circumscribed demyelination in the inferior temporal gyrus and adjacent white matter. Fatal case of a gunshot wound with overwhelming rapid infection. Death on the fourth day. Note absence of local cerebral displacements (arrows!). Myelin stain

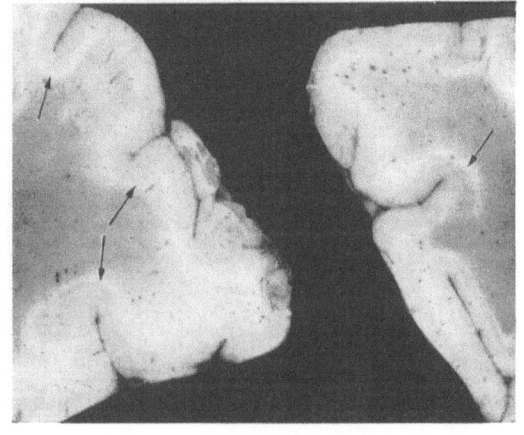

Fig. 355. Marked brownish-green edema in the white matter in a case of a metastatic malignant melanoma. The U-fibers are again particularly well seen (arrows!)

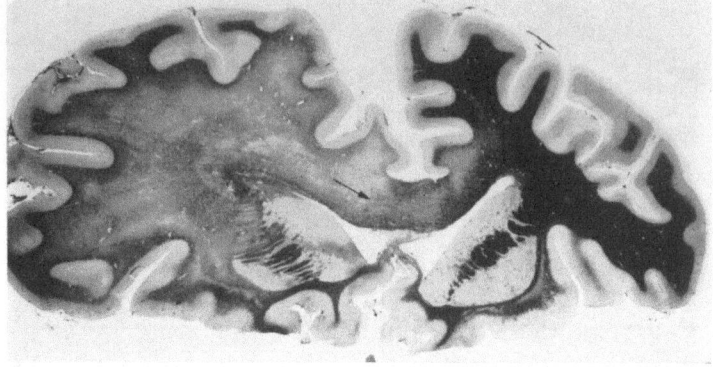

Fig. 356. Swelling and broadening of the frontal white matter of one cerebral hemisphere including the corpus callosum with shift to opposite side (arrow!). Death followed by 3 days a frontal lobectomy for an oligodendroglioma. Myelin-stain

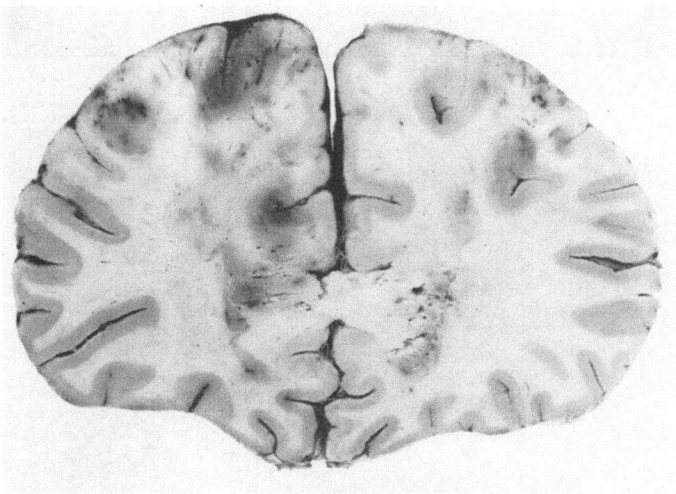

Fig. 357. Occlusion of the superior sagittal sinus. The sections show a hemorrhagic infarction in the appropriate distribution, which is similar to that of the anterior cerebral artery. Note, however, that the white matter is relatively more involved and the veins and venules more engorged than in the infarct of the anterior cerebral

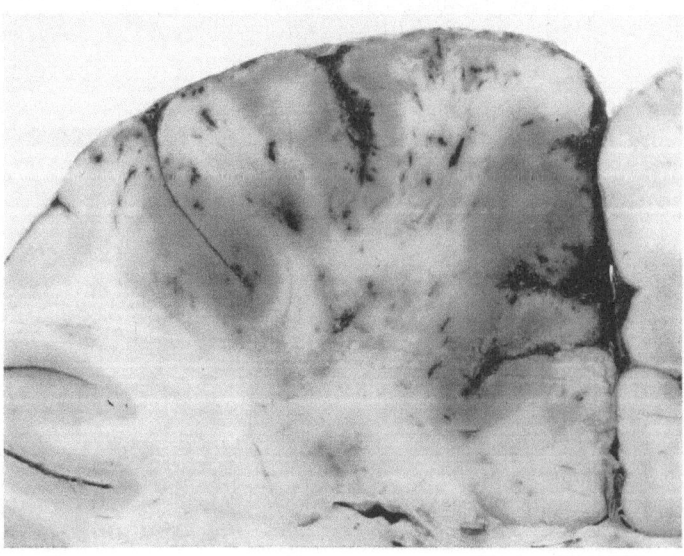

Fig. 358. Close-up view of frontal section after occlusion of the superior sagittal sinus (see Fig. 357)

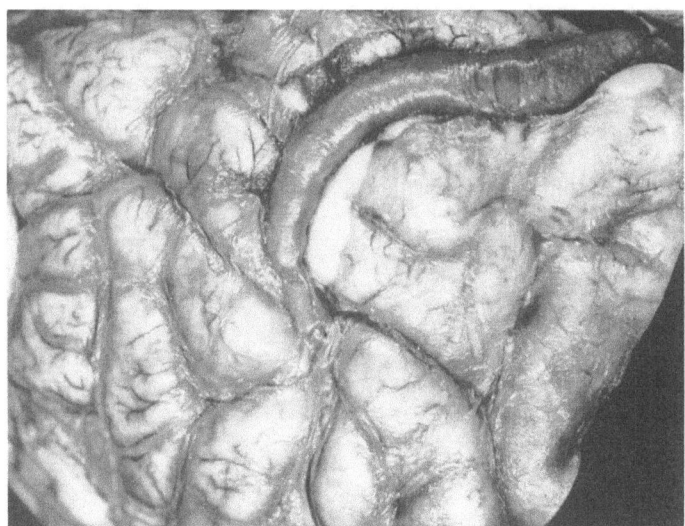

Fig. 359. Thrombosis of the superior sagittal sinus with propagation of clot to the bridging veins

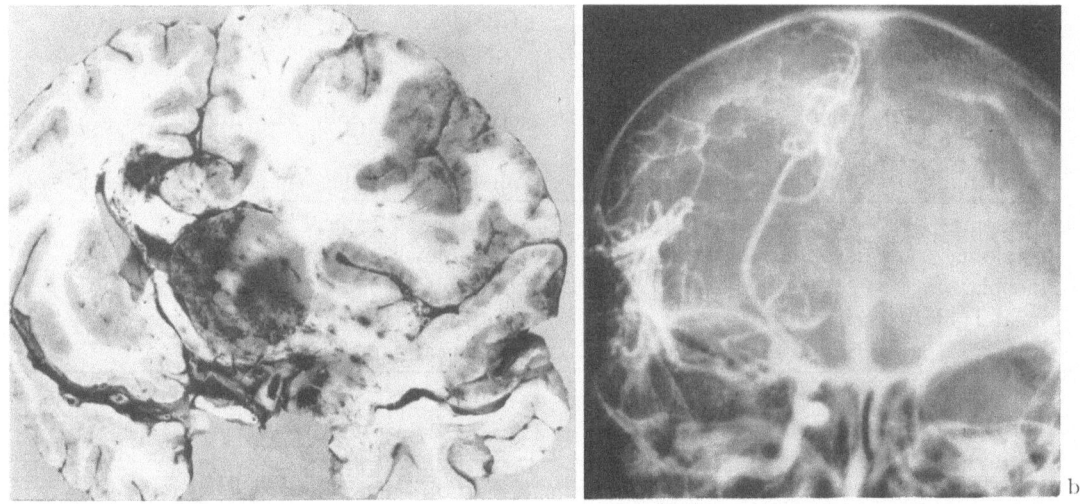

a   b

Fig. 360a and b. Extreme cerebral edema on the third day after an infarct in the territory of the anterior and posterior cerebral artery with marked mass shift towards the opposite side. a) Brain section with a partly hemorrhagic infarct. b) "Negative angiogram" of tissue displacements. Angiography was performed on the wrong side for the exclusion of a subdural hematoma because of the "wrong", homolateral neurological signs due to the pressure against the opposite tentorial edge (see Fig. 32)

Classification of the principal groups, based on UICC nomenclature	Probable nomenclature of subgroups in future
Gangliocytomas	Gangliocytomas Gangliogliomas Neuroblastomas
Gangliocytomas, polymorphous	Gangliocytomas and Gangliogliomas, anaplastic (malignant)
Ependymomas	Ependymomas; variants: myxopapillary, papillary; Subependymomas
Ependymomas, polymorphous	Ependymomas, anaplastic (malignant)
Plexuspapillomas	Choroid Plexus Papillomas
Plexuspapillomas, polymorphous	Choroid Plexus Papillomas, anaplastic (malignant)
Astrocytomas	Astrocytomas; fibrillary, protoplasmic, gemistocytic
Astrocytomas, polymorphous	Astrocytomas, anaplastic (malignant)
Oligodendrogliomas	Oligodendrogliomas; typical; mixed
Oligodendrogliomas, polymorphous	Oligodendrogliomas, anaplastic (malignant)
Glioblastomas	Glioblastomas, typical; with sarcomatous component
Spongioblastomas	Astrocytomas, pilocytic (piloid)
Spongioblastomas, polymorphous	Astrocytomas, pilocytic, anaplastic (malignant)
Medulloblastomas	Medulloblastomas, typical; desmoplastic
Pinealomas	Pinealomas, typical
Pinealomas, polymorphous	Pinealomas, anaplastic (malignant)
Pineoblastomas	Pineoblastomas
Pineal Tumors, variants	Germinomas, Embryonal Carcinomas, Choriocarcinomas
Neurinomas	Neurinomas, Schwannomas, Neurilemmomas
Neurinomas, polymitotic	Neurinomas, malignant
Neurinomas, variants	Neurofibromas Neurofibromas, malignant
Meningiomas	Meningiomas: meningotheliomatous, fibroblastic, mixed, psammomatous, angiomatous, hemangioblastic, hemangiopericytic
Meningiomas, polymitotic	Meningiomas, anaplastic (malignant)
Angioblastomas	Hemangioblastomas (capillary)
Sarcomas	Sarcomas: Fibrosarcomas; primary meningeal sarcomatosis; polymorphic cell sarcomas; monstrocellular sarcomas; reticulosarcomas (microgliomas), periadventitial diffuse sarcomas and other primary malignant forms of lymphoma
Pituitary Adenomas	Pituitary Adenomas, acidophil, basophil, mixed, chromophobe
Pituitary Adenomas, polymorphous	Adenocarcinomas
Craniopharyngiomas	Craniopharyngiomas

2. Obstructive Hydrocephalus

An obstruction in the cerebrospinal fluid pathways occurring anywhere from the choroid plexus to the arachnoidal granulations results in the development of an obstructive hydrocephalus (Fig. 361) of the ventricles lying behind the block, provided the choroid plexus continues to function. However, all cases of hydrocephalus are completely reversible at the beginning and in part later on. This can be explained by the initial expansion of the ventricles and the "inflation" of the brain—an expansion that takes place at the cost of the subarachnoid space; the sulci disappear with the increase in intracranial pressure (Fig. 2). If the increased pressure disappears, the enlargement of the ventricles vanishes and the subarachnoid space is re-established. If the hydrocephalus persists, it is no longer reversible, and the brain is compressed into a thin mantle (Fig. 14)—most drastically exemplified by the paper-thin third ventricular floor (Figs. 57, 144, 162). Secondary to hydrocephalus, herniations of the frontobasal parts into the middle fossa occur (Fig. 24) which displace the middle cerebral artery in the same direction (angiogram, see M_2 segment of the artery). In addition to these well-recognized processes, certain particular hydrodynamic mechanisms which have recently been discussed should be mentioned. In occlusion of the aqueduct, the suprapineal recess can expand (Fig. 76) to the size of a chestnut; it pushes its way under the tentorium against the superior cerebellar vermis. The brain substance may perforate at various places, most frequently on the medial wall of the trigonum (Figs. 362,) of the lateral ventricle, and the cerebrospinal fluid escapes through the opening and forms a subarachnoid cyst the size of a chestnut (Fig. 362). This cyst may extend into the cisterna ambiens in the direction of the anterior lobe of the cerebellum. When, by means

of this rare mechanism, a connection is reestablished between the ventricles and the subarachnoid space a spontaneous cure ensues; this may also be accomplished surgically (ventriculocisternotomy, atrio-ventricular shunt, etc.).

The distinction between the communicating and obstructive forms of hydrocephalus is not entirely logical because both are in fact "obstructive"—in the former the obstruction is usually located external to the ventricular system (Fig. 331) and its outlets, whereas in the latter it occurs within the ventricular system or at the foramina of the fourth ventricle. However, a "communicating" hydrocephalus by convention usually results either from failure of the spinal fluid to make its way over the cerebral hemispheres (Fig. 361) or from failure of absorption once it gets there.

Potential sites of obstruction and the resulting types of hydrocephalus are illustrated in Fig. 361 and are commented on below.

1. A unilateral obstructive hydrocephalus is seen after occlusion of a single foramen of Monro secondary to either a well-situated tumor near the foramen itself (Figs. 54, 55) or at the base of the frontal horn or secondary to a lateral cerebral displacement resulting from a mass effect. Occlusion of both foramina of Monro occurs in association with the so-called colloid cysts of the third ventricle (Fig. 73), as well as with the fronto-basal midline tumors [olfactory meningiomas (Fig. 193), large falx meningiomas (Fig. 190), and even "butterfly" glioblastomas (Fig. 125)].

2. Similarly, an obstructive hydrocephalus often follows third ventricular tumors which may be primary—ependymomas, plexus papillomas (Fig. 81), meningiomas of the velum interpositum—or secondary. These latter tumors impinge on the lumen of the third ventricle

from without and include the spongioblastomas (Fig. 150), the craniopharyngiomas (Figs. 258, 259), and the pituitary adenomas (Fig. 250).

3. Occlusion at the level of the aqueduct may also occur and is most commonly caused by tumors, by cicatrices (Figs. 363, 364) and ependymal membranes (Fig. 76), and by other space-occupying lesions, such as arachnoidal cysts (Fig. 332). Again, the tumors may be primarily aqueductal in origin—spongioblastomas (Figs. 152, 159), astrocytomas, ependymomas—or secondary. The secondary lesions arise from the pineal region—teratomas, pinealomas (Figs. 242, 244), pineoblastomas (Figs. 245, 246)—or from the vicinity of the quadrigeminal plate [astrocytomas of the tectum or spongioblastomas (Figs. 153, 154)].

4. Obstruction within the fourth ventricle or at its outlets is seen secondary to tumors (Figs. 62, 147, 162), to cicatrices (Fig. 365), or to arachnoiditis with cyst formation (Figs. 329, 330). Frequently responsible tumors are the ependymoma (Fig. 62), the angioblastoma (Fig. 224), the plexus papilloma, the medulloblastoma (Figs. 162, 167), the spongioblastoma (Fig. 147), dermoids (Fig. 274) and teratomas. Partial occlusion is more usual with the extra-cerebellar tumors, such as the torcular meningiomas (Fig. 206), the clivus chordomas, the cerebellopontine angle tumors (Figs. 172–175, 200–203), and the craniospinal meningiomas (Fig. 207).

5. Hydrocephalus may also follow paramedian masses if they obstruct or at least temporarily impede the CSF pathway.

6. Blockage of the CSF pathways external to the ventricular system commonly follows cicatrization after meningitis (tuberculous meningitis in particular with obliteration of the peri-mesencephalic cisterns and cyst formation) (Fig. 331), but is most frequently seen in "congenital" hydrocephalus in association with the Arnold-Chiari malformation. This group corresponds to the clinical "communicating" hydrocephalus and also includes cases where the pathways along the sulci have become obliterated or even where the Pacchionion granulations are blocked.

Very rarely hypersecretion of the spinal fluid may occur in association with plexus papillomas of the lateral ventricles as deduced from the autopsy specimen. The patients are usually very young and are sometimes born with the disease. Here, the external CSF pathways are rarely outlined by virtue of the exaggeration of the normal channels which has taken place—the cisterns are grooved by the increased flow and the sulci (between the Sylvian fissure and the arachnoidal granulations) are widened and deepened.

Occlusive hydrocephalus is accompanied by varying degrees of ventricular dilatation (Figs. 366–375 a–c) depending on the completeness of the obstruction—intermittent hydrocephalus, for example, is less marked than the more persistent forms. In long-standing hydrocephalus, pressure-atrophy of the brain substance ensues (Figs. 369, 370). In children the brain mantle is sometimes only a few centimeters thick (Figs. 371, 375) and the floor of the third ventricle paper-thin (Figs. 57, 144). However, in its early stages the effects of the hydrocephalus are nearly always partially or totally reversible. The rapid decrease in dilatation following either surgical removal of the block or a shunting procedure, can be explained by the fact that the brain possesses an inherent elasticity and the dilatation process is mainly one of compression, with the ventricular system being initially "blown up" like a rubber balloon, the spinal fluid in the sulci and cisterns is forced out and the convolutions are flattened, stretched out, and pressed against the calvarium. After early release of the obstruction, the whole process simply reverses itself, often without adverse clinical sequelae.

Any eccentric form of hydrocephalus may cause a lateral displacement of brain substance (see Fig. 361). The midline type of obstruction, however, with ensuing bilateral hydrocephalus causes generalized increased intracranial pressure and eventually an "axial" shift.

Some particularities of formation of hydrocephalus can be briefly mentioned (Figs. 376–379).

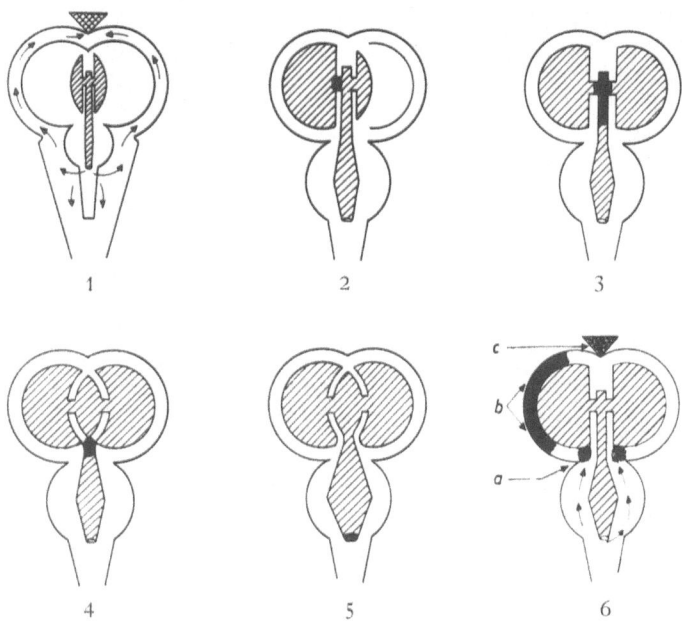

Fig. 361. The different forms of occlusive hydrocephalus and the underlying blocks
1 Pathway of normal CSF flow; *2* Unilateral block of the foramen of monro; *3* Third ventricular block; *4* Block of the aqueduct; *5* Block of the outlets of the fourth ventricle; *6* Block within the external CSF pathways, *a* Ambient cisterns, *b* Sylvian fissure and over convexity, *c* Pacchionian granulations, sagittal sinus

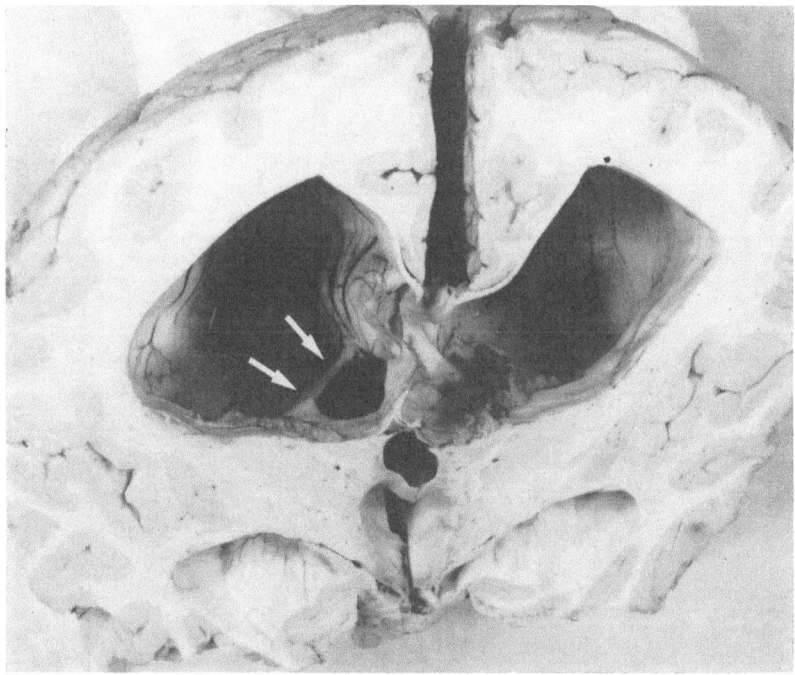

Fig. 362. The medial wall of the right trigonum (arrows!) has ruptured. Marked obstructive hydrocephalus consequent to an aqueductal blockage (c.f. Fig. 361) and an arachnoidal cyst was trapped in the quadrigeminal area

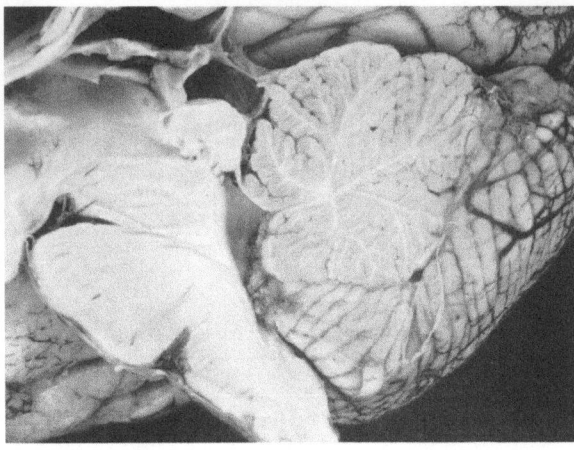

Fig. 363. Trabecular scars from chronic ependymitis obstructing the lumen of the aqueduct

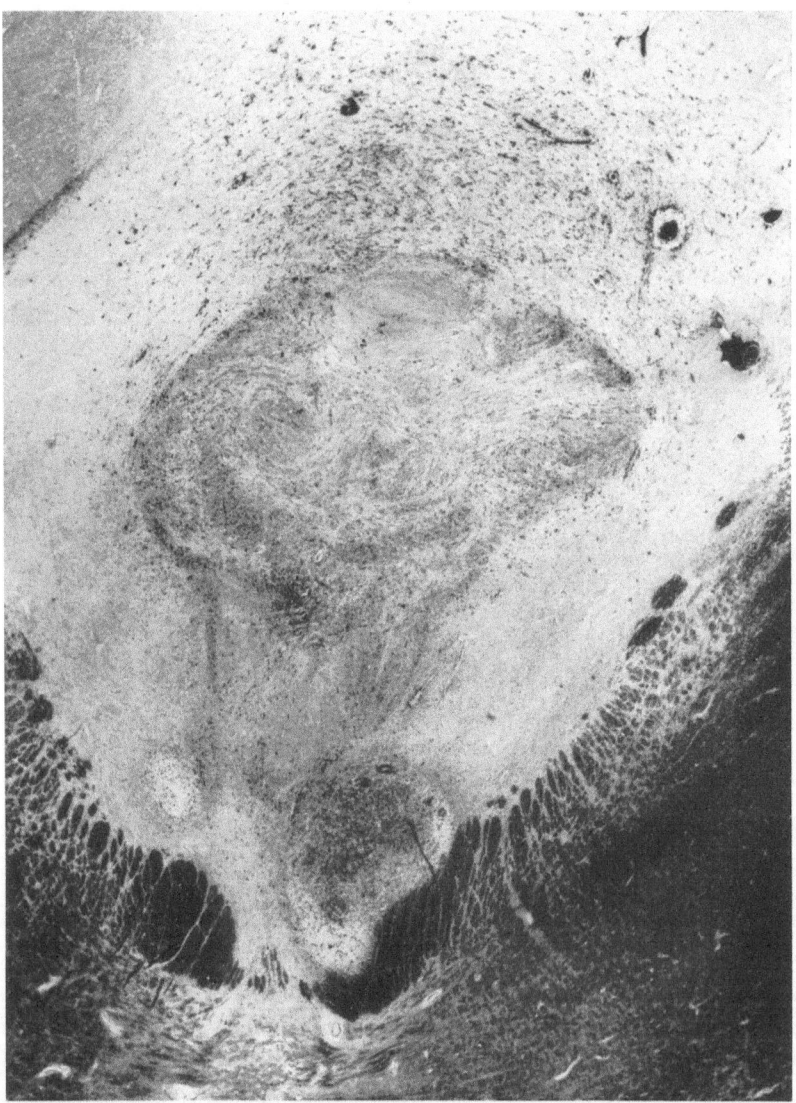

Fig. 364. Obstruction of the aqueduct consequent to chronic luetic ependymitis. Numerous Rosenthal fibers have been formed as a result of the inflammatory reaction in the periaqueductal grey

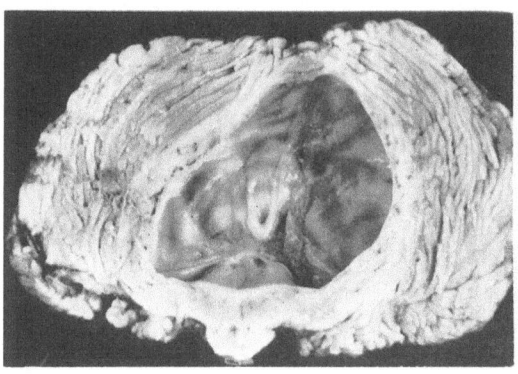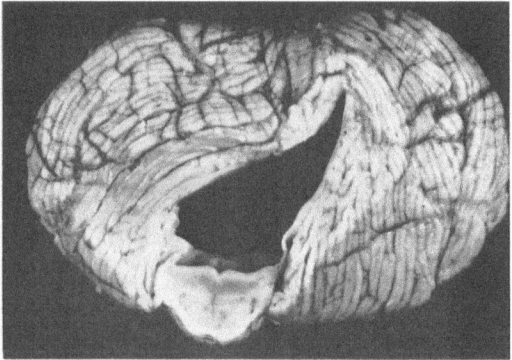

Fig. 365. Scar formation in the basal leptomeninges blocking the outlets of the fourth ventricle. Note the enormous dilatation of the fourth ventricle

Fig. 366. Obstructive hydrocephalus (Grade I) in a case of cerebellar angioblastoma

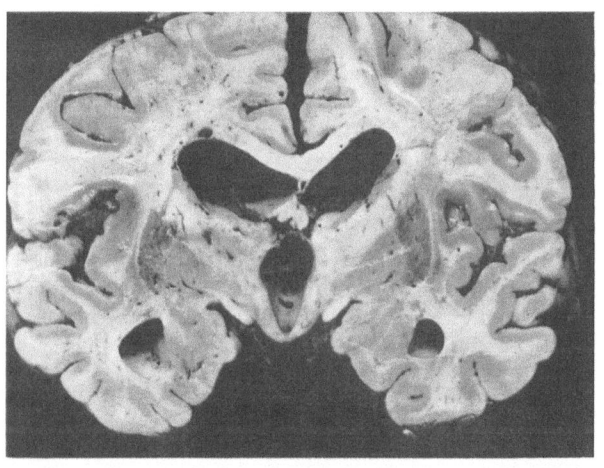

Fig. 367. Occlusive hydrocephalus due to a tumor in the posterior fossa. Note the marked dilatation of the third ventricle and the tips of the temporal horns (Grade II)

213

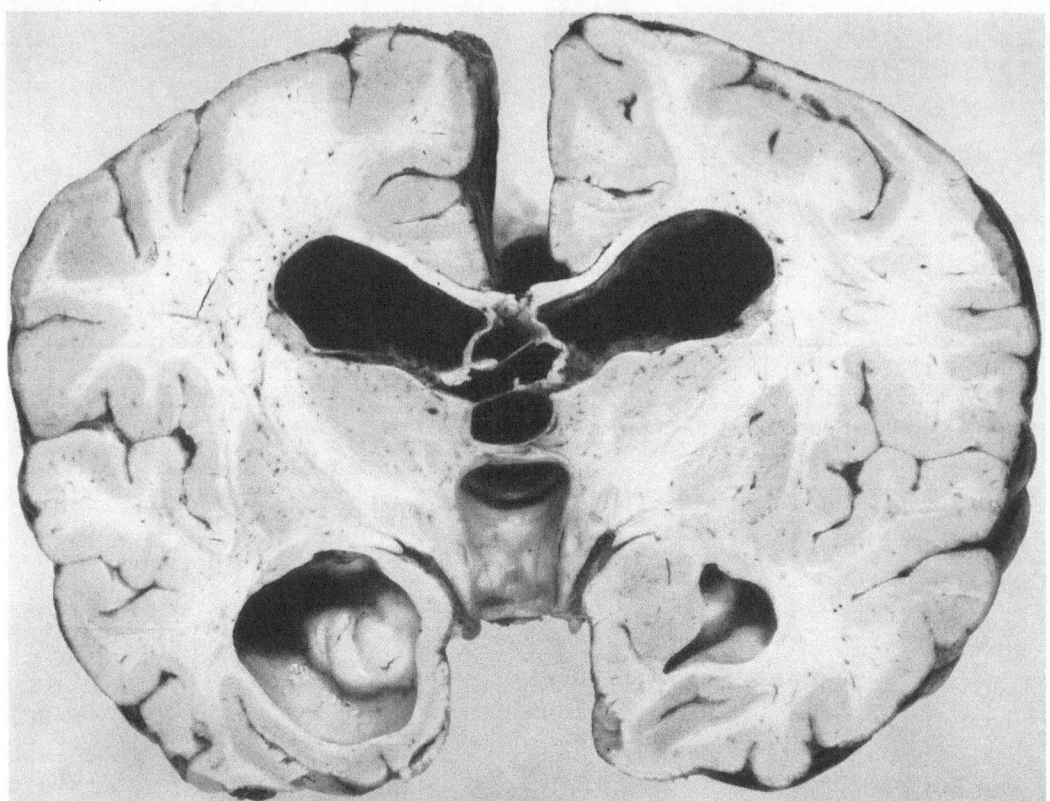

Fig. 368. Case of massive obstructive hydrocephalus secondary to a lesion in the posterior fossa. The enlargement of the frontal horns is well demonstrated; the corpus callosum is torn. Note the round configuration of the ventricles and the tips of the temporal horns. The two forniceal columns and the anterior commissure are particularly well seen

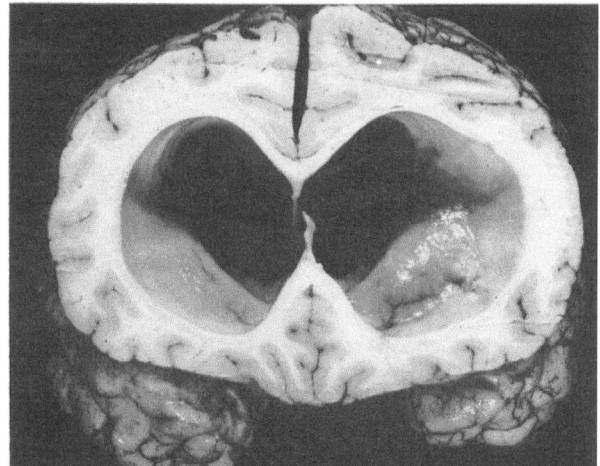

Fig. 369. Obstructive hydrocephalus in a case of a lesion of the posterior fossa. Note the enormous enlargement of the frontal horns (Grade III)

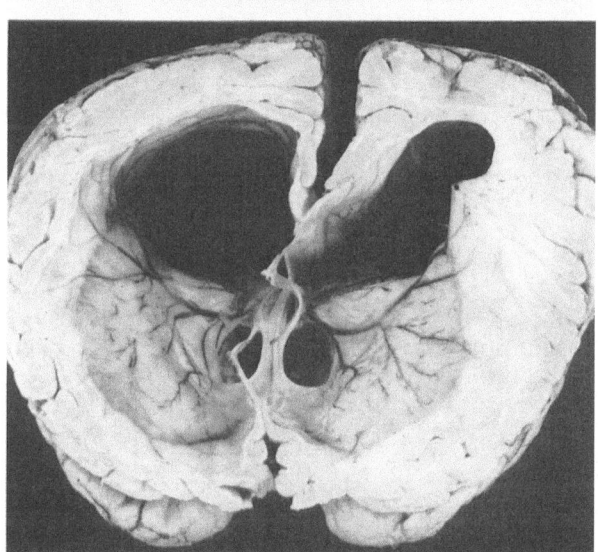

Fig. 370. Enormous ventricular dilatation in obstructive hydrocephalus. Note the enlarged foramina of Monro

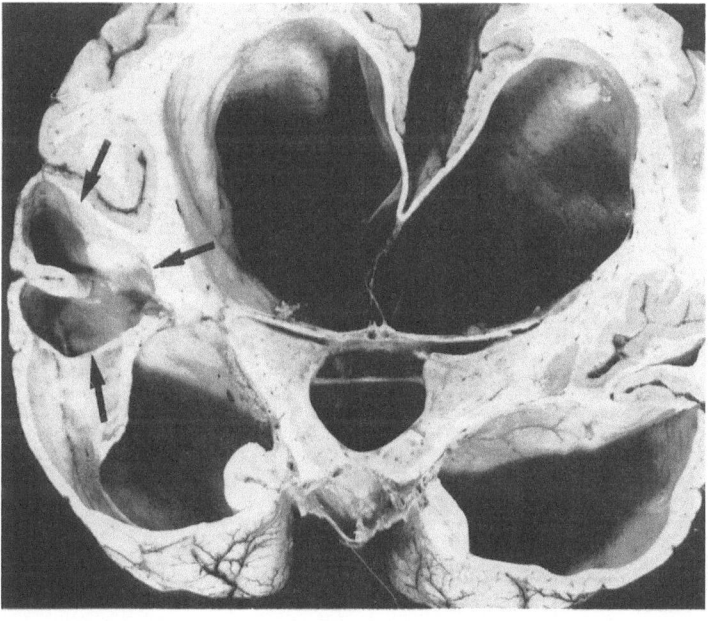

Fig. 371. In the temporal convolutions on both sides degeneration of the white matter with cyst formation has occurred (arrows!). Note the spherical dilatation of the third ventricle in this case of obstructive hydrocephalus

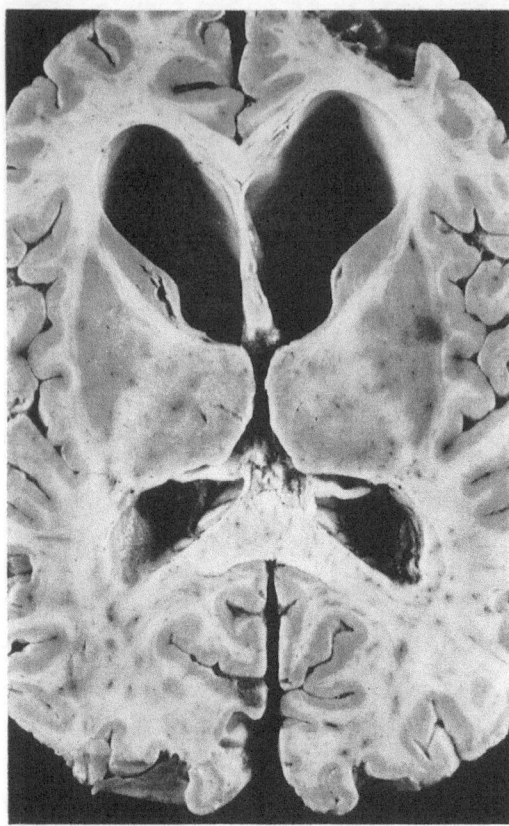

Fig. 372. Obstructive hydrocephalus in a case of total occlusion of the foramen of Magendi and the lateral recesses (see Fig. 373)

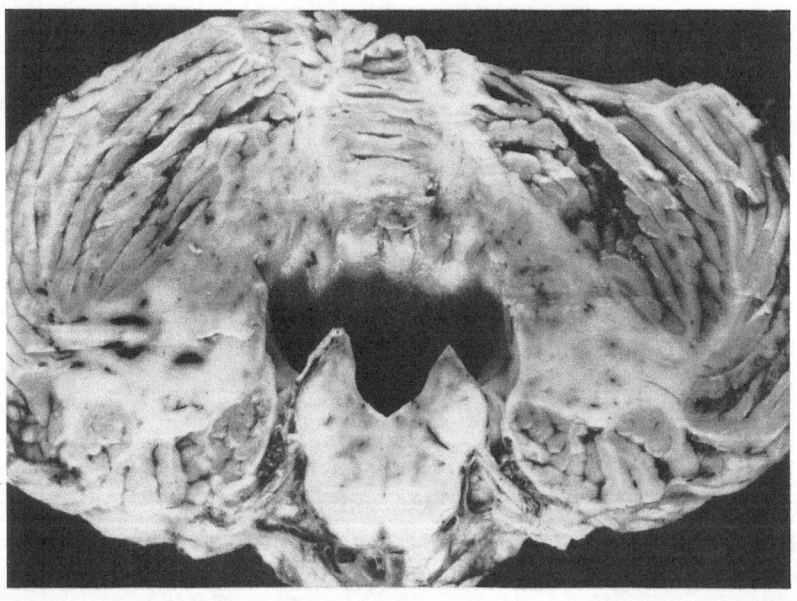

Fig. 373. Scar formation in the arachnoidal spaces blocking the foramen of Magendi and the lateral recesses. Note the dilatation of the latter

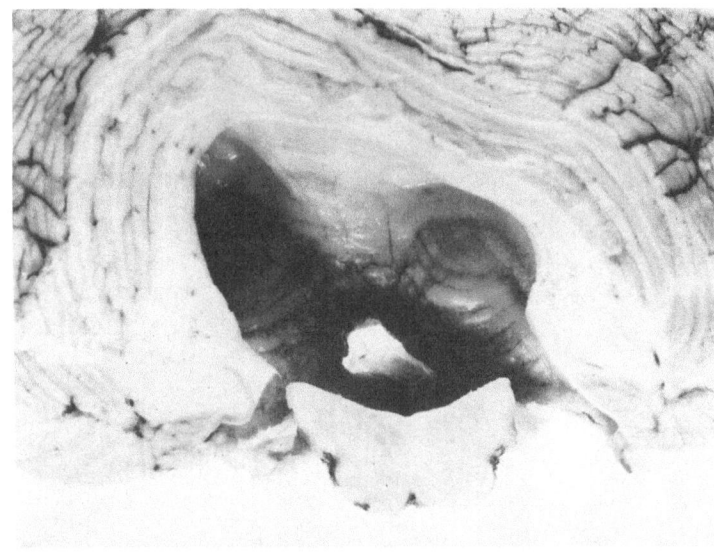

Fig. 374. Enormous dilatation of the fourth ventricle and the foramina of Magendi and Luschka in a case of congenital membranous occlusion of the foramina of Luschka and Magendi combined with cerebellar hypoplasia

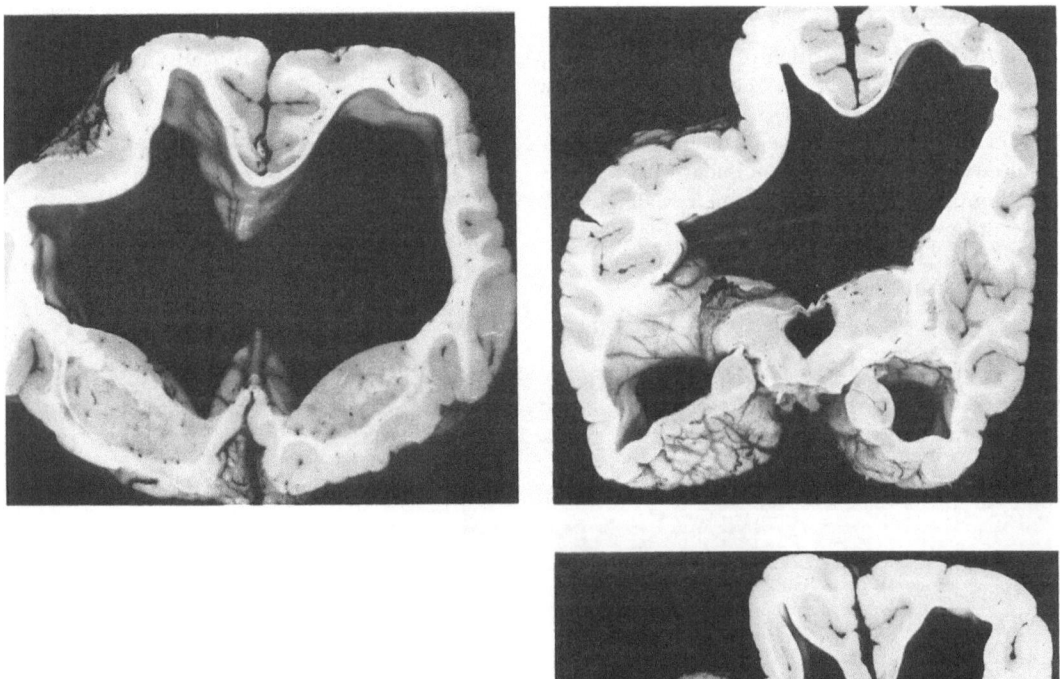

Fig. 375. a—c. Massive obstructive hydrocephalus with fenestration and tearing of the septum pellucidum

217

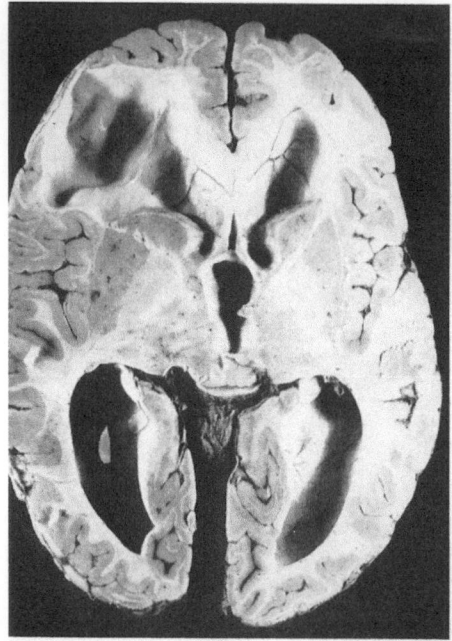

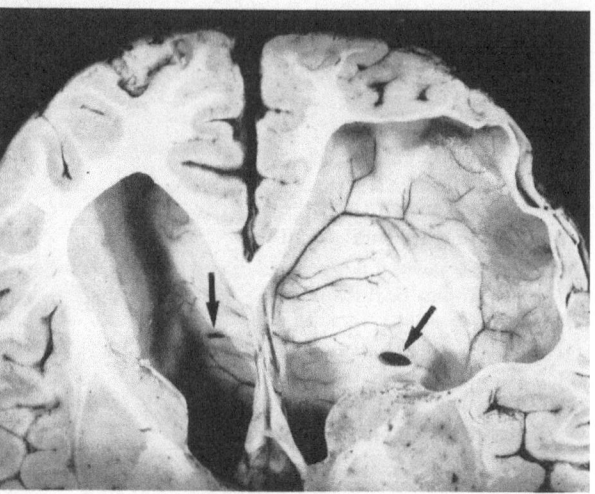

Fig. 376. Horizontal section of a brain in obstructive hydrocephalus. Marked degeneration of white matter with cyst formation in the left frontal lobe. This finally resulted in one huge cavity confluent with the frontal horn. The ventricular wall has ruptured in two locations (see Fig. 377), thus forming a communication with the subarachnoid space

Fig. 377. See Fig. 376: the two ruptures are marked by arrows

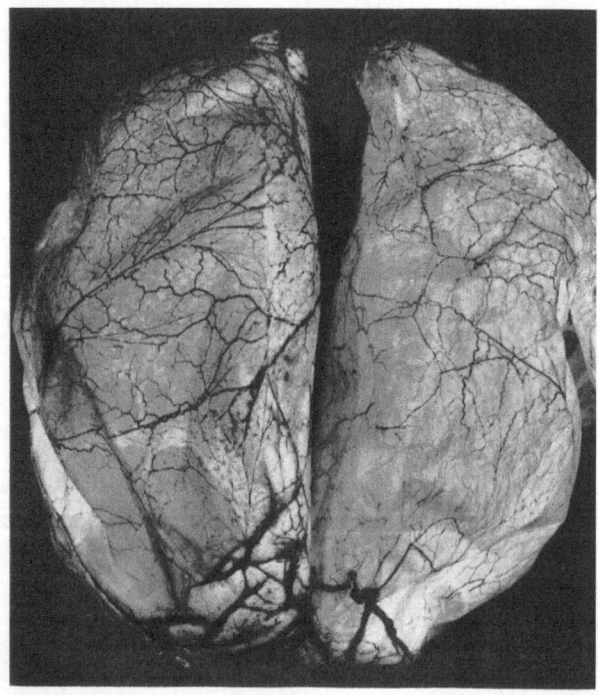

Fig. 378. Case of complete obstruction of the aqueduct. Curious transformation of the posterior parts of both hemispheres into large bulli. View from above

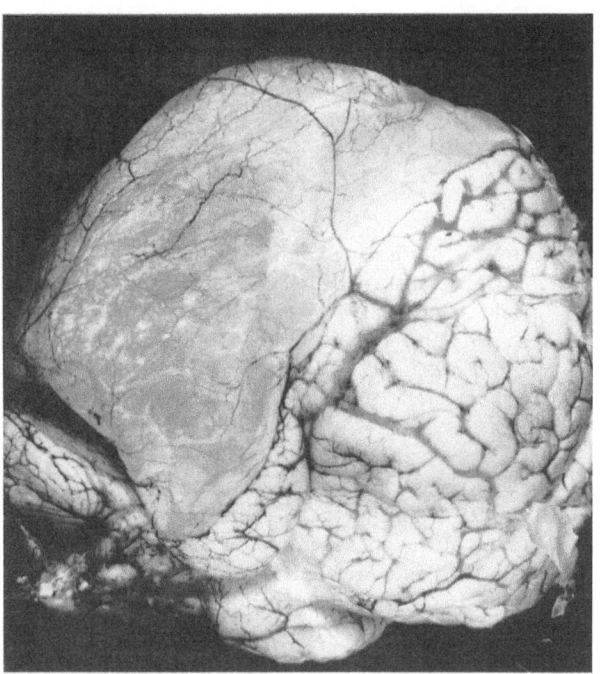

Fig. 379. See Fig. 378, lateral view

References

of authors cited in the Atlas

ARENDT, A.: Histologisch-diagnostischer Atlas der Geschwülste des ZNS und seiner Anhangsgebilde. Jena: VEB Fischer, 1964.

BAILEY, P.: Intracranial tumors. London: Baillière, Tindall and Cox 1933.

BAILEY, P.: Die Hirngeschwülste. Stuttgart: Enke 1951.

BAILEY, P., CUSHING, H.: Medulloblastoma cerebelli. Arch. Neur. 14, 192–223 (1925).

BAILEY, P., CUSHING, H.: A classification of the tumors of the glioma group on a histogenetic basis with a correlated study of prognosis. Philadelphia: J. B. Lippincott & Co. 1926.

BAILEY, P., CUSHING, H.: Die Gewebsverschiedenheit der Gliome und ihre Bedeutung für die Prognose. Jena: Fischer 1930.

BRODERS, A. C.: Carcinoma: Grading and Practical Application. Arch. Path. Laborat. Med. 2, 376–381 (1926).

CASTELLANO, F., GUIDETTI, B., OLIVECRONA, H.: Pterional meningiomas "en plaque". J. Neurosurg. 9, 188–196 (1952).

CUSHING, H.: The meningeomas. The Cavendish lecture. Brain 45, 282–316 (1922).

CUSHING, H.: Experiences with the cerebellar medulloblastomas. Acta path. scand. (Copenh.) 7, 1–86 (1930).

CUSHING, H.: Experiences with the cerebellar astrocytomas. Surg. Gyn. Obstetr. 52, 129–204 (1931).

CUSHING, H.: Intracranial tumors. Springfield: Ch. C. Thomas 1932.

CUSHING, H.: Intrakranielle Tumoren. Berlin: Springer 1935.

CUSHING, H., BAILEY, P.: Tumors arising from the blood vessels of the brain. Springfield: Ch. C. Thomas 1928.

CUSHING, H., EISENHARDT, L.: Meningiomas: Their classification, regional behavior, life history, and surgical end results. Springfield: Ch. C. Thomas 1938.

DANDY, W. E.: Surgery of the brain. In: Lewis's Practice of Surgery. Hagerstown: W. F. Prior Co. 12, 1–682, 1932.

DEL RIO HORTEGA, P.: Estructura y systematisacion de los gliomas y paragliomas. Arch. Espan. Oncol. 2, 411–677 (1932).

DEL RIO HORTEGA, P.: Nomenclatura y clasificacion de los tumores del sistema nervioso. Buenos Aires: Lopez & Etchefoyen 1945.

FINDEISEN, L., TÖNNIS, W.: Über intrakranielle Epidermoide. Zbl. Neurochir. 2, 301–315 (1937).

FINKEMEYER, H., PFINGST, E., ZÜLCH, K. J.: The astrocytomas of the cerebral hemispheres. In: Handbook of Clinical Neurology, Vol. 18, eds. VINKEN and BRUYN. North Holland Publ. Comp., Amsterdam 1974.

FOERSTER, O., GAGEL, O.: Das umschriebene Arachnoidalsarkom des Kleinhirns. Z. Neur. 164, 565–580 (1939).

GAGEL, O.: Über Hirngeschwülste. Z. Neurol. 161, 69–113 (1938).

GURDJIAN, E. S.: Operative Neurosurgery, 2nd Edition. Baltimore: The Williams and Wilkins Comp. 1964.

HENSCHEN, F.: Tumoren des ZNS und seiner Hüllen. In: Handbuch der speziellen pathologischen Anatomie und Histologie, Bd. XIII/3. Berlin-Göttingen-Heidelberg: Springer 1955.

INGRAHAM, F. D.: Medulloblastoma cerebelli: Diagnosis, Treatment and Survivals. With Report of 56 Cases. New Engl. J. Med. 238, 171 (1948).

KEMPE, L. G.: Operative Neurosurgery, vol. I: Cranial, Cerebral and Intracranial Vascular Diseases. Berlin-Heidelberg-New York: Springer 1968.

KEMPE, L. G.: Operative Neurosurgery, vol. II: Posterior Fossa, Spinal Cord and Peripheral Nerve Disease. Berlin-Heidelberg-New York: Springer 1970.

KERNOHAN, J. W., MABON, R. F., SVIEN, H. J., ADSON, A. W.: A simplified classification of the gliomas. Symp. on a new simplified concept of gliomas. Proc. Staff Meet. Mayo Clin. 24, 71–75 (1949).

KERNOHAN, J. W., SAYRE, G.: Tumors of the central nervous system. Washington: Armed Forces Institute of Pathology 1952.

KERNOHAN, J. W., UIHLEIN, A.: Sarcomas of the brain. Springfield: Ch. C. Thomas 1962.

KRAYENBÜHL, H.: Anamnese und Klinik des Glioblastoma multiforme. Acta Neurochir., Suppl. VI, 31–39. Wien: Springer 1959.

McCRAIG, W., KEITH, H. M., KERNOHAN, J. W.: Tumors of the brain occurring in childhood. Acta psychiat. (Copenh.) 24, 375–390 (1949).

220

NONNE, M.: Über diffuse Sarkomatose der Pia mater des ganzen Zentralnervensystems. Dtsch. Z. Nervenheilk. **21**, 396 (1902).

OLIVECRONA, H.: Die chirurgische Behandlung der Hirntumoren. Berlin: Springer 1927.

OLIVECRONA, H.: The surgical treatment of intracranial tumors. Handbuch der Neurochirurgie, Bd. IV/4. Berlin-Heidelberg-New York: Springer 1967.

OSTERTAG, B.: Grundsätzliches über die Einteilung der Hirngeschwülste und deren praktische Bedeutung. Zbl. Neur. 67, 266–271 (1932).

OSTERTAG, B.: Einteilung und Charakteristik der Hirngewächse. Jena: Fischer 1936.

PENFIELD, W.: The classification of gliomas and neuroglia cell types. Arch. Neurol. Psychiat. **26**, 745 (1931).

PENFIELD, W.: A paper on the classification of brain tumors and its practical application. Brit. Med. J. **1**, 337–342 (1931).

PENFIELD, W.: Tumors of the sheaths of the nervous system. In: Cytology and cellular pathology of the nervous system; edit. by W. Penfield. New York: Hoeber 1932.

PENFIELD, W.: Principles of the pathology of neurosurgery. Chapter VI, 303–347. New York: Nelson & Sons 1927 (Suppl. 1932).

RECKLINGHAUSEN, F. v.: Über die multiplen Fibrome der Haut und ihre Beziehungen zu den multiplen Neuromen. Festschrift für Virchow. Berlin: Hirschwald 1882.

RINGERTZ, N.: Grading of gliomas. Acta path. scand. (Copenh.) **27**, 51–64 (1950).

RINGERTZ, N., REYMOND, A.: Ependymomas and choroid plexus papillomas. J. Neuropath. **8**, 355–380 (1949).

ROUSSY, G., OBERLING, CH.: Atlas du cancer. Paris: Felix Alcan 1931.

RUBINSTEIN, L. J.: Atlas of Tumor Pathology. Tumors of the Central Nervous System. II. Series. Fasc. 6. Washington: Armed Forces Institute of Pathology (AFIP) 1972.

RUSSELL, D. S., RUBINSTEIN, L. J.: Pathology of tumours of the nervous system, third Edition. London: E. Arnold 1971.

SAYRE, G. P.: The concept of grading gliomas of the central nervous system. J. Internat. Coll. Surgeons, Chicago XXVI, 440–447 (1956).

SAYRE, G. P.: The system of grading of gliomas. In: Classification of Brain Tumors, edit. by K. J. Zülch and A. L. Woolf. Acta Neurochir., Suppl. X, 98–106. Wien: Springer 1964.

SCHMIDT, M. B.: Über die Pacchionischen Granulationen und ihr Verhalten zu den Sarkomen und Psammomen der Dura mater. Virch. Arch. **170**, 429 (1902).

SCHWARTZ, PH.: Anatomische Typen der Hirngliome. Nervenarzt (Berlin) **5**, 449–456 (1932).

SCHWARTZ, PH.: Anatomische Typen der Hirngliome. Mitt. II. Kongr. f. Krebsforsch., 257–260 (1936).

TÖNNIS, W.: Über Hirngeschwülste. Z. Neur. *161*, 114–149 (1938).

TÖNNIS, W.: Diagnostik der intrakraniellen Geschwülste. Handbuch der Neurochirurgie, Bd. IV/3. Berlin-Göttingen-Heidelberg: Springer 1962.

Unio Internationalis Contra Cancrum (UICC): Histologische Nomenklatur menschlicher Tumoren. Zschr. Krebsforsch. **63**, 75–98 (1959).

Unio Internationalis Contra Cancrum (UICC): Illustrated Tumor Nomenclature. Berlin-Heidelberg-New York: Springer 1965.

ZÜLCH, K. J.: Hirngeschwülste im Jugendalter. Zbl. Neurochir. **5**, 238–274 (1940).

ZÜLCH, K. J.: Die Hirngeschwülste in biologischer und morphologischer Darstellung, third Edition. Leipzig: Joh. Ambr. Barth 1958.

ZÜLCH, K. J.: Biologie und Pathologie der Hirngeschwülste. Handbuch der Neurochirurgie, Bd. III. Berlin-Göttingen-Heidelberg: Springer 1956.

ZÜLCH, K. J.: Brain Tumors. Their Biology and Pathology, second Edition. New York: Springer Publ. Comp. Inc., 1965; Italian Edition: Padova, Piccin Editore, 1974.

ZÜLCH, K. J.: Störungen des intrakraniellen Druckes. Handbuch der Neurochirurgie, Bd. I/1, pp. 208–303. Berlin-Göttingen-Heidelberg: Springer 1959.

ZÜLCH, K. J.: The present state of the classification of intracranial tumors and its value for the neurosurgeon. In: The Biology and Treatment of Intracranial Tumors, edit. by Field and Sharkey, pp. 157–177. Springfield: Ch. C. Thomas 1962.

ZÜLCH, K. J.: Atlas of the Histology of Brain Tumors. Berlin-Heidelberg-New York: Springer 1971.

ZÜLCH, K. J., MENNEL, H. D.: The biology of brain tumours. Handbook of Clinical Neurology, Vol. 16. Amsterdam: North-Holland Publ. Comp. 1974.

ZÜLCH, K. J., MENNEL, H. D., ZIMMERMANN, V.: Intracranial hypertension. In: Handbook of Clinical Neurology, Vol. XVI, eds. VINKEN and BRUYN. Amsterdam: North Holland Publ. Comp. 1974.

ZÜLCH, K. J., WECHSLER, W.: Pathology and classification of gliomas. Progr. Neurol. Surg. II, 1–84. Basel-New York: S. Karger 1968.

ZÜLCH, K. J., WOOLF, A. L.: Classification of Brain Tumours. Symposium on the classification of brain tumours in collaboration with the World Federation of Neurology and the Deutsche Forschungsgemeinschaft, Köln 1961. Wien: Springer 1964.

References

Further References on General Aspects of Brain Tumors and Selected Original Papers

ANTONI, N.: Tumoren des Rückenmarks, seiner Wurzeln und Häute. In: Handbuch der Neurologie, Hrsg. BUMKE-FOERSTER, Bd. 14. Berlin: Springer 1936.

BATZDORF, U., MALAMUD, N.: The problem of multicentric gliomas. J. Neurosurg. **20**, 122 (1963).

BAYREUTHER, K.: Chromosomes in primary neoplastic growth. Nature (Lond.) **186**, 6 (1960).

BENEDICT, B. F., PORTER, I. H., BROWN, C. H. D., FLORENTIN, R. A.: Cytogenetic diagnosis of malignancy in recurrent meningioma. Lancet **1970 I**, 971—973.

BERGSTRAND, H.: Über das sogenannte Astrocytom des Kleinhirns. Virchows Arch. path. Anat. **287**, 538 (1932).

BORST, M.: Die Lehre von den Geschwülsten. Wiesbaden: Bergmann 1902.

CALVO, W.: Tumores encefalomedulares. Estudio morfologico y biologico. Arch. esp. Morfol. (Suppl.) V (1954).

CANTI, R. G., BLAND, J. O. W., RUSSELL, D. S.: Tissue culture of gliomata. Ass. Res. nerv. Dis. Proc. **16**, 1 (1935).

COSTERO, I.: Pathology of glial neoplasms. In: The biology and treatment of intracranial tumors, ed. by FIELDS and SHARKEY, p. 178. Springfield/Ill.: Charles C. Thomas 1962.

COSTERO, I., POMERAT, C. M.: Standard cellular morphology of gliomas in vitro as compared with explanted normal brain cells. Proc. II. Intern. Congr. Neuropath., London 1955. Excerpta med. Neur. Psych. 2, 273.

COURVILLE, C. B.: Intracranial tumors. Notes upon a series of three thousand verified cases with some current observations pertaining to their mortality. Bull. Los Angeles neurol. Soc. **32**, Suppl. 2/II (1967).

EARLE, K. M., REUTSCHLER, E. H., SNODGRASS, S. R.: Primary intracranial neoplasms. Prognosis and classification of 513 verified cases. N. Neuropath. exp. Neurol. **16**, 321 (1957).

FIELDS, W. S., SHARKEY, P.: The biology and treatment of intracranial tumors. Springfield/Ill.: Charles C. Thomas 1962.

GLUZCZ, A.: Grouping of supratentorial gliomas according to their dominant biomorphological features. Acta neuropath. (Berl.) **22**, 110—126 (1972).

HARVALD, B., HAUGE, M.: On the heredity of glioblastoma. J. Nat. Cancer Inst. **17**, 289 (1956).

JÄNISCH, W., SCHREIBER, D.: Experimentelle Geschwülste des Zentralnervensystems. Jena: VEB Gustav Fischer 1969.

KATSURA, S., SUZUKI, J., WADA, T.: A statistical study of brain tumors in the neurosurgical clinics in Japan. J. Neurosurg. **16**, 570 (1959)

KAUTZKY, R., ZÜLCH, K. J.: Neurologisch-neurochirurgische Röntgendiagnostik und andere Methoden zur Erkennung intrakranieller Erkrankungen. Berlin-Göttingen-Heidelberg: Springer 1955 (2nd edition in preparation).

KERSTING, G.: Die Gewebszüchtung menschlicher Hirngeschwülste. Berlin-Göttingen-Heidelberg: Springer 1961.

KHOMINSKY, B. S.: Histologische Diagnostik der Geschwülste des Zentralnervensystems. Moskau: Verlag Medizin 1969 [Russian].

KIRSCH, W. M., GROSSI PAOLETTI, E., PAOLETTI, P.: The experimental biology of brain tumors. Springfield/Ill.: Charles C. Thomas 1972.

KOCH, G.: Beitrag zur Erblichkeit der Hirngeschwülste. Acta Genet. med. (Roma) **3**, 170 (1954).

KUHLENDAHL, H., MILTZ, H., WÜLLENWEBER, R.: Die Astrozytome des Großhirns. Untersuchung zur Gruppierung und Prognose. Acta neurochir. (Wien) **29**, 151—162 (1973).

LUGINBÜHL, H., FANKHAUSER, R., McGRATH, J. T.: Spontaneous neoplasms of the nervous system in animals. Progr. neurol. Surg. **2**, 85 (1968).

LUMSDEN, C. E.: Tissue culture in relation to tumours of the nervous system. In: The pathology of tumours of the nervous system, ed. by RUSSELL and RUBINSTEIN, p. 272. London: Arnold 1959.

LUSE, S. A.: Electron microscopic studies of brain tumors. Neurology (Minneap.) **10**, 881 (1960).

MARK, J.: Origin of the ring chromosome in a human recurrent meningioma studied with G-band technique. Acta path. microbiol. scand. **81**, 591—592 (1973).

MÜLLER, W., SCHRÖDER, R.: Zur Diagnostik der Gliome. Neurochirurgia (Stuttg.) **11**, 30 (1968).

MURRAY, M. R., STOUT, A. P.: The classification and diagnosis of the human tumors by tissue culture methods. Tex. Rep. Biol. Med. **12**, 898 (1954).

POLAK, M.: Blastomas del Sistema Nervioso Central y Periferico, Pathologia y Ordenacion Histogenética. Buenos Aires: Lopez Libreros Edit. 1966.

SCHARENBERG, K., LISS, L.: Neuroectodermal tumors of the central and peripheral nervous system. Baltimore: Williams & Wilkins Co. 1969.

SCHIFFER, D., FABIANI, A.: Patologia dei Tumori Cerebrali. Rom: Il Pensiero Scientifico Editore 1970.

SCHRÖDER, R., BONIS, G., MÜLLER, W., VORREITH, M.: Statistische Beiträge zum Grading der Gliome. I. Acta neurochir. (Wien) **18**, 43—56 (1968).

SCHRÖDER, R., BONIS, G., MÜLLER, W., VORREITH, M.: Statistische Beiträge zum Grading der Gliome. II. Acta neurochir. (Wien) **18**, 186—200 (1968).

SCHRÖDER, R., MÜLLER, W., BONIS, G., VORREITH, M.: Statistische Beiträge zum Grading der Gliome. III. Acta neurochir. (Wien) **23**, 1—29 (1970).

SINGER, H., ZANG, K. D.: Cytologische Untersuchungen an Hirntumoren. Hum. Genet. **9**, 172—184 (1970).

STOUT, A. P.: Atlas of Tumor Pathology. Sect. II-Fasc. 6: Tumors of the peripheral nervous system. Washington: Armed Forces Institute of Pathologie 1949.

STROEBE, H.: Über Entstehung und Bau der Hirngliome. Beitr. path. Anat. (Jena) **18**, 405 (1895).

WIEL, H. J. VAN DER: Inheritance of gliomas. Amsterdam - London - New York - Princeton: Elsevier 1960.

ZIMMERMAN, H. M.: The nature gliomas as revealed by animal experimentation. Amer. J. Path. **31**, 1 (1955).

Author Index

Subject Index

Page numbers type-set in *italics* indicate principal discussion of each subject

Subject Index

K. J. Zülch:

Atlas of the Histology of Brain Tumors

Title and text in six languages
(English, German, French, Spanish,
Russian, and Japanese)
100 figures. XVI, 261 pages. 1971
Cloth DM 88,—; US $35.90
ISBN 3-540-05274-7

Distribution rights for Japan:
Nankodo Co. Ltd., Tokyo

This atlas shows the growth pattern of
the intracranial tumors, their frequent
variations and the typical changes occurring as a result of regressive changes.
Therefore, it guides one in the art of
making a correct classification. There is
also a discussion concerning the prognosis based on "genuine growth" in
which KERNOHAN'S grading system is
further developed and adapted for daily
use. It is hoped that this atlas forms a
solid basis for the morphological diagnosis of brain tumors.

S. L. Palay, V. Chan-Palay:

Cerebellar Cortex

Cytology and Organization
267 figures including 203 plates
X, 348 pages. 1974
Cloth DM 156,—; US $63.70
ISBN 3-540-06228-9

Distribution rights for Japan:
Igaku Shoin Ltd., Tokyo

Contents: Introduction. — The Purkinje
Cell. — Granule Cells. — The Golgi Cells.
— The Lugaro Cell. — The Mossy Fibers.
— The Basket Cell. — The Stellate Cell.
— Functional Architectonics without
Numbers. — The Climbing Fiber. — The
Neuroglial Cells of the Cerebellar Cortex.
— Methods.

Prices are subject to change
without notice

J. M. van Buren, R. C. Borke:

Variations and Connections of the Human Thalamus

In two parts, not sold separately

Part 1:
The Nuclei and Cerebral Connections of
the Human Thalamus
Part 2:
Variations of the Human Diencephalon
98 figures, 187 plates. XXI, 587 pages
1972
Cloth DM 670,—; US $273.40
ISBN 3-540-05543-6

Distribution rights for Japan:
Igaku Shoin Ltd., Tokyo

The first part reevaluates the morphology
and cerebral connections of the human
thalamus using a wide variety of exclusively human material. Part 2 provides
a three-plane variation atlas of the brain
with a special study of the thalamus for
the stereotaxic surgeon.

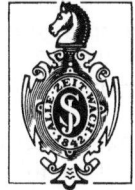

Springer-Verlag Berlin Heidelberg NewYork

München Johannesburg London Madrid
New Delhi Paris Rio de Janeiro Sydney
Tokyo Utrecht Wien

Classification of Brain Tumours

Report of the International Symposium at Cologne
30 August – 1 September, 1961
Sponsored by The Max-Planck-Gesellschaft, The Deutsche
Forschungsgemeinschaft, The World Federation of Neurology. Editors: K. J. Zülch, A. L. Woolf

First Edition 1964 – reprinted 1965
71 figures. X, 218 pages. 1965
(Acta Neurochirurgica, Supplementum X)
DM 70,–; US $28.60
Reduced price for subscribers to "Acta Neurochirurgica"
DM 63,–; US $25.70. ISBN 3-211-80712-8

L.G. Kempe: Operative Neurosurgery

Vol. 1: **Cranial, Cerebral, and Intracranial Vascular Disease**

335 figures, some in color. XIII, 269 pages. 1968
Cloth DM 190,–; US $77.60. ISBN 3-540-04208-3
Distribution rights for Japan: Nankodo Co. Ltd., Tokyo

This volume presents the major neurosurgical procedures
involving the anterior and middle cranial fossa.
The precise detailed operative technique shown in this book
is intended to illustrate the basic techniques of the major
neurosurgical procedures and to give guidance and the
necessary flexibility which is in constant demand for the
execution of every surgical procedure. This book should
also be of interest to general surgeons who may be called
upon primarily to handle some of the emergency neurosurgical procedures. The description is so detailed that the
nonspecialist will also find guidance for these emergency
procedures.

Vol. 2: **Posterior Fossa, Spinal Cord, and Peripheral Nerve Disease**

290 figures, some in color. VIII, 281 pages. 1970
Cloth DM 190,–; US $77.60. ISBN 3-540-04890-1
Distribution rights for Japan: Nankodo Co. Ltd., Tokyo

The text describes and the figures illustrate the step-by-step
surgical technique. Emphasis is placed on anatomical topo-
graphic views of the operative exposure as seen by the
surgeon. The contents have been arranged on the basis of
anatomical location rather than etiology.

Prices are subject
to change
without notice

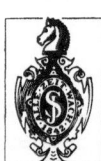

Springer-Verlag
Berlin Heidelberg New York
München Johannesburg London Madrid New Delhi Paris
Rio de Janeiro Sydney Tokyo Utrecht Wien